A JERRY BAKER GOOD HEALTH BOOK

TOP 25
Homemade
HEALERS

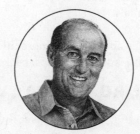

www.jerrybaker.com

TOP 25
Homemade
HEALERS

2,173 DIY HEALTH AND BEAUTY SOLUTIONS
Featuring Vinegar, Honey, Castor Oil, and 22 More!

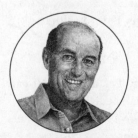

by Jerry Baker

Published by American Master Products, Inc.

NOTICE—All efforts have been made to ensure accuracy. This is a reference volume only, not a medical manual. Although the information presented may help you make informed decisions about your health, it is not intended as a substitute for prescribed medical treatment. If you have a medical problem, please seek competent medical help immediately. Jerry Baker assumes no responsibility or liability for any injuries, damages, or losses incurred during the use of or as a result of following this information.

Herbal research is still in its infancy, and the interaction between herbs and pharmaceutical products remains largely unknown. Herbal remedies and nutraceuticals can have effects similar to those of pharmaceutical products. As a result, they are not without risk. They can interact with each other or with conventional medications, and some people may experience an allergic reaction or other adverse effects when starting an herbal or nutraceutical regimen. That's why you should always check with your doctor before you use them.

Women who are pregnant or breastfeeding and children under age 18 should not use herbal or nutraceutical products without their doctor's specific recommendation.

IMPORTANT—Study all directions carefully before taking any action based on the information and advice presented in this book. When using any commercial product, always read and follow label directions. When reference is made to any trade or brand name, no endorsement by Jerry Baker is implied, nor is any discrimination intended.

Executive Editor: Kim Adam Gasior
Managing Editor: Cheryl Winters-Tetreau
Copy Editor: Nanette Bendyna
Interior Design and Layout: Sandy Freeman
Indexer: Nan Badgett

Publisher's Cataloging-in-Publication
(Provided by Quality Books, Inc.)

Baker, Jerry.
    Top 25 homemade healers : 2,173 DIY health and beauty
solutions featuring vinegar, honey, castor oil, and 22
more! / Jerry Baker.
    pages cm. -- (A Jerry Baker health book)
    Includes index.
    ISBN 978-0-922433-70-4

    1. Health. 2. Beauty, Personal. 3. Self-care,
Health. 4. Traditional medicine.   I. Title.
II. Title: Top twenty-five homemade healers. III. Series:
Jerry Baker health book.

RA776.B1925 2014   613
        QBI13-2478

Printed in the United States of America
2 4 6 8 10 9 7 5 3 hardcover

Contents

Contents

Introduction

Today you can buy a special remedy to treat just about every health and beauty problem under the sun, from sunburned skin to strained muscles, skeeter bites to sleepless nights, and dry hair to dingy teeth. But until the Fabulous Fifties, most of these miraculous cure-alls (that we now take for granted) didn't even exist. Instead, folks relied on the same methods their ancestors had used for centuries to heal their wounds, cure their ills, and improve their looks.

Well, guess what? Here in the 21st century, everything old is new again. Study after study is showing just how effective those homemade healers can be—at a fraction of the cost of commercial concoctions and with none of the potential side effects.

In this book, I've gathered the top 25 health and beauty megastars, all of which you'll find in your kitchen, garden, or local supermarket (or, often on the Internet). For ease of use, each chapter is divided into two sections. One presents scads of time-tested—or, in some cases, cutting-edge—health remedies, while the other zeros in on superbly simple beauty secrets.

In addition, I've rounded up close to 100 more heroic healers in the "Best of the Rest" sections in each chapter. This supporting cast is closely related to the stars of our show, and they provide a boatload of additional ways to tap into the amazing power of Mother Nature's medicine chest and beauty kit.

These pages are crammed full of terrific tips and tricks that show you how to prevent, cure, or heal your most annoying health and beauty dilemmas—quickly, safely, and cheaply. For instance, you'll learn how to:

- Banish arthritis pain with honey and vinegar.

- Cure carpal tunnel syndrome with chamomile tea.

- Ditch the itch of hemorrhoids with a baking soda mix.

- Make age spots fade with onion juice.

- Deflate puffy eyes with a DIY salt solution.

- Detox your overstylized hair with carrots.

- Look years younger with a delicious Smooth-Skin Smoothie.

CAUTION ⚠

While all of the homemade healers featured in these pages are among the healthiest substances you can put on or into your body, there are some things you need to keep in mind:

- None of the information in this book is intended to replace professional medical care. Always consult your doctor before you use any of the remedies presented here. That's especially important if you are taking drugs of any kind or if you are pregnant or think you might be pregnant.

- Even the safest products may irritate your skin, so before you try any topical health or beauty remedy, always test it on a small patch of skin before you use it on a larger area.

- When a tip or a potion calls for a specific amount of any ingredient, don't assume that more is better. Follow the directions and stick to the proportions given in the text. (The exception, of course, is food recipes, where artistic tinkering is the hallmark of a creative cook!)

- Essential oils, which are used throughout this book, are very potent. So always dilute them in water or another carrier oil before you apply them to your skin.

- This goes without saying (I hope!), but when any remedy specifies hot water, always make sure it is comfortable to the touch—not burning hot.

But that's not all! You'll also find fantastic features like **You Don't Say!**, which contain the fascinating and sometimes bizarre stories behind some of our most potent homemade healers. Just to pique your curiosity, here are a couple of fabulous factoids that you can toss around at your next neighborhood barbecue: The United States is the only country in the world where moo juice is the most popular kind of milk (page 355), and

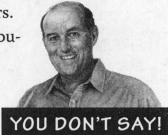

YOU DON'T SAY!

until the 1920s, avocados were considered such powerful aphrodisiacs that most respectable folks refused to eat them (see page 21).

In **Healthful Hints**, I'll show you hundreds of super-simple—and super-cheap—ways to improve your health. Sneak preview: When you peel onions, hang on to the skins. Then toss them into soups, stews, or rice (wrapped in a cheesecloth pouch) to tap into what's been called a "medicinal gold mine" (see page 253).

Beauty Secrets deliver the same kind of out-of-the-box tricks as *Healthful Hints*, but with a cosmetic twist. For instance, I'll clue you in on making a carroty facial

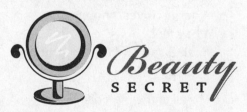

mask that'll fight off wrinkles and improve the texture of your skin better than fancy commercial creams (see page 68).

POTENT POTION

Potent Potions include fast, fun, and foolproof formulas for making health and beauty remedies, ranging from cough syrups to skin toners, and muscle liniments to mouthwash. A quick sampling: You'll learn how to ease the itch of eczema, hives, or a

Fabulous Food Fix

FIVE-MINUTE ALL-STAR MARINADE

This delicious marinade will not only enhance the flavor of your favorite meat or poultry, but will also deliver the powerful health and beauty benefits of more than a half dozen of the Top 25 Homemade Healers.

½ cup of red-wine vinegar
2 tbsp. of chopped fresh oregano
2 tbsp. of chopped fresh rosemary
2 tbsp. of olive oil
4 garlic cloves, chopped
1 bay leaf
Kosher salt and freshly ground black pepper

Mix all of the ingredients in a shallow bowl, and pour over your meat or poultry. Let the meat sit, covered, in the refrigerator for 30 minutes to eight hours. Then carry on with your usual grilling or broiling routine.

YIELD: ENOUGH FOR 1½ TO 2 POUNDS OF MEAT OR POULTRY

poison-plant rash by soaking in a "cocktail" made from green-tea bags and a trio of common essential oils (see page 303).

Finally, **Fabulous Food Fixes** consist of easy-to-prepare recipes that not only taste great, but can also improve your health or your looks—or both! Just to whet your appetite, you can whip up this Five-Minute All-Star Marinade that can turn even the toughest steak or chicken into the most tender Cordon Bleu–plate special. And while you're at it, check out the Fettuccine Sweet and Hot dish (page 89) that delivers a potent load of disease-busting antioxidants, the Get-Up-and-Go Honey Bars (page 157) that give you a powerful energy boost, and the tasty Curried Yogurt Dip (page 353) that'll make your skin softer, smoother, and younger looking.

With all this good stuff inside, what are we waiting for? Time's a wastin', so let's hit the road to good health and good looks!

1

Apples

When Eve handed Adam the world's most famous apple, she was offering him a lot more than an entrée into a life of wedded bliss. Although she couldn't have known it at the time, that tempting, tasty treat was a true health-food superstar. Of course, it still is. But, unlike Eve (thanks to modern nutritional research), we now know why this common fruit performs such powerful feats for our good health—and our good looks.

An Apple a Day

✔ Fiber on the Double

It seems that every time you turn around, you hear some nutritional guru talking about how important dietary fiber is to good health. Well, that essential fiber happens to come in two types: soluble and insoluble, and apples deliver a sizable load of both kinds. So what's the difference between the two? Just this:

SOLUBLE FIBER dissolves in water and combines with other substances to form a gel-like material that prevents fats and sugars from being absorbed into your body, which can help control diabetes and lower LDL (bad) cholesterol. (See the following pages for the specifics.)

INSOLUBLE FIBER does not dissolve in water (surprise!). Rather, it absorbs bile and cholesterol in your intestines and carries them out of your body. Insoluble fiber can also help prevent constipation.

✔ A Popular Portable Powerhouse

According to the folks who study food consumption, the average American eats approximately 45 pounds of apples each year, which makes Eve's offering number one on the list of our most consumed fruits. In part, that's due to the fact that besides being delicious, apples are pretty much available year-round in supermarkets throughout the country. But there are a host of other reasons for their popularity, including:

■ They're sturdy and easily portable—just the ticket for tucking into a lunch box, backpack, or pocket.

■ They provide satisfying bulk at a low calorie count (roughly 80 calories for a medium-size apple).

■ Their content is 85 to 95 percent water, so they quench your thirst as well as fill your tummy.

■ They're versatile. Apples pack the same healthy wallop whether you eat them fresh, dried, frozen, or cooked—or drink them in the form of 100 percent apple juice or cider.

HEALTHFUL HINT

An Apple Shopper's Guide

Whether you buy your apples in the supermarket or from a farm stand, these tips will help you find the best-tasting and longest-lasting fruit:

THINK FIRM. Hold the fruit in your hand and give it a gentle squeeze with your fingers. If your digits produce dents, it means the apple has passed its peak of freshness.

THINK SMALL. Some varieties of apples naturally grow bigger than others, but within categories, smaller is generally better.

THINK PRETTY. Choose apples that have nice color for their type, tight skins, and no cuts or bruises.

STORE THEM RIGHT. As soon as you get your apples home, stash them in the fridge, where they'll keep for up to six weeks. If you leave them out at room temperature, they'll go downhill fast.

✔ Pick a Peck of Pectin

Every time you eat an apple, you consume the richest source of pectin—a natural fiber that not only controls diarrhea, but also decreases the likelihood of colon cancer, reduces high blood pressure, and helps prevent or even dissolve gallstones. What's more, it slows the absorption of nutrients into the bloodstream, thereby helping to keep blood sugar under control. (Diabetics, take note!)

✔ Wait—There's More!

Pectin aside, apples contain a truck-size load of other nutrients, enzymes, and biochemical compounds that are essential to good health. Numerous studies have found that eating apples on a regular basis can help most folks by relieving or preventing a whole lot of common health problems—like these, for instance:

- Asthma
- Cardiovascular disease
- Colds
- Coronary heart disease
- Seasonal allergies
- Stroke

✔ Boot Out Bad Cholesterol

If you have high levels of LDL (bad) cholesterol, an increase in apple intake is just what the doctor ordered. Studies show that eating two large apples a day can reduce LDL cholesterol levels by as much as 23 percent. If you want to eat more, go for it! After all, you'd have to be chomping on apples day and night to eat too many.

✔ Clear Up Conjunctivitis

A lot of things can cause red, watery, or itchy eyes. But if your orbs are really irritated, it could indicate that you're coming down with conjunctivitis, a.k.a. pinkeye. If you act fast, an apple poultice just may stop the infection in its tracks. To make it, first dampen a piece of soft, all-cotton fabric that's about 12 inches square. Next, grate a large, peeled apple. Spread the pulp in the center of the cloth, and fold the sides over to form a rectangular mask. Then lie down, lay

Fabulous Food Fix

HEIRLOOM FLU STOPPER

In the days before flu vaccines came along, folks relied on home remedies like this one to keep trouble at bay. And you know what? It still works to fend off viruses that cause colds and flu. So even if you get your yearly flu shot faithfully, keep this recipe close at hand, and reach for it at the first sign of symptoms.

1 large, tart, juicy apple
1 qt. of water
2 shots of whiskey
½ tsp. of lemon juice
Honey (optional)

Cut the apple into quarters and boil it in the water until the apple falls apart in pieces. Strain out the solids, and add the whiskey and lemon juice to the remaining apple liquid. Sweeten to taste with honey, if you like. Then get in bed and drink the toddy. If you've acted in time, by morning, those germs should be history!

the poultice over your closed eyes, and relax for half an hour. Within a day or two, your eye problem should clear up. If it doesn't, then get prompt medical help.

✔ Send Artery Plaque Packin'

Arteriosclerosis, a.k.a. clogging of the arteries, is caused by plaque, a combination of LDL (bad) cholesterol, calcium, fatty food substances, and other matter. It builds up over many years as a result of smoking, lack of exercise, and poor diet. If that description fits your lifestyle (but you haven't been diagnosed with the condition), keep clogs at bay with this old Slavic folk remedy: Once a day, drink a glass of apple cider boiled with a clove of garlic. And for heaven's sake, clean up your act!

✔ Stretch Your Stamina

In addition to relieving runny noses and watery eyes, the quercetin in apples enhances physical endurance by making oxygen more available to

An Apple for Every Purpose

Although all varieties of apples offer plenty of health and beauty benefits, in terms of good eating, they are *not* all created equal. This handy guide will help you choose the kinds that deliver the best flavor and texture for the job at hand.

PURPOSE	BEST VARIETIES
Eating fresh	Braeburn, Empire, Granny Smith, Jonagold, Jonathan, Macoun, Mutsu/Crispin, Raritan, Winesap, York Imperial
Mixed in salads	Braeburn, Cortland, Golden Delicious, Granny Smith, Jonagold, Winesap
Applesauce	Braeburn, Gala, Golden Delicious, Granny Smith, Melrose, Mutsu/Crispin, Newtown Pippin, Winesap
Baking (whole or in non-dessert recipes)	Braeburn, Granny Smith, Ida Red, Jonathan, Melrose, Mutsu/Crispin, Northern Spy, York Imperial
Pies and cobblers	Braeburn, Granny Smith, Ida Red, Jonathan, Melrose, Newtown Pippin, Northern Spy, York Imperial

the lungs. So if you eat an apple before you hop on the treadmill at the gym, take off on your bike, or hit the hiking trail, you may find that you have a lot more staying power.

✔ Boost Your Brainpower

Diseases aside, no matter what your age, you'll do the old gray cells a big favor if you add more apples to your diet. That's because these fabulous fruits contain plenty of boron, a potent mineral that stimulates brain cells, thereby helping you stay active, alert, and in tip-top mental condition.

✔ Ease Your Achin' Joints

The next time your knees, elbows, or other joints start hurting—or better yet, before the pain starts—eat a few apples. Their boron, the same trace element that kicks brain cells into high gear, can relieve joint pain and stiffness and actually seems to protect against arthritis.

✔ Lower Your Blood Pressure

Excess fluid levels in your arteries can elevate your blood pressure—pronto! Apples can help keep things on an even keel because they pack an impressive amount of potassium, which works in conjunction with sodium to regulate your body's fluid levels.

✔ Easy on a Queasy Stomach

The next time you come down with a bout of stomach flu, reach for a big glass of 100 percent apple juice, and drink up. Apples contain compounds that help to fight flu and other viruses, so that tummy bug won't be a bother for long.

Fabulous Food Fix

GOUT-BE-GONE PRESERVES

Gout is a form of arthritis that results from the buildup of uric acid in the blood. As you know, if you're prone to this nasty disease, the symptoms can strike with the speed of lightning. This ultra-simple recipe can help relieve the pain and swelling by neutralizing the acid.

4 apples (any kind will do)
Water

Peel, core, and slice the apples, put them in a pan, and add just enough water to cover the slices. Simmer them for three hours or more, until they turn thick, brown, and sweet, adding more water as necessary. Store the mixture in the refrigerator. Spread it on toast or bagels, use it as a condiment with chicken or ham—or simply put it in a bowl and dig in with a spoon!

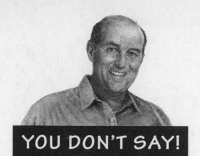

✔ Fight Alzheimer's

I think it's safe to say that for most folks, there is no more dreaded disease than Alzheimer's. Well, here's some good news: Eating at least two apples a day may cut your risk of getting this most common form of dementia. Research shows that the quercetin in the fruit helps protect brain cells from oxidation damage caused by free radicals that can lead to the onset of Alzheimer's. If that doesn't give you the incentive to up your apple intake, I don't know what will!

✔ Create Health-Giving Treasure

One of the best ways to tap into the healing power of apples is to turn them into apple cider vinegar. Sure, you can buy this vinegar in any supermarket, but when it comes to solving health and beauty problems, nothing beats the kind you make yourself. It does take time to "brew," but the six-step process couldn't be simpler:

STEP 1. Round up 12 ripe apples (any variety, but preferably organic), one package of active dry yeast, and a quart or so of pure spring water.

STEP 2. Peel and dice the apples, and toss them (including cores, but not peels) into a stoneware crock, or a deep glass or ceramic bowl.

STEP 3. Add the yeast, and pour in enough spring water to cover the apples.

STEP 4. Cover the bowl with a piece of cheese-cloth, and secure it with a rubber band. Put the container in a warm place (ideally where the temperature will stay at roughly 80°F), and let it sit for three to four months, or until the natural sugars have been converted to alcohol. (You'll know by the taste that you now have hard cider.)

STEP 5. Strain out the apples, and pour the liquid into a fresh crock or bowl. Cover the top with a clean piece of cheesecloth or other cotton fabric. Then set the container back in its warm place, and leave it for another three to four months.

STEP 6. Pour the vinegar into a glass bottle or jar. Store it at room temperature, and use it in any of the terrific healthful tips, tricks, and tonics you'll find in Chapter 23.

Fabulous Food Fix

APPLE TUNA WRAPS

A wrap is a quick, easy lunch to prepare—and a great way to enjoy a healthy dose of apples at home or at work.

2 flour tortillas, 8-inch diameter
2 tbsp. of herbed cream cheese spread
1 large apple, washed, cored, and thinly sliced
1 can (6½-oz.) of white tuna in water, drained*
½–1 tbsp. of mayonnaise to taste
Freshly ground black pepper
Mild curry powder (optional)
2 scallions with tops, chopped

Lay the tortillas on plates and spread each one with half the cream cheese spread. Arrange the apple slices down the center of each tortilla, leaving the edges clear. In a small bowl, mix the tuna with mayonnaise and pepper, and spoon the mixture over the apple slices. Dust with curry powder if you like, add the scallions, and roll up the wraps. Serve immediately, or wrap them up and pop them into lunch boxes with an ice pack to keep cold.

* Or substitute leftover cooked salmon, chicken, or turkey.

YIELD: 2 SERVINGS

✔ Cool Your Hot Flashes

Attention, ladies of a certain age! Apples can also come to your aid when your internal furnace starts blasting away. That's because they contain naturally occurring plant sterols called phytoestrogens. Although they're not as powerful as human estrogens, they have a similar effect, so they can help cool down hot flashes that are triggered by fluctuating hormones.

✔ Put a Damper on Diarrhea

When your problem is the opposite of constipation, bring on the BRAT: bananas, rice, applesauce, and toast. Stick to that diet for a day or so, and your diarrhea should hit the skids. Remember, a bout of diarrhea could dehydrate a rain forest, so be sure to drink plenty of water. The more the better, but try to down at least eight glasses a day.

✔ Get a Move On

Apples are known far and wide as one of Mother Nature's most effective laxatives. How you use that gentle power to get things moving is up to you. Here's a trio of classic choices:

EAT 'EM. Simply munch on a few apples with the peels on. That insoluble fiber should jump-start things in a jiffy.

DRINK UP. Enjoy a glass or two of 100 percent apple juice or apple cider. Many folks find that this does the trick quite nicely.

MAKE A COCKTAIL. Try the classic hospital remedy: Just mix four to six chopped prunes and 1 tablespoon of bran with ½ cup of apple–sauce. Eat the mixture just before you go to bed, and by morning your "plumbing" should be back to normal.

> **CAUTION !**
>
> Although apples with their peels on rank among the healthiest foods on the planet, they also appear high on the "Dirty Dozen" list of fruits and vegetables that retain huge amounts of herbicides and pesticides. So whether you plan to eat the fruits or use them for cosmetic purposes, scrub the skins thoroughly. Better yet, whenever possible, buy organically grown apples.

✔ Keep Your Cool

On a steamy summer day, there's no better way to beat the heat than reaching for a nice cold beer, right? Wrong! Downing a brewski or another chilly treat (like ice cream or an ice pop) will give you temporary relief, but in the long run, cold substances can actually inhibit your body's natural cooling system by interfering with digestion and sweating. You'll get longer-lasting results if you munch on a nice juicy apple. Aside from the high water content that quenches your thirst, apples contain compounds that help release heat from your body and regulate your hydration levels.

✔ Munch to Lose

Believe it or not, eating apples actually subtracts calories from your diet. That's because the calories your body uses to break down the fiber in the apple exceed those contained in the fruit. Bottom line: The more apples you eat, the more weight you lose. Just don't get carried away—after all, man (or woman) cannot live by apples alone.

✔ Drink to a Thinner You

Legions of folks have been able to shed excess pounds painlessly with this tasty—and healthy—apple cocktail: Mix 64 ounces of 100 percent organic apple juice, ½ cup of unfiltered apple cider vinegar, and ½ teaspoon of liquid stevia (either plain or your favorite flavor) in a pitcher that has a tight-fitting lid. Store it in the refrigerator, and drink an 8-ounce glass of the tangy-sweet beverage before each and every meal.

The Apple of Your Eye

✤ Perk Up Your Pearly Whites

Sure, you can spend a small fortune on those fancy tooth-whitening treatments—and they work, too. But munching on an apple will also help polish away tooth stains safely, and for a lot less money than your dentist will probably charge.

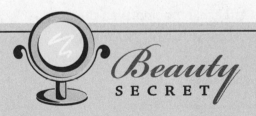

COSMETIC APPLESAUCE

Applesauce that's chock-full of tasty spices is great for eating, but for cosmetic purposes, you want pure, no-frills sauce. To make your own supply, peel and core two medium-size apples, put them in a small baking dish, and pour about ⅛ cup of water over them. Bake them in a 350°F oven for 15 minutes, or until they're slightly mushy. Puree the apples in a blender or food processor, and use the sauce to wash your hair or to whip up any facial mask that calls for applesauce. Store any leftovers in the refrigerator.

Beauty S E C R E T

POTENT POTION

APPLE HAIR RINSE

Are your once-gleaming tresses starting to lose their shine? If so, it's time for a dose of this clarifying rinse. It will help restore your scalp's normal pH level and remove built-up residue from hair sprays and gels.

1 large apple, peeled, cored, and diced
2 tbsp. of apple cider vinegar*
2 cups of water

Put all of the ingredients in a blender or food processor and liquefy. Strain the mixture into a clean container. After shampooing, pour the rinse over your hair. Work it into your hair well, and rinse thoroughly with cool water.

* If you have very dry hair or a sensitive scalp, use only 1 tablespoon of vinegar.

✤ Freshen Your Breath

When hefty helpings of onions or garlic give you a case of dragon breath, sink your teeth into a fresh, crisp apple. It'll dilute the pungent aroma in a flash.

✤ And Banish Coffee Mouth, Too

Even for gung ho coffee lovers, the aftertaste of coffee can be unpleasant. What to do? Eat an apple, of course!

✤ Firm Your Face

Skin-firming facial masks don't come much easier than this one: Mix 1 tablespoon of 100 percent applesauce (no additives!) with 1 tablespoon of wheat germ. Apply the mixture to your skin, and leave it on for 15 minutes. Then rinse it off with warm water and follow up with your usual moisturizer.

✤ Firm Your Face, Take 2

For a sweeter, moister firming experience, peel and core an apple, and puree the pulp with a teaspoon of honey. Smooth the concoction onto your face, wait 15 minutes, and rinse it off with lukewarm water.

✤ Whip Up a Nifty Night Cream

A high-quality night cream can do wonders for your skin's health and elasticity. But the commercial ones—especially those made for sensitive skin—can cost a bundle. So instead of forking over big bucks, march right into your kitchen and follow this five-step procedure:

STEP 1. Gather your supplies. You'll need an apple (any kind will do), 1 cup of olive oil, and 1 cup of rose water*, along with a blender or food processor, and a double boiler.

STEP 2. Wash and dry the apple thoroughly (don't peel it!), then cut it in half, removing the core, seeds, and stem. Cut the fruit into small pieces, and toss them into the blender or food processor.

STEP 3. Start the blender and slowly add the olive oil until a paste forms.

STEP 4. Put tap water in the bottom of the double boiler and the apple-oil mixture in the top part; heat it until it's just lukewarm. (If you don't have a double boiler, substitute a saucepan and a heat-proof bowl.) Don't let the apple cook—if it does, the key ingredient (malic acid) will dissipate.

STEP 5. Set the mixture aside until it cools to room temperature, then add the rose water and stir until the ingredients are thoroughly combined.

Store the cream in a plastic jar in the fridge, where it will keep for up to six days. Use it every night before you go to bed, and within a week or so, you should see softer, more supple skin.

* You can buy rose water in health-food stores and herb shops and (of course) from the Internet.

✤ Wash Your Hair

When you're fresh out of shampoo—or you simply want to get your hair shiny, healthy, and deep-down clean—all-natural applesauce will do the trick. Scoop a handful out of the jar and scrub it deeply into your hair and scalp. Leave it on for 10 minutes, then rinse thoroughly. There's no need

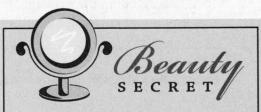

Beauty S E C R E T

FADE AWAY

An apple-lemon potion can help fade age spots gently and naturally. To make it, mix a large, grated apple with 2 teaspoons of lemon juice and ¼ cup of orange flower water (available in herb and health-food shops). Once a day, smooth the mixture over your face, leave it on for 10 minutes, and rinse with clear, cool water.

to add conditioner. **Note:** It may take several minutes to get all the sauce out of your hair, but the results will be well worth the time and effort.

✤ Rub Out Wrinkles

Before you go out and drop a bundle on another fancy anti-wrinkle treatment, give this trick a try: Every morning, core an apple, slice it in half, and rub your face with the cut side. Enzymes in the fruit help your skin retain its moisture and also have a smoothing, firming effect. You should start to see a difference in a week or so.

✤ Try a Triple-Threat Toner

The gentle, but powerful acids and enzymes in apples keep your pores clean and free of bacteria, shield your skin from environmental toxins, and remove dead skin cells and surface dirt. To pull off your own triple play, simply mix ¼ cup of 100 percent apple juice (either homemade or a store-bought organic brand) with 4 tablespoons of witch hazel in a clean bottle. Use a cotton pad to wipe your freshly washed face with the formula, avoiding the eye area. Perform this routine every morning and evening if you have oily skin. If your skin is dry, stick to just once a day.

Best of the Rest

★ Ease Menstrual Woes with Apricots

Most women of childbearing age suffer some degree of menstrual discomfort. But even if you breeze through your monthly periods, it's important to replace the iron that you lose through bleeding. One excellent way to do that is to munch on dried apricots. They're among the most iron-rich—and easily portable—foods you can find.

★ Don't Get SAD

No one is quite sure why some folks are troubled by seasonal affective disorder (SAD) while others are not, but we do know what triggers it: The absence of light during winter's gray days and long nights causes the pineal gland to turn the hormone serotonin into melatonin. The absence of serotonin disrupts normal sleep patterns and causes depression and a craving for sweets and starches. One of the best ways to alleviate those debilitating symptoms is to eat plenty of apricots, pears, plums, and apples. All of these tree fruits gradually raise serotonin levels and help keep them there—so you'll lose your desire to crawl into bed and hibernate.

★ Rout Out Gout with Cherries

They help clear toxins from your body and clean your kidneys, which puts them at the top of the gout-relief list. Eat 10 to 12 fresh or frozen cherries a day, or a handful of dried cherries. You can also drink 100 percent cherry juice to ease gout pain.

Fabulous Food Fix

LIGHT CHERRY CLAFOUTIS

Clafoutis is a pretty fancy-sounding word for what is actually a simple, economical, and healthy dessert. Try it—you and your family will love it!
Note: You can make this recipe in a 9- or 10-inch round baking pan or an 8- or 9-inch square one.

⅔ cup of flour
Pinch of salt
3 large eggs
⅓ cup of sugar
1 cup of 1 percent milk
1 tbsp. of pure vanilla extract
2 tbsp. of butter, melted
1 lb. of fresh cherries, washed, pitted, and dried*
¼ cup of confectioners sugar (optional)

Mix the flour and salt in a large bowl. Beat in the eggs one at a time, then beat in the sugar. Gradually add the milk and vanilla, stirring until the batter is smooth. Pour the butter into the pan, and coat the surface. Add about ¼ inch of batter, and bake at 350°F until lightly set. Remove from the oven, spread the cherries evenly over the batter, and cover them with the remaining batter. Return the pan to the oven. Bake for about 50 minutes, or until the clafoutis is puffed and brown. It will fall, but that's what it is supposed to do. Serve warm or at room temperature. You can dust it with confectioners sugar just before serving.

* Or substitute frozen, pitted cherries that have been thawed and drained, or use another fruit like sliced apples, peaches, or pears.

YIELD: 8 SERVINGS

★ Beat Boils with Figs

You biblical scholars may remember the passage in 2 Kings where Isaiah recommends relieving boils with "a lump of figs." Well, it worked then, and it still works today to draw out the pus and inflammation. Just roast a fresh fig, cut it in two, and lay one half, mushy side down, on the boil. Secure it in place with a bandage or strip of cloth, and leave it on for a couple of hours. Then remove it, warm up the other fig half, and repeat the procedure. **Note:** If the pain of a boil gets progressively worse, or if you see a red streak in it, get medical help pronto. The pus-filled bump may need to be drained surgically.

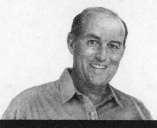

YOU DON'T SAY!

When most folks remove pits from cherries, they toss the things in the trash. But back in 1974, Michigan cherry farmer Herb Teichman had a better idea: He launched a competition to see who could spit the pits the farthest. What was once a neighborhood get-together has now blossomed into the International Cherry Pit-Spitting Championship, which attracts pit spitters from throughout the United States and abroad. Each year in July, they compete for honors at the Teichman family's Tree-Mendus Fruit Farm in Eau Claire, Michigan. The current record holder, Ron Matt of Chicago, spat his pit a whopping 69 feet in 2012!

★ Whip Windburn with Peaches

On a sunny winter day, cold, dry breezes can deliver a nasty windburn before you know it. To ease the pain, slice a peach in half, and rub the juicy surface over your afflicted skin. You'll feel better in no time!

★ Pear Away IBS

Irritable bowel syndrome (IBS) ranks right along with the common cold as a major reason people miss work or school. Fortunately, IBS is not an actual disease, it does not lead to other, more serious intestinal conditions—and there are plenty of gentle, natural remedies that can relieve the painful spasms. One of the best is pears. Either eating the fresh, ripe fruit, or drinking 100 percent pear juice can go a long way toward easing your discomfort.

★ A Plum Good Way to Fight Ulcers

As recently as 10 years or so ago, everyone (the medical community included) thought that ulcers were caused by stress or a hard-charging Type A lifestyle. Well, scientific research has proven that's not the case at all. Nearly all ulcers result from infection of the stomach or duodenum by a bacterium called *Helicobacter pylori*. Whether you've been diagnosed with an ulcer or simply want to avoid one, you can't go wrong eating plenty of plums. Along with other red- and purple-colored foods, they have been shown to inhibit the growth of *H. pylori*.

★ More Prunes for More Immunity

You may think of dried plums, a.k.a. prunes, as just a handy tool to get your internal "plumbing" working smoothly. Well, think again. Prunes rank among the best sources of antioxidants, one of your body's prime weapons in the fight against diseases.

★ Lighten Up with Cherry Juice

Did you know that cherries have terrific skin-lightening properties? It's true! And here's a simple way to put their power to work. In a bowl, mix 2 teaspoons of honey into ¼ cup of 100 percent cherry juice, and stir in ½ cup of sugar (to slough off dead skin cells). Using a soft paintbrush, apply the mixture to discolored areas of your skin. Leave it on for 20 minutes, and then wash it off with warm water.

★ Smooth Your Skin with Peaches

No matter what type of skin you have, peaches can make it look and feel better. Just whip a ripe peach (peeled and pitted) in a blender with the white of one egg. Gently pat the mixture onto your face, leave it on for half an hour, and rinse it off with cool water.

POTENT POTION

A PEACHY-KEEN FACIAL

Here's a mask that will leave your skin feeling soft, smooth, and supple—but only if you can keep from eating it before you get it onto your face!

1 large peach, skinned
1 tbsp. of honey
2 tbsp. of plain yogurt

Mash the peach and honey together. Then stir in the yogurt until you have a paste. Pat the mixture evenly over your face, including the eye area. Leave it on for about 10 minutes. Rinse it off with warm water, pat dry, and apply your normal toner and moisturizer.

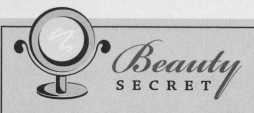

DRINK TO A CLEAR COMPLEXION

*Don't get me wrong—I'm not suggesting that downing a few brewskis or a dry martini will end your skin problems! I'm talking about fruit smoothies—to my mind one of the most pleasant ways of all to enjoy the many cosmetic (and health) benefits of fruit. To make one, just pull out your blender, and blend 1½ to 2 cups of diced, fresh fruit with 1 cup of frozen yogurt and ½ cup of 100 percent fruit juice, pure fruit nectar, or milk. Use any flavor combinations that suit your fancy or accomplish the mission(s) you have in mind. **Note:** If you use frozen fruit for your smoothie, you can use unfrozen yogurt.*

★ Figs Fight Dark Circles

If you've got dark circles under your eyes, and you do care a feather *and* a fig about it, treat yourself to this rejuvenating routine. Simply cut a fresh fig in two, then lie down and put one fig half over each eye for about 10 minutes.

★ Pick a Peach of a Toner

This formula is specially designed for dry, flaky skin. Peel two peaches, remove the stones, and mash the fruit in a bowl with a teaspoon of heavy cream. Mix in enough olive oil to make a smooth paste. Then smear the mixture onto your face, wait 10 minutes, and rinse it off with lukewarm water. The result: smooth, fresh, and clear skin!

★ Pears Promote Pretty Skin

If an apple a day keeps the doctor away, what does a pear a day keep away? Skin problems of all kinds! Pears are loaded with lots of essential nutrients that you need to keep your skin beautiful and healthy. So gobble 'em up!

★ Eat Acne Away

In the ongoing fight against acne (for teenagers and adults), four fabulous tree fruits rank as true heroes. What are they? Apricots, cherries, pears, and the star of this chapter, apples. They all contain vitamins and minerals that flush toxins out of your system and help banish the bacteria that cause acne. So we'll finish where we started—An apple a day . . . helps keep acne away!

2 Avocados

Not so long ago, when folks were avoiding fatty foods like the plague, avocados wound up on dietary no-no lists nationwide. But now we know that while avocados (a.k.a. alligator pears) are high in fat, 80 percent of it offers both health and beauty benefits galore. What's more, these creamy green treats exceed every other fruit in certain plant compounds that may help prevent cancer and heart disease. And avocado oil packs the same powerful load of goodness for the inside *and* outside of your body!

A Sunbelt Superstar

✔ Fast Fat Facts

So how can a food that's high in fat be good for you? Well, most of the fat in avocados is the unsaturated kind, which helps lower levels of LDL (bad) cholesterol, while maintaining supplies of HDL (good) cholesterol. It's as simple as that.

✔ Fruity First Aid

You're slicing into an avocado, the knife slips, and you slice into your finger. What do you do? Count your lucky stars, that's what—because you've got first aid at your fingertips. Just break off a little piece of the avocado flesh, and apply it to the cut. The fruit has antibiotic properties that will start working right away to heal the wound. Plus, the soft, mellow pulp will help ease the pain.

✔ Fight Fat with Fat

Trying to drop a few pounds? Avocados can help you reduce your calorie intake painlessly if you put them to work in two ways:

1. SPREAD IT ON. Just mash an avocado and mix it with lemon or lime juice and your choice of herbs. Then use it to replace higher-calorie spreads and toppings (see "Hasty-Tasty Avocado Spread," below).

2. BAKE WITH IT. Puree an avocado in a blender (or mash it thoroughly with a fork). Then replace either all or half the amount of butter called for in your recipe with the mashed avocado. Just a few words of warning: Although you should notice little if any difference in flavor, the finished product will have a lighter texture and may have a slight greenish tinge.

✔ Lose the Blues

Whether the problem is caused by your monthly bout with PMS, a wintertime SAD attack, or a simple case of the blahs, avocados can cheer you up fast. They contain potent supplies of serotonin and tryptophan, two compounds that help boost your brain's natural mood-lifting chemicals. **Note:** If you're battling prolonged depression, rather than just a short period of the

Fabulous Food Fix

HASTY-TASTY AVOCADO SPREAD

You couldn't ask for an easier—or more delicious—way to cut calories. This versatile condiment takes only minutes to make, and each 2-tablespoon serving contains just 53 calories, compared to 215 for the same amount of butter or mayonnaise, and 105 for cream cheese.

1 medium avocado, peeled and pitted
2 tbsp. of lemon or lime juice
2 tbsp. of fresh, chopped basil*

In a medium bowl, mash the avocado, and stir in the lemon or lime juice and basil. Cover, and chill the mixture for an hour or so to blend the flavors. Then use it instead of your usual toppings on baked potatoes, sandwiches, bagels, or crackers.

* Or substitute your favorite herbs or herb combos. Cumin, coriander, garlic, and hot red-pepper flakes all complement the flavor of avocado.

YIELD: 6 (2-TABLESPOON) SERVINGS

gloomy-doomies, don't fuss with dietary remedies—get professional help pronto!

✔ Deliver a Dynamic Duo

In addition to their beneficial fat, avocados contain healthy amounts of many essential vitamins and minerals. But the fruit's true superstar status lies in the fact that it contains much larger supplies of two powerful plant compounds than you'll find in any other commonly eaten fruit—in some cases, up to seven times as much!

BETA-SITOSTEROL inhibits the absorption of cholesterol from your intestines into your bloodstream, thereby reducing your risk of heart disease. Research has also shown that beta-sitosterol can reduce inflammation, boost the immune system, and may hinder the growth of cancerous tumors.

GLUTATHIONE is a powerful antioxidant that, among other feats, boosts the immune system, encourages a healthy nervous system, slows the aging process, and may help prevent heart disease, as well as cancers of the mouth and pharynx.

✔ Soothe Your Sunburn . . .

And minor kitchen burns, too. How? Just rub a little avocado oil over the affected area. Or scoop the flesh out of an avocado, and rub it onto your ailin' skin. Either treatment will provide cooling, healing relief in a hurry.

✔ Relieve Psoriasis and Eczema

Avocado oil contains compounds called sterolins that moisturize the skin, keeping it soft and hydrated. That's why it's a prime choice for treating the pain and itching of skin disorders like psoriasis and eczema.

Can the Calluses

HEALTHFUL HINT

If you use a cane, walker, or crutches, then you're well acquainted with the calluses that often develop in the palms of your hands from the constant pressure and rubbing. To remove those painful, annoying bumps, simply mix 1 tablespoon of mashed avocado with 1 to 2 tablespoons of cornmeal to form a paste. Take the mixture in the palm of one hand, and rub both hands together, working the gritty stuff into the calluses and around your fingers. Then rinse your hands with warm water and pat dry. Repeat once or twice a week, and soon your skin will be soft and smooth again.

POTENT POTION

AVOCADO ANTIFUNGAL CREAM

Folks who use this powerful concoction claim it fights athlete's foot, eczema, and other skin irritations as well as or better than any commercial product they've found. Give it a try, and see if you don't agree.

4 oz. of shea butter
2 tbsp. of avocado oil
2 tbsp. of olive oil
15 drops of tea tree oil

Combine the shea butter, avocado oil, and olive oil in a double boiler or heat-proof bowl, and heat until the shea butter melts. Remove from the heat, and stir in the tea tree oil. Pour the mixture into a lidded container like a small clamp-top canning jar or a 6-ounce herb-storage tin. Refrigerate to cool. Once the cream is firm, take it out of the fridge, and store it at room temperature. Scoop some out of the jar as the need arises, and smooth it over your affected skin.

YIELD: APPROXIMATELY ⅔ CUP

✔ Eat a Sports "Drink"

Avocados contain approximately 60 percent more potassium than bananas, which makes them heavyweight champs when it comes to relieving muscle cramps. So when your next marathon—or cutthroat badminton match—leaves you with a charley horse, don't down a Gatorade®; grab a 'gator pear, and chow down instead. (My favorite fast fix for this purpose is to simply chop a small avocado or half of a large one, and toss the pieces with a half-and-half mixture of olive oil and balsamic vinegar.) Your muscles will say "Thanks!"

✔ Oil's Well Massage Formula

When it comes to lowering stress levels, boosting energy, or easing the aches and pains of overworked muscles, nothing beats a good rubdown with a high-quality massage oil. You can buy plenty of excellent ones, but it's easy—and a whole lot cheaper—to make your own. Simply mix equal parts of avocado oil and almond oil in a glass bottle with a tight-fitting cap, and store it in the refrigerator. Then, whenever your body or spirits feel the need, pour 1 tablespoon of the oil in a small dish and warm it up slightly in the microwave (test a drop on your forearm; it should feel comfortably warm, not hot). Add a few drops of essential oil that's right for the job at hand, and you're good to go. You'll find scads of scents in herb and aromatherapy shops, but here's a sampling of good choices:

LAVENDER delivers a calming, relaxing effect.

ORANGE, LEMON, AND GRAPEFRUIT rev up your spirits and renew your energy.

PEPPERMINT refreshes tired or sore muscles. (It makes a fabulous foot rub!)

✔ More Power from Potassium

You don't have to be a weekend warrior to benefit from the potassium avocados offer up. Eating plenty of these creamy green fruits can help solve some of your most nagging health problems. Like these, for instance:

FLUID RETENTION. The potassium will counter-balance the sodium in your body and help reduce the excess fluids.

HIGH BLOOD PRESSURE. Potassium prevents the thickening of your artery walls and also helps regulate your body's fluid levels, which are crucial to regulating your blood pressure.

INSOMNIA. Having trouble sleeping through the night? Eat avocados (and other potassium-rich foods) on a regular basis. This mighty mineral encourages deep, restful sleep.

✔ Easy Does It

When you're recovering from surgery, or suffering from an illness that reduces your appetite level to near zero, pureed avocado is just what the doctor ordered. It packs a boatload of the nutrients you need to build up your strength and get your system working smoothly again, yet its flavor and texture are mild enough to sit easy in oh-so-sensitive stomachs.

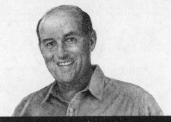

YOU DON'T SAY!

Avocados are native to Central and South America, where they've been cultivated for more than 10,000 years. The Aztecs considered them to be powerful aphrodisiacs—so much so that, according to lore, folks would lock their nubile daughters indoors during the harvesting season. When the conquistadors and early colonists arrived on the scene, they were horrified at the mere thought of consuming the fruits. Their unsavory reputation continued well into the 20th century. It was not until the 1920s, when commercial growers launched a major ad campaign to dispel the old myth, that avocados started to gain real traction as a delicious, healthful—and respectable—treat.

CAUTION ⚠️

Although avocados are a health boon to us humans, the same is not true for our four-footed and fine-feathered friends. According to the *Merck Veterinary Manual,* feeding avocado fruit, seeds, or leaves to dogs, cats, and birds—as well as horses, cattle, goats, and rabbits—can result in their severe illness or even death.

✔ Eat Up, Baby!

The high-powered nutrients and easygoing flavor make pureed avocado a natural choice for the infant in your life. In fact, in its native tropics, the smooth, green fruit is pretty much a staple in every new mother's pantry.

✔ Leverage the Leaves

Attention, Sunbelt dwellers (or you Northerners who grow avocado trees as indoor-outdoor potted plants)! An avocado leaf poultice is one of the most effective "weapons" you can have in your first-aid arsenal. It's a simple way to ease the pain of muscle strains and sprains, and headaches. To make a poultice, just heat six or eight avocado leaves in water until they're warm, but not hot, and lay them in the middle of a piece of soft, all-cotton cloth that's about 12 inches square. Fold the sides in to form a rectangular pouch, and lay it on your achin' body part. Leave the poultice in place until it cools down. Repeat several times a day as needed.

✔ Avocados Produce More Amore

Over time, the vagina's natural lubrication tends to diminish, and even slight dryness can make intercourse unpleasant or even downright painful. The simple solution: Apply avocado oil to the affected area. It'll solve the problem at a fraction of the cost of commercial products. P.S.: Many women also find that having a massage with soothing oil helps them relax prior to intercourse—and avocado oil is an ideal mood maker!

The Avocado Attraction

✤ Banish Bad Breath

Avocados rank among Mother Nature's most effective breath fresheners. That's because they don't simply remove the residual aroma of food you've just eaten. Instead, compounds in the fruit help remove decomposing residue in your intestines, which can contribute to bad breath. There is no specific dosage required to perform this useful feat—so making avocados a regular part of your diet will go a long way toward clearing the air.

✤ Fight the Frizzies

The battle couldn't be any easier: Simply peel and mash a ripe avocado, work it into your hair, and leave it on for 15 minutes. Rinse it out with cool water, and your hair will be smooth, not frazzled.

POTENT POTION

AVOCADO BODY BUTTER

The same vitamins, minerals, and protein that make avocados an A1 choice for facial treatments work just as well to soften and nourish the skin on the rest of your body. That's why avocado-"flavored" body butters are selling like hotcakes. But why spend your hard-earned bucks, when it's a snap to make your own supply?

9 oz. of cocoa butter

9 oz. of avocado oil

**50 drops of your favorite
    essential oil***

3 tsp. of cornstarch

Ice water

Sterilized wide-mouth jars**

In the top of a double boiler, melt the cocoa butter over medium heat until it's just warm. Add the avocado oil, essential oil, and cornstarch, and mix thoroughly. Remove from the heat, and set the bowl into a larger one filled with ice water. Using an electric mixer, whip the mixture until it reaches the consistency of whipped cream and forms stiff peaks. Spoon the butter into the jars. It'll keep for about two months at room temperature. After a shower, scoop out a handful, smooth it all over your body, and say "Ahhh. . ."

* Lemon, orange, lavender, and mint are excellent skin-friendly choices.

** To sterilize jars (and lids), put them in a pot with enough water to cover them by at least 1 inch, and boil for about 10 minutes.

YIELD: 2 TO 2½ CUPS

✤ Beat the Smoggy Heat

Hot, smoggy weather can take a major toll on your hair. If you live in an area where humid heat and pollution reign supreme in the summertime, there is nothing you can do to change the climate—but you can protect your hair from the damage it inflicts. Every month or so, mash half of an avocado with ¼ cup of mayonnaise (the real stuff, with plenty of eggs and oil in it, not the low-fat kind). Massage the mixture into your scalp, and comb it out to the ends of your hair. Cover your hair with a shower cap, and wrap a hot, wet towel around your head. Leave it on for at least 30 minutes, and then rinse thoroughly.

✤ Ditch the Itch

A scalp that's chronically dry and itchy can be a real nightmare. But here's a simple way to solve that problem once and for all: Once or twice a month, massage your scalp with a teaspoon or so of avocado oil (more if you need it). Rinse it out thoroughly, and say bye-bye to that bad dream.

Fabulous Food Fix

AVOCADO-MANGO SALAD

Nutritional gurus rank avocados number one on the list of foods that help your skin maintain its good health and good looks. This ultra-simple recipe pairs avocados with mangoes—another health and beauty wonder worker.

2 large avocados, halved, peeled, pitted, and chilled
2 large mangoes, halved, peeled, pitted, and chilled
Cayenne pepper to taste
Salt to taste
¾ cup of plain low-fat yogurt
Juice of 2 large limes
3 tbsp. of honey
4 mint sprigs, for garnish

Cut the avocado and mango halves lengthwise into ½-inch slices. Arrange them on four individual salad plates, alternating the green and yellow fruits. Mix equal parts of cayenne pepper and salt, and lightly sprinkle over the fruit slices. Stir the yogurt, lime juice, and honey in a bowl. Just before serving, spoon 2 to 3 tablespoons of dressing over each salad. Garnish with the mint sprigs.

YIELD: 4 SERVINGS

❧ Shine Your Tresses

For the softest, shiniest hair in town, mix a mashed avocado with 1 tablespoon each of olive oil and honey (either by hand or in a blender). Massage the green paste into your damp hair, working from the roots out to the tips. Cover your head with a shower cap, and go about your business for 20 minutes or so. Rinse the concoction out, then follow up with shampoo and conditioner.

❧ Supercharge Your Shampoo

To keep your hair moisturized with no muss and no fuss, pour a teaspoon or two of avocado oil into your regular bottle of shampoo. Shake the bottle well before each use, and then wash your tresses as usual. Your hair will be smooth as silk.

❧ Fortify Creams and Lotions

Want to get the full softening power of upscale skin-care products without the hefty price tags? Then just mix a few drops of avocado oil into your favorite commercial brand(s). Bingo: More beautifying action for a lot less money!

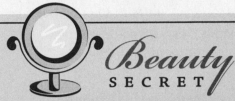

Beauty SECRET

DEEP-CLEAN AND SOFTEN

Deliver dual results with this facial mask: Mix half an avocado, 2 tablespoons of orange juice, and 1 teaspoon each of molasses and honey in a blender. Smooth the mixture onto your skin, and wait 30 to 40 minutes. Remove the mask using a damp, warm washcloth. Store any leftovers in a covered container in the refrigerator; it will keep for two or three days.

❧ Soften Dry Skin

The healthy fats in avocados can work wonders to moisten and soothe dry skin. To give your face a treat, simply mix half of a mashed avocado with half of a mashed banana, and spread the "cream" on your face and neck. Wait 15 minutes, rinse with lukewarm water, and pat dry.

❧ Nourish Not-So-Dry Skin

If your skin is normal to oily, this facial formula is the one for you. Mix 2 tablespoons of mashed avocado with 1 tablespoon of crushed almonds

POTENT POTION

INTENSIVE AVOCADO HAND TREATMENT

When work or play leaves you with sore, chapped hands, treat them to this super-soothing routine.

¼ **avocado, peeled and pitted**
1 egg white
2 tbsp. of uncooked oatmeal
1 tsp. of lemon or lime juice

Mash the avocado in a bowl, add the remaining ingredients, and mix thoroughly. Rub the mixture into your skin, leave it on for 20 minutes, then rinse with warm water.

and ½ teaspoon of honey until the mixture is creamy. Smooth it onto your face with your hands, and leave it on for 30 minutes or so. Rinse with lukewarm water, and pat dry.

✤ An All-Type Titan

To work softening wonders for any type of skin—dry, oily, or normal—mix 2 tablespoons of mashed avocado in a bowl with 2 tablespoons of honey and 1 egg yolk. Apply the mixture to your face and leave it on for 30 minutes. Rinse with warm water, and pat dry.

✤ A Tough Customer Delivers Soft Skin

Avocados got their nickname, alligator pears, from their thick, leathery coverings. But those rough and tough skins can actually provide a couple of kind and gentle ways to soften yours:

■ **GIVE YOURSELF A FACIAL.** Grab an avocado peel with a thin layer of fruit left on it, and rub the rind over your face. Its gritty texture will slough off dead skin, while the pulp that stays on your face moisturizes it. Wait 10 minutes, then rinse with cool water.

■ **SMOOTH YOUR HEELS, KNEES, AND ELBOWS.** Scrape an avocado peel clean of any fruit, and sprinkle a few drops of lemon juice on the surface. Then rub it across your rough body part. It'll feel a little strange at first, but your dry skin will love it—guaranteed!

✤ A Super-Simple Softener

For a one-step moisturizing routine, rub a little avocado oil on your face and neck. Leave it on for about 10 minutes, then rinse with warm water, and pat dry.

✤ Bag the Bags

When cosmetic trouble strikes in the form of sagging skin under your eyes, don't just stand there—take it lying down! Cut two thick slices from a peeled avocado, lie down, and lay a wedge under each eye. Leave the fruit in place for about 20 minutes, then rinse off the residue. The potassium in the avocado will tighten your skin and help reduce that "baggy" look.

✤ Punch Up Your Cleansing Cream

The gritty texture and high nutrient content of avocado pits make them just the ticket for intensifying the power of facial cleansers. To add them to your beauty arsenal, simply remove the pits from three or four avocados, making sure to get all the fruit off. Then proceed as follows:

STEP 1. Put the pits in a heavy-duty, ziplock plastic bag, and smash them with a hammer until the pieces are about the size of peas. Then spread the little chunks out on a baking sheet to dry for a few days.

STEP 2. When they're completely dry, put them into a coffee grinder or food processor, and grind them into a powder (about the consistency of ground coffee).

STEP 3. Again, spread them out to dry, then store them in an airtight container (a clamp-top canning jar is perfect). When you wash your face, add a teaspoon or so of the ground pits to your favorite liquid soap or cleansing potion for a fantastic finish.

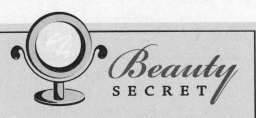

A Speedy, Seedy Massage

Beauty SECRET

Nothing relieves tired, stiff muscles like a good massage. But if don't have time for a rubdown, reach for an avocado seed. Rinse off all of the fruit, and dry the pit. Then rub it over your arms, legs, hips, and as much of your back as you can reach. It'll improve your circulation and make you feel good all over. (Some folks also claim it helps conquer cellulite.)

✤ Heal Cracked Cuticles

Dry, damaged cuticles aren't merely unattractive—they're as painful as all get-out! Here's a super-simple trick that'll have them looking and feeling better in a jiffy. Just mix 1 tablespoon of avocado oil and 5 drops of tea tree oil in a small bottle with a flip spout. Once or twice a day, dampen the skin on your affected fingers and/or toes. Then apply a drop of the mixture to each cuticle, and massage the oil in thoroughly. Use a cuticle stick to gently push the cuticle back from the nail. You should start seeing rather dramatic results within a few days.

Best of the Rest

★ An A-Peeling Healing Solution

To look at a banana peel, you'd never take it to be a first-class first-aid worker. But it is! In fact, these super skins are world champs at solving a number of common mishaps. **Note:** In each use below, apply the peel inner side down, with the moist side on your skin:

FIRE ANT BITES. Place the peel on the bite, and leave it on for 20 minutes. Wash the area, and apply a new peel if symptoms persist.

MINOR CUTS AND SCRAPES. Just put a piece of peel on the wound, and secure it in place with a bandage or strip of cloth. Change the peel every three to four hours until the "owie" is no longer "Wowie!"

PLANTAR WARTS. At bedtime, tape a piece of peel over the wart. Cover the peel with a bandage or

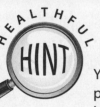

HEALTHFUL HINT

A First-Aid Kit in a Jar

You'll always be prepared for sudden bruises, sore joints, and insect stings with this surefire painkiller. Fill a jar with chopped banana peels, pour in enough rubbing alcohol to cover the peels, and put the lid on the jar. Stash it in your medicine cabinet (without straining out the solids), and let the mixture "brew" for two weeks before you use it. Then, whenever trouble strikes, dip a cotton ball or pad into the solution, and dab it on wherever you're sore, swollen, or stung.

a tight sock, and leave it on overnight. Repeat the procedure each night until the wart is gone—it shouldn't take more than two or three treatments.

POISON IVY. Lay peels all across the rash-covered area, keeping the skins in place with bandages or pieces of cloth. Before you know it, the rash will begin to dry up, and the itch will be history.

Fabulous Food Fix

MANGOSICLES

In tropical climes, folks rely on mangoes and their juice to help fend off heatstroke. But no matter where you live, on a hot summer day, these icy pops are just the ticket to keep your internal temperature down and your energy level up.

2 cups of chopped mangoes
¾ cup of water
½ cup of evaporated skim milk
¼ cup of frozen pineapple juice
   concentrate, thawed

Puree the fruit in a blender until smooth. Add the remaining ingredients, and blend thoroughly. Pour the mixture into freezer molds or paper cups, and insert wooden sticks. Cover the surfaces, and pop the pops into the freezer. Then, when you crave a cool (and healthy) treat, unmold a 'sicle and enjoy!

YIELD: 4 SERVINGS

★ Peel Away Pounds
Trying to lose weight? Then wake up and smell the bananas! Studies have shown that dieters who sniffed a banana whenever they felt like munching on food lost an average of 30 pounds in six months.

★ Keep Your Eye on Mangoes
But don't just look at the pretty yellow-orange fruits—eat 'em as often as you can. Just 1 cup of sliced mangoes supplies 25 percent of your minimum daily requirement of vitamin A, which promotes good eyesight and helps fend off both night blindness and dry eyes.

★ Dodge Indigestion with Papayas
Papayas break down the food compounds in your stomach that cause indigestion. So if you have a chronically slow digestive system, give it a

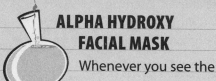

POTENT POTION

ALPHA HYDROXY FACIAL MASK

Whenever you see the words *alpha hydroxy* on a commercial skin-treatment label, you'll also see big numbers on the price tag. Well, this kitchen-counter cosmetic gives you the same results at a fraction of the price.

1 cup of fresh pineapple
½ fresh (slightly green) papaya
2 tbsp. of honey

Puree the fruits in a blender, pour the mixture into a bowl, and stir in the honey. Apply the concoction to your just-washed face and neck, avoiding the eye area. Leave it on for five minutes (no longer!), and rinse it off with cool water. Repeat with a fresh batch once a week. The enzymes in the fruit help firm your skin, even out your skin tone, and make tiny lines less apparent, while the honey provides deep-down moisture.

jump-start each morning by eating half a papaya or drinking a glass of 100 percent papaya juice. Or, if you feel discomfort only after you've eaten rich food, down a glass of the juice half an hour or so before you indulge.

★ Papaya the "Plumber" to the Rescue

The same papaya enzymes that ease your digestive discomfort can also stimulate bowel movements. The next time you need to loosen things up, eat some papaya fruit or drink a glass of juice to get things moving.

★ Tropical Booty for Black Eyes

Got a shiner? Eat plenty of fresh papaya and/or pineapple for two or three days. How much is enough? The more the better, but aim for at least 2 to 3 cups every 24 hours. The enzymes in these fruits will help you lose the bruise.

★ Pineapple: A Gentle Dental Helper

As soon as you've scheduled a dental appointment, start packing in the pineapple. Eat a cup or so of the fruit every day—either fresh or canned in its own juice, not sugary syrup—and drink at least 8 ounces of 100 percent pineapple juice. After your dental work is completed, continue this routine for several days. The enzymes in the fruit should ease any pain and discomfort, and also hasten the healing process.

★ Ward Off Wrinkles with Bananas

Chances are your face has already collected some, um, signs of "experience." To discourage more from joining the crowd, mash a ripe banana, and mix in a few drops of peanut oil. Smooth it onto your face using an upward and outward motion, and leave it on for at least 30 minutes. Then rinse it off with lukewarm water.

★ Scrub-a-Dub-Dub . . .

With mangoes in the tub. Use this super-moisturizing body scrub in your next bath, and your skin will feel smooth and supple from head to toe. To make it, put a peeled and seeded mango into a blender with 1 tablespoon of honey, 2 tablespoons of whole milk, and ½ cup of sugar. Blend thoroughly, pour the mixture into a bowl, and rub the scrub vigorously all over your body. Rinse with warm water, followed by cold water.

★ Cure a Suntan "Hangover"

Papaya is a fabulous remedy for dry, flaky, or rough skin—especially when it's the result of a fading suntan. Just mash the fruit, and apply it in a thin layer to your face, neck, and chest. Wait 10 to 20 minutes, then rinse with cool water and pat dry.

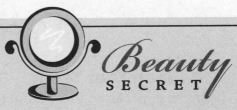

PAPAYAS FIGHT FRECKLES

Beauty SECRET

If you've been spending your hard-earned cash on commercial spot-removal products, here's good news: The key ingredient in those creams, papain, comes from papayas. To get the same skin-lightening results at a fraction of the price, puree a peeled, seeded papaya in a blender. Wash and gently dry your face and any other areas of your body that you want to de-freckle. Smooth the paste-like mash onto your skin, avoiding the eye area. Leave it on for 15 minutes or so, then rinse it off with warm water, pat dry, and apply your usual moisturizer. Repeat three times a week. Within about three weeks, you should start to see major results.

3

Baking Soda

When French chemist and surgeon Nicolas Leblanc first formulated soda ash in 1791, he intended it as a leavening agent to be used in baking bread. But others were experimenting, too, and used his discovery as the stepping-stone to creating baking soda. Little did any of the early tinkerers know that this handy kitchen helper would gain worldwide fame as one of our most versatile and effective health and beauty helpers.

A Medicine Chest in a Box

✔ Clean Your Teeth

In the days before commercial toothpastes came along, folks kept their teeth and gums healthy by brushing twice a day with a little baking soda on a wet toothbrush. Guess what? That simple (and cheap) routine works just as well today!

✔ Douse Your Dentures

Keep your dentures clean and germ-free by soaking them each night in a glass of water with 2 teaspoons of baking soda added to it.

✔ Say "So Long" to Canker Sores

Get rid of painful canker sores by rinsing your mouth with a solution of ½ teaspoon of baking soda in half a glass of warm water. Repeat every few hours, as necessary, until the bothersome bumps are gone.

✔ Fight Gum Diseases

To combat the bacteria that cause gum diseases, brush two or (whenever possible) three times a day with a paste made from 3 parts baking soda and 1 part hydrogen peroxide. To perk up the flavor, add your choice of tasty extracts, such as lemon, almond, or cherry.

✔ Fend Off Flea Bites

Flea bites cause just as much pain and itching in humans as they do in dogs and cats. The blood-sucking little buggers are most likely to strike if you've recently moved into an abode where a flea-ridden dog or cat used to dwell—and it's all but guaranteed that you'll find them lingering in the carpet. Send them to their just rewards with this procedure:

STEP 1. Sprinkle the rug thickly with a half-and-half mixture of baking soda and table salt.

STEP 2. Let it sit overnight, then vacuum well.

STEP 3. Repeat the procedure two more times on dry days, and you'll be flea-free!

✔ Give Hives the Heave-Ho

All kinds of things can make your skin break out in hives and rashes. But no matter what caused the itchy, red blotches, this old trick will send 'em packin' in no time at all. Just add ½ cup of baking soda to a tub of warm water, and settle in for a long, soothing soak (cool drink, glowing candle, and non-serious reading matter are optional).

✔ Banish Bug-Bite Woes

When the bug bites or the bee stings, there are a whole lot of ways to reduce

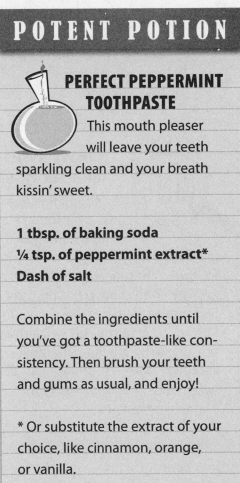

POTENT POTION

PERFECT PEPPERMINT TOOTHPASTE

This mouth pleaser will leave your teeth sparkling clean and your breath kissin' sweet.

1 tbsp. of baking soda
¼ tsp. of peppermint extract*
Dash of salt

Combine the ingredients until you've got a toothpaste-like consistency. Then brush your teeth and gums as usual, and enjoy!

* Or substitute the extract of your choice, like cinnamon, orange, or vanilla.

the pain, itch, and swelling, but this old-timer can't be beat: Dissolve 1 teaspoon of baking soda in 1 cup of water. Then dip a soft, clean cloth into the solution, and hold it on the bite for 20 minutes or so. Problem solved! **Note:** If the culprit was a bee, then you'll need to remove the stinger before you apply the soda.

✔ Ditch the Itch of Hemorrhoids

For many hemorrhoid sufferers, the pain of these swollen rectal veins can't hold a candle to the constant itch that can't be scratched. But it *can* be relieved in other ways, and this is one of the best: Mix 1 cup of baking soda with 5 to 10 drops of chamomile oil (available in herb shops and natural-food stores). Add the mixture to a tub of warm water, get in, and soak for about 15 minutes or so. You'll feel much better—guaranteed!

✔ Cool Your Sunburn

When you've spent too much time under the hot summer sun, reach for that familiar bright orange box. What you do after that depends on where you are, and what parts of your body are burned. You have two options:

1. Add ½ cup of baking soda to a tub of lukewarm water, then soak in it for 15 to 20 minutes. When you get out, don't towel off. Instead, let your body air-dry, and leave the soda residue on your skin so it continues to provide cooling relief.

2. If you're not near a bathtub—or the burn "victim" is your face—saturate a washcloth with a solution of 4 tablespoons of baking soda in 1 quart of lukewarm water. Gently apply the compress to your afflicted skin, and hold it there until you start to feel relief. **Note:** If you experience chills or a fever, or if you develop blisters or a rash on top of your sunburn, get medical help immediately—you may have sun poisoning.

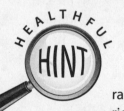

HEALTHFUL HINT

Down with Diaper Rash!

Although diaper rash may not be a serious health hazard, it *is* a major pain in the you-know-what for the infant sufferer—and for parents trying to comfort the tiny tyke. Fortunately, help is as close as your kitchen cupboard. Gently wipe baby's bottom with a solution of 4 tablespoons of baking soda per quart of warm water. The rash will dry up—and so will the tears.

✔ Sidestep Heatstroke

Even if you've slathered yourself with sunscreen, covered yourself from head to toe in UV-protective clothing, or you're indoors with no air-conditioning, sweltering summer heat can take a serious (and even deadly) toll. Well, don't take any chances: Lower your internal temperature by soaking for 15 to 20 minutes in a cool bath with 2 cups of baking soda added to the water. While you're at it, sip a tall glass of cold water to really chill out.

✔ Unstuff Your Nose

Nasty head cold got you all but glued to a vaporizer? This simple additive will clear things up in a hurry. Just pour 1 teaspoon of baking soda into the water inside. It'll unblock your nasal passages and keep your vaporizer clean, to boot!

✔ Relieve Indigestion and Heartburn

Whenever you feel those annoying symptoms coming on, drink a glass of water with 1 teaspoon of baking soda dissolved in it. The alkaline properties of the soda will neutralize the overactive acids in your stomach and soothe the burn.

✔ Ease Ulcer Pain

The same properties that relieve indigestion—namely, the ability to reduce your system's acidity—make baking soda a natural for treating ulcers. In this case, the dose is 1 to 2 teaspoons in a glass of water whenever you feel discomfort.

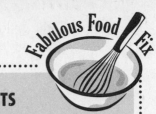

Fabulous Food Fix

DIY SPORTS DRINK

Sports drinks are not just for serious athletes. Anyone who works or plays in the hot sun needs to keep fluids, glucose, and electrolytes flowing through his or her system. You can accomplish this by downing one of many commercial products—or you can make your own elixir at a small fraction of the cost. **Note:** Do not give this potion to children under the age of 12.

½ tbsp. of sugar
½ tsp. of baking soda
½ tsp. of table salt
¼ tsp. of potassium-based salt substitute*
1 qt. of water
Unsweetened Kool-Aid® powder or other flavoring to taste (optional, but highly recommended)

Mix all of the ingredients thoroughly, and drink up frequently.

* Such as Morton® Lite Salt™ Mixture or Morton® Salt Substitute.

YIELD: 4 (8-OUNCE) SERVINGS

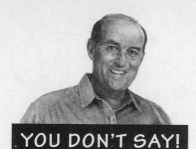

✔ Say "So Long, Splinter!"

Got a sliver in your finger? Whatever you do, don't start digging into your skin! Instead, mix 1 tablespoon of baking soda in a small glass of warm water, and soak your digit for about 10 minutes. Repeat twice a day until the splinter pokes far enough out of your skin that you can grasp it with tweezers and gently ease it out.

✔ Give Colds and Flu the Cold Shoulder

Old-timers knew a secret that the modern medical community has only recently rediscovered: Your body is best able to fend off health woes of all kinds, including infectious diseases, when your system is highly alkaline. Back in the 1920s, doctors routinely prescribed a solution of ½ teaspoon of baking soda mixed in a glass of cool water for patients who had come down with colds and flu (known in those days as the grippe). It works every bit as well today if you follow this schedule:

DAY 1. Take one dose of the drink at roughly two-hour intervals to total six doxes.

DAY 2. Take one dose of the drink at roughly two-hour intervals to total four doses.

DAY 3. Take one dose each morning and evening.

Thereafter, drink a glass of the solution each morning until your symptoms are gone.

✔ Auxiliary Action

In addition to the oral prescription, old-time docs recommended soaking in a hot baking soda bath, so the health-giving alkali could penetrate your system from the outside. So just before bedtime, fill your bathtub with water that's as hot as you can stand, and mix in ½ to 1 pound of baking soda. Ease your achin' body into the tub, stay there for about 15 minutes, then immediately dry off and hit the sack. How much better you feel in the morning will depend on how advanced your symptoms are—but you should feel a lot more chipper than you did when you went to bed!

✔ Cut Gas Production

Are some of your favorite foods the kind that tend to make you feel gassy and bloated after you've eaten them? If so, then simply sprinkle a little baking soda on the gas producers. You'll be able to dig in and enjoy your meal with no worries about unwelcome after effects.

✔ Heal Fever Blisters

There are few more miserable skin afflictions than fever blisters (a.k.a. cold sores) on your ultra-sensitive lips. To clear up the painful bumps in a hurry, mix 2 tablespoons of baking soda with enough water to make a thick paste, and cover the blister with a heavy coat of it. Reapply throughout the day as needed until the blister is history.

✔ Alleviate Anxiety

Dreading an upcoming visit to the dentist? Or maybe your annual performance review at work? Well, getting all hot and bothered won't help you avoid the experience. But this simple trick will help you face it in a calmer mood. The morning of the big day, get up a bit earlier than usual so you can mix ⅓ cup of baking soda and ⅓ cup of powdered ginger in a tub of warm water and soak in it for 15 minutes or so. Your anxiety level will plummet.

Fabulous Food Fix

DIARRHEA REHYDRATION FORMULA

This tried-and-true folk remedy can help stop the runs—and fight the dehydration that often accompanies a bout of diarrhea.

¼ tsp. of baking soda
8 oz. of water
8 oz. of 100 percent orange or apple juice
½ tsp. of honey or corn syrup
Pinch of salt

Mix the baking soda and water in a glass. In another glass, mix the juice, honey or corn syrup, and salt. Take alternate swigs from both glasses until you've downed everything. Within a short time, you should be feeling in fine fettle again.

CAUTION ⚠️

Baking soda has a very high sodium content. So if you're on a low-sodium diet, are over age 60, or are treating a child under the age of 5, consult your doctor before using any oral remedy that contains baking soda. **Note:** Topical potions are perfectly safe for use by people of any age.

✔ Nix the Nicotine

Trying to quit smoking? Congratulations! Here's a tip that could help speed your success: With each meal, drink a glass of cool water with 2 tablespoons of baking soda mixed in it. The solution will reduce your cravings for those cancer sticks.

✔ Scrub Pesticide Worries Away

The skins of many fruits and vegetables pack boatloads of essential nutrients. Unfortunately, they may also contain huge amounts of residue from pesticides and herbicides. Even organically grown produce can carry stuff that you don't care to consume—good old garden-variety dirt, for instance. Your best plan of action: Mix a pinch or two of baking soda in a quart or so of water, and scrub the produce clean with a good stiff brush.

Out-of-the-Box Beauty Magic

✤ Deodorize—Naturally

Fresh out of deodorant? Don't panic. Just dust a little baking soda on your underarm skin. It'll absorb the perspiration (thereby eliminating odors), making you feel cooler and drier—and prevent stains on your clothes.

✤ Clean Your Nails . . .

And soften your cuticles at the same time. How? Just dip a moistened nail-brush into some baking soda, and scrub-a-dub-dub!

✤ Deep-Clean Your Face

Keep a jar of baking soda by your bathroom sink, and use it to lift out the traces of oil, dirt, and makeup that even the best cleansers can leave behind. Here's the game plan: Wash your face with your regular soap or cleanser. Then add 3 parts baking soda to 1 part water, and gently massage the mixture into your damp skin. Rinse with clear, cool water, and pat dry.

❖ Axe the Acne

Whether you or your resident teenagers are suffering from these facial blemishes, you can rise to the occasion with this quick trick: Mix equal parts of baking soda and wheat germ with enough water to make a paste. Rub the mixture onto the zits, wait about 10 minutes, rinse with warm water, and pat dry.

❖ Eliminate Acne "Hangover"

Many acne sufferers find that once they've cleared up the annoying zits, they're faced with a problem that's just as unpleasant, if not more so: "souvenirs" in the form of discolorations and unbalanced skin tones. This three-step routine will help remove acne scarring and give you clear, smooth skin:

STEP 1. Mix ¼ cup of baking soda with just enough water to make a soft paste. Apply it to wet skin, and massage it in for 30 to 60 seconds, then rinse it off with lukewarm water. This procedure will remove dead and discolored skin cells.

STEP 2. Mix 1 teaspoon of baking soda with 1 cup of water in a spray bottle. Spritz your facial skin thoroughly, and let it air-dry.

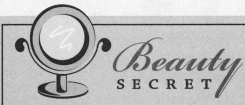

Beauty S E C R E T

BANISH BREAKOUTS

*Here's a super-simple way to keep your face blemish-free: Mix a pinch of baking soda with a bit of coconut oil the size of a pencil eraser, and use it to wash your face in gentle, circular motions. Rinse thoroughly with lukewarm water. Repeat every week or two, and your zits will soon be forgotten nightmares. **Note:** Your face may seem oily at first, but within minutes, the oil will be absorbed and your skin will be glowing.*

STEP 3. Make the same paste described in Step 1, and spread it onto your face. Leave it on for four to five minutes, then rinse it off.

Repeat the process daily until you like the face that's smiling back at you in the mirror.

POTENT POTION

OUTDOORSY BATH SALTS

For those who prefer the scents of the great outdoors to the perfumey aromas commonly found in bath salts, this soothing mixture is just what Mother Nature ordered.

1 cup of baking soda
1 cup of kosher salt or sea salt crystals
5 drops of pine oil*
3 drops of bergamot oil*
3 drops of sandalwood oil*

Mix the baking soda and salt in a bowl, breaking up any clumps. Stir in the oils, and spread the mixture out on a plate or tray for a few hours, until it's completely dry. Store the salts in a wide-mouth jar with a tight-fitting lid. (Make sure the jar is good and dry; otherwise, the salts will harden into a rock-solid clump!) To use, pour ½ cup of the salts under the spigot while you fill the tub with warm water.

* Available in herb and aromatherapy shops and in many health-food and bed and bath stores.

YIELD: ENOUGH FOR 4 BATHS

✤ Whiten Your Choppers

Baking soda is a key ingredient in most toothpastes that boast potent whitening power. But it works just as well straight out of the box to help lighten coffee, tea, and other surface stains on your teeth. Plus, you'll save your hard-earned dollars by making your own whitening toothpaste. Just pour a little soda in your hand, add a drop or two of water, and dip your wet toothbrush into the powdery paste.

✤ Say "Bye-Bye" to Razor Burn

Attention, guys! If your facial skin is on the sensitive side, here's a little secret that you ought to know: Baking soda can end your razor burn woes once and for all. Simply mix 1 tablespoon of baking soda per cup of water, and splash the solution onto your face, either before or after you shave (or even both, if you like).

✤ Nix the Shaving Cream, Gals!

Instead of coating your legs with shaving cream or gel before you shave them, use a solution of 1 tablespoon of baking soda per cup of water. Your razor will glide right over your skin, leaving it satiny smooth—at a fraction of the price of those expensive commercial products.

✤ A Handy Odor-Eater

Whether your paws picked up an unpleasant aroma from peeling onions, filleting fish, or puttering in your workshop, the same simple treatment will send that odor packin' pronto. Just add a little baking soda to the soapy water before you scrub away.

✤ Wash Warts Away

Make a solution of a heaping teaspoon of baking soda per quart of water. Wash your wart-plagued hand or foot with the potion, then let the appendage air-dry. Repeat several times a day until the ugly bump has bugged off.

✤ Freshen Up

If you can't hop into the shower or take a bath—whether the reason is recent surgery, a cast-bound broken limb, or simply the fact that you're rushing off to catch a plane—use this old-time routine: Give yourself a "sponge bath" with a washcloth dipped in a solution of 4 tablespoons of baking soda per quart of water.

✤ Freshen Your Feet, Too

Whether your dogs are simply dog-tired and achy, or they're doggone itchy, your action plan is the same: Soak those tootsies for 10 to 15 minutes in a basin of hot water with about ¼ cup of baking soda mixed in. Dry your feet thoroughly, slip on your shoes, and you're good to go!

✤ Revive Winter-Weary Skin

Wintry winds and indoor heat can leave your skin feeling so dry and itchy that you want to

> **CAUTION** ⚠️
>
> Warts are caused by the human papillomavirus (HPV). Warts don't pose a serious health threat, but the virus can spread like crazy through even tiny breaks in your skin. For that reason, never try to remove a wart by cutting it off. Also, avoid all temptation to scratch or touch one of the bumps, be extra careful when you're shaving, and whatever you do, don't bite your nails!

climb the walls—or hop a plane bound for a tropical island. If a warm-weather escape isn't possible, try this more practical solution: Add 1 cup of baking soda and 1¼ cups of baby oil to a tub of warm water, and soak your discomfort away.

✤ Clean Brushes Brush Clean

No matter how often you shampoo your hair, it won't stay clean if you use hairbrushes and combs that are full of residue from sprays and gels. So every week or so, soak your grooming tools overnight in a solution of 4 tablespoons of baking soda per quart of water. Rinse them with cool water and let them air-dry.

✤ Eliminate Hair-Product Residue

In just a short time, styling gels, sprays, and even conditioners can build up in your hair and make those locks look dull, drab, and dingy. But it's easy to keep the bright lights shining. At least once a week, pour about 1 teaspoon of baking soda into the palm of your hand, and mix it with your regular shampoo. Then wash your hair as usual, and rinse thoroughly.

POTENT POTION

SHAMPOO FOR HARRIED SWIMMERS

When it comes to "hair pollution," styling products can't hold a candle to the high doses of chlorine and other chemicals used in public swimming pools. So dunk the gunk with this intensive treatment.

¼ cup of fresh-squeezed lemon juice
2 tbsp. of baking soda
1 tsp. of mild shampoo

Mix all of the ingredients thoroughly. Wet your hair with water, and work the mixture into your scalp and hair, clear down to the tips. Cover your locks with a shower cap or plastic bag, and go about your business for about half an hour. Rinse well, and shampoo as usual. Repeat the process as necessary. (The frequency depends on how often you swim, and how thoroughly you rinse your hair after each dip.)

Best of the Rest

★ Make Heat Rash Take a Powder

Most problems in life are a whole lot easier to prevent than they are to solve, and heat rash is no exception. Whether the potential victim is a child or an adult, your prevention plan is ultra-simple: On hot summer nights, just sprinkle your bedsheets with baking powder. You'll stay cool, calm, and collected.

★ Corny Cramp Relief

Cornmeal can ease internal woes. The next time you're struck with a severe case of stomach cramps, use this American Indian folk remedy: Put 1 teaspoon of cornmeal in a mug, and add 1 cup of boiling water to it. Let it sit for five minutes, then stir in salt to taste, and drink the potion slowly.

★ Cornstarch Goes Three for Three

If you spend much time working or playing in the great outdoors, you're bound to pick up your share of poison-plant rashes, bee stings, and insect bites. Regardless of which mishap befalls you, mix cornstarch with enough lemon juice to make a paste. (The amounts will depend on how large the afflicted areas are, but for a single insect bite, 1 or 2 teaspoons of cornstarch will do the trick.) Rub the paste gently onto the problem spots. Presto—end of pain and itch! **Note:** If the rash is from poison oak, ivy, or sumac, wash your hands thoroughly to avoid spreading your trouble.

Fabulous Food Fix

CAJUN POPCORN TOPPING

Bet you never thought of popcorn as a health food. Well, it can be when you toss it with this tasty condiment—thanks to the star player, brewer's yeast, which packs a hefty load of B vitamins, minerals, and essential amino acids.

1 tbsp. of brewer's yeast flakes
1 tsp. of dried onion flakes
1 tsp. of Old Bay® seasoning
1 tsp. of red-pepper flakes

Mix all of the ingredients in a big bowl, add your favorite popcorn (buttered or not, as you prefer), and toss until thoroughly coated. Then dig in, and enjoy!

YIELD: 2 TABLESPOONS

★ A Traditional Remedy for Boils

Talk about really old-time remedies! This one for relieving the pain and discomfort of boils comes straight from the Aztecs and Cherokees: Bring ½ cup of water to a boil, and stir in enough cornmeal to make a thick paste. Apply it to the boil, and cover it with a cloth or bandage. Repeat every one to two hours until the painful bump comes to a head and drains away.

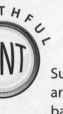

HEALTHFUL HINT

Sunburn Help for Overlooked Skin

Sunburn often strikes the areas at the edges of your bathing suit—the easy-to-forget but oh-so-tender areas that you've neglected to smear with sunscreen or tanning lotion. Unfortunately, those burn spots will have to suffer daily irritation from bras and underwear. To reduce chafing, dust the area(s) thoroughly with cornstarch. And whatever you do, don't mix the cornstarch with petroleum jelly or oil of any kind; that will only make the burn worse by blocking your sore pores.

★ Dry Feet Are Happy Feet

Do you always seem to get blisters on your feet, even though your shoes fit fine? Well, it may be that your feet are too sweaty. If you notice that your socks are frequently soggy, splash a dash of cornstarch into them before you put them on. Dust some between your toes, too, and you'll step a lot more lively! **Note:** This same routine also helps to prevent athlete's foot.

★ Cornstarch Eases Hemorrhoid Pain

When internal pain has you climbing the walls, a cornstarch enema can bring quick relief. Just mix 1 tablespoon of cornstarch in enough water to make a paste. Gradually add more water, stirring, until you have a pint of liquid. Boil the mixture for a few minutes, let it cool, and pour it into an enema bag.

★ Halt Hives with Cream of Tartar

A friend of mine who is prone to breaking out in hives for no apparent reason swears by a remedy she found in her great-grandma's cookbook: Before breakfast, mix 1 teaspoon of cream of tartar in an 8-ounce glass of water, and drink up. In no time flat, you should be itch-free. **Note:** This trick works best if you use it as soon as the hives first appear.

★ Cure UTIs with C of T

In the days before antibiotics, cream of tartar was a popular "drug" for combating urinary tract infections. To relieve your woes, dissolve 1 tablespoon of cream of tartar in 8 ounces of lukewarm water, and drink the potion three times a day. You can multiply the recipe and store it in the refrigerator for up to 48 hours. Give it a good stir before pouring a drink. **Note:** This formula is not meant to replace medical treatment. If you suspect that you have a urinary tract infection, see your doctor ASAP!

★ Lower Your Numbers

Here's a cream of tartar remedy that may help lower your blood pressure. Three times a day (with each meal), drink a potion made from ½ teaspoon of cream of tartar mixed with ½ teaspoon of lemon juice in 8 ounces of water. You can multiply the recipe and store it in the refrigerator for up to 48 hours. Stir the mixture thoroughly before pouring. **Note:** This regimen is not meant to replace medical treatment. If you have high blood pressure, check with your doctor before you use this potion.

★ Put Brewer's Yeast on the Outside

Fight wrinkles with this simple routine: Twice a week, mix equal parts of brewer's yeast and plain yogurt, and apply the mixture to your face. Let it dry thoroughly, then gently wash it off with lukewarm water, and pat dry.

★ Scent-Sational Bath Powder

To make an inexpensive scented body powder, mix a few drops of your favorite perfume or scented oil with cornstarch. If a spicy scent is more your style, add 1 tablespoon of cinnamon per ½ cup of cornstarch.

POTENT POTION

RELAXING BATH BLEND
Make up a batch of this magical mixture, and keep it on hand for instant relief whenever you've had one of *those* days.

2½ cups of baking soda
2 cups of cream of tartar
½ cup of cornstarch

Mix all of the ingredients, and store the blend in a covered container. When you feel the need, fill your bathtub with warm water, and stir in ¼ cup of the mixture. Then settle in, and soak your worries away.

YIELD: ENOUGH FOR 20 BATHS

★ Serve Oily Skin a Corn Meal

Does makeup seem to slide off your face? Try this fix before you get |dolled up: Pour a little liquid castile soap into the palm of your hand, and add about 1 teaspoon of cornmeal. Massage it into your face until it lathers, being careful to avoid your eyes. Rinse with warm water, and pat dry. Now you're ready to "put on your face" and hit the town!

★ Drink to Fewer Wrinkles

Most anti-wrinkle treatments—whether commercial or homemade—are applied directly to your skin. But this brewer's yeast beverage contains potent supplies of nutrients that just may help you lessen your external signs of "experience." Start with 1 teaspoon of brewer's yeast mixed in a glass of 100 percent fruit juice (any kind will do). Then each day, add another teaspoon of brewer's yeast until you've worked your way up to 6 teaspoons (2 tablespoons) per day. **Note:** Some people experience a gassy feeling at first, but natural-health gurus say that this means your body really needs the nutrients, and once the requirements are met, the gassiness will pass.

★ Powder Your Nose

Fresh out of face powder? Then use either baking powder or cornstarch as a substitute. But don't get carried away—if you use too much, you'll end up looking like Clarabel the Clown!

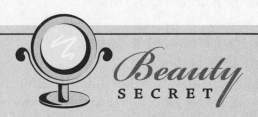

REFRESHING SKIN SCRUB

*K*iss *dead skin cells good-bye with this powerful, but gentle exfoliator: It's quick and easy to whip up. Simply blend ½ cup of uncooked oatmeal and 1 tablespoon of cornmeal in a food processor until you get a fine powder, and store the mixture in an airtight* container. *Then two or three times a week, add ½ teaspoon of the mix to your favorite cleanser. It'll help even out your skin tone, diminish fine lines, and make your skin feel softer, smoother, and refreshed.*

Beauty SECRET

4

Berries

It's almost impossible to believe that anything as sweet and delicious as berries could rank among the healthiest foods on the planet. But it's true! It seems that every day scientists learn more about the beneficial substances in berries that perform feats ranging from fending off debilitating diseases to keeping your weight down, your vision sharp, and your brain humming right along. Of course, berries—and berry juices—can work the same kind of wonders for the outside of your body as they do for the inside. And just think: This berried treasure is as close as your local supermarket!

To Your Berry Good Health!

✔ Color Them Healthy

The same compounds that give berries their beautiful colors—namely anthocyanins—also earn them their standing in the superfood category. All berries pack mega-supplies of anthocyanins, which have been shown to reduce the risk of chronic diseases by protecting the body's cells from damage. What's more, they improve eyesight and help ward off cancer and coronary heart disease.

✔ Feed Your Brain

Anthocyanins are not only beneficial for your body—they're also a boon for your brain. A recent study in the *Annals of Neurology* suggests that eating berries regularly may improve your memory, enhance general brain function, and possibly reduce your risk of developing Parkinson's disease. But that's not all! Researchers have also found that eating two or more servings of blueberries and strawberries a week may delay cognitive aging by as much as two and a half years.

✔ Berries Battle Athlete's Foot

There's nothing that athlete's foot fungus hates more than vitamin C, which blueberries and strawberries just happen to be loaded with. Again, there is no minimum or maximum dose—just pack 'em in!

✔ Berries Ease Bursitis Pain

The flavonoids found in all dark-colored berries, including blackberries, blueberries, boysenberries, and black raspberries, reduce inflammation and can ease the pain of bursitis—as well as arthritis and muscle strains. As for the amount, the more the better! With berries (or any other kind of fruit), there's no such thing as an overdose. Just make sure you regularly include them in your recommended minimum of five fruit and veggie servings per day.

Fabulous Food Fix

RASPBERRY-LEAF TEA

This old-time beverage is one of the most versatile—and effective—remedies you'll ever find for treating a number of internal and external health woes.

4 cups of water
6 tbsp. of dried raspberry leaves*

Bring the water to a boil, remove it from the heat, and add the raspberry leaves. Steep for 40 minutes. Then either drink the tea hot, put it in the fridge to chill (it will keep well over-night), or pour it into ice-pop molds, and freeze them. As for how to use your medicinal treasure, see "Dr. Raspberry Is In" starting on page 52.

* Available in health-food stores or herb shops and from herbal websites. You can also harvest wild or cultivated raspberry leaves in spring or midsummer (when the healthful compounds are most potent). Dry them indoors, away from light, to prepare them for use.

YIELD: 4 CUPS

✔ Black Out Hay Fever

Blackberries are jam-packed with quercetin, a plant compound that halts the production of histamine. This is the substance that makes people with seasonal allergies sneeze, wheeze, and generally feel miserable. Fortunately, blackberries ripen just as hay fever season starts, so get 'em while they're fresh and gobble 'em up to your heart's—rather, your nose's—content!

✔ Blackberries Cure the Big Ds

Since biblical times, folks have been using blackberries in one form or another to cure diarrhea and dysentery. How you take your tasty medicine is up to you, but you should drink one of these lovely libations every four hours:

- 1 shot glass (2 tablespoons) of blackberry brandy

- 2 ounces (4 tablespoons) of blackberry wine

- 6 ounces of 100 percent blackberry juice

> ### The Eyes Have It
>
> HEALTHFUL HINT
>
> Fresh bilberries are hard to come by in supermarkets, but they are widely available via the Internet in both dried and frozen forms—and they're well worth seeking out if you have eye problems of any kind. These blueberry relatives are especially renowned for their power to sharpen your vision and help your eyes adjust quickly from light to darkness. In fact, they're so effective that during World War II, the British Royal Air Force included generous supplies of bilberry jam in its pilots' ration kits.

If the diarrhea sufferer is an infant or a young child, nix the alcoholic beverages and instead give the tot 2 or 3 tablespoons of 100 percent blackberry juice four times a day.

✔ Help for Hemorrhoids

Are painful hemorrhoids driving you up the wall? Cranberries can help put your problems behind you. Here's the routine: Finely chop ¼ cup of cranberries (fresh or frozen) in a blender or food processor. Wrap 1 tablespoon of the chopped berries in a piece of cheesecloth, and place the pouch "where the sun don't shine." Leave it there for about an hour, and replace it with a fresh pouch for another hour. After the two-hour treatment, your sitting area should feel a whole lot better.

✔ Drink Up, Ladies!

Drinking plenty of 100 percent cranberry juice can help cure and/or prevent two common female woes: urinary tract infections and water retention. Drinking 10 ounces of juice a day should prevent bacteria from building up in your urethra (the tube that empties urine from the bladder), and it will also keep fluids flowing freely out of your body. You can't ask for a more tasty way to stay healthy.

✔ Heal Cuts

In olden days, American Indians used cranberry poultices to pull toxins from arrow wounds. Chances are you won't get too many arrow injuries as you go about your day, but the antibacterial properties of cranberries work just as well to disinfect modern-day cuts, scrapes, and puncture wounds. Simply blend or chop ¼ cup or so of whole cranberries, apply the mash to the cut, and cover it with a bandage. Change the dressing every few hours until the wound has healed.

Cranberry Juice to the Rescue!

Pure, unsweetened cranberry juice is just what the doctor ordered for relieving a number of nagging health conditions. Just remember to use 100 percent cranberry juice (not juice combos) with no sugar or preservatives added. And, as always, consult with your doctor before using any of these treatments.

CONDITION	DOSAGE
Asthma	2 tablespoons ½ hour before each meal and at the onset of an asthma attack
Canker sores	One 8-ounce glass between meals
Cystitis	One 8-ounce glass in the morning before breakfast, and one in the late afternoon*
Kidney and bladder infections	6 ounces, 3 times a day
Nausea and vomiting	Frequently throughout the day to replenish lost fluids and nutrients

* Make sure the juice is at room temperature, not chilled.

✔ Give Bruises the Blues

Blueberries are rich in bioflavonoids, which are essential for repairing blood vessels. Eating ½ cup of the tasty blue fruits each day will not only speed the healing of your current bruises, but also strengthen your blood vessels so they're better able to fend off future damage. **Note:** A serving of blueberries can also help reduce swollen varicose veins.

✔ Swig Some Sore Throat Relief

Plenty of beverages can ease the pain of a sore throat, but one of the most effective comfort givers is good old blueberry juice. If you can't find 100 percent juice at your local supermarket or health-food store, liquefy a handful of the berries in a juicer, blender, or food processor, and drink up. (Add a little water to taste if the flavor is too intense to suit you.)

✔ Give Shingles Pain the Raspberries

Few skin afflictions are more painful than shingles. But if you grow raspberries or have friends who do, this truly ancient remedy can help ease the discomfort. Put about 1 cup of raspberry blossoms in a blender or food processor, and blend in enough honey to make a paste. (A tablespoon or so should do the trick.) Apply it very gently to the afflicted skin. **Note:** To keep the sticky stuff from getting all over your sheets or furniture, put on loose, clean, all-cotton pajamas or a baggy T-shirt.

POTENT POTION

RASPBERRY SORE THROAT SOLUTION
This fruity gargle is the worst enemy a scratchy sore throat ever had!

2 cups of ripe red raspberries
2½ cups of white-wine vinegar
1 cup of sugar

Put the whole berries in a bowl, and add the vinegar. Cover, and refrigerate for three days. Then pour the mixture into a saucepan, stir in the sugar, and bring to a low boil. Simmer for 15 minutes, stirring occasionally, and remove from the heat. When the mixture has cooled almost to room temperature, strain it through a sieve or cheesecloth, pressing on the berries to extract as much juice as possible. Pour the potion into a glass bottle with a tight-fitting lid, store it in the refrigerator, and then gargle with it as needed.

YIELD: ABOUT 18 USES

✔ Soothe Your Achin' Eyes

You can use the same raspberry-blossom paste (see page 51) to relieve burning, strained, or inflamed eyes. Just smooth it over your closed lids, and cover the area with a warm, slightly damp washcloth. Lie down in a comfortable spot, and relax for 10 to 15 minutes. Then rinse the paste off with lukewarm water. You'll be bright-eyed and bushy-tailed, quick as a wink!

✔ Dr. Raspberry Is In

You couldn't ask for a more valuable home-health ally than raspberry-leaf tea. Lots of folks I know drink it on a regular basis—or eat it in the form of ice pops—just to keep their systems on an even keel (see page 48 for the recipe). Here are guidelines for using it to treat specific conditions:

BLOODSHOT EYES. Let freshly brewed tea cool to a temperature that's comfortable to the touch. Soak a soft, clean cloth in the solution. Then lie down in a comfortable spot,

Fabulous Food Fix

CHILLED BERRY SOUP

This ultra-simple soup provides a boatload of berries' health-giving benefits for both your body and your mind. In my book, it doesn't get any better than that!

3 cups of fresh mixed berries*
2 tbsp. of sugar
1 tbsp. of orange juice
1 tsp. of finely grated lemon zest
1 tsp. of fresh-squeezed lemon juice
1 tsp. of fresh-squeezed lime juice
1 sprig of fresh mint
Small mint leaves for garnish
Vanilla ice cream or frozen yogurt (optional)

Combine the first seven ingredients in a medium-size heat-proof bowl, and toss to coat. Cover with plastic wrap. Set the bowl over a large saucepan of simmering water, and cook for 10 minutes, stirring occasionally. Remove from the heat and let cool for 15 minutes. Chill in the refrigerator for about four hours before serving. Divide the soup among four bowls and garnish with mint leaves. Top each serving with a scoop of ice cream or frozen yogurt if you like. **Note:** You can make the soup one day ahead of time and keep it in the refrigerator.

* If you're using strawberries, cut them into ½-inch pieces.

YIELD: 4 SERVINGS

and lay the cloth over your closed eyes. Relax for 10 minutes or so. If your peepers are still red, repeat the procedure.

CHILDBIRTH. To reduce the longevity and pain of labor and ease the delivery, drink 1 cup of cool tea each day throughout your pregnancy. If you experience morning sickness, up the dose to 2 cups each day. Then, just before you go into the hospital (or you're about to give birth at home), drink 4 cups of strong, hot tea.

DIARRHEA. Drink the tea cool or warm, or eat ice pops as desired throughout the day until the runs have stopped running. When the patient is a baby under one year of age, the dose is ½ teaspoon of room-temperature tea four times a day. For children one year old and over, give 2 teaspoons four times a day.

HIGH BLOOD PRESSURE. Drink 1 cup per day, hot or cold, for one week. Then check the results to see how you're doing.

LEG CRAMPS. Drink 1 cup in the morning and 1 cup at night until your cramp attacks end.

MOTION SICKNESS. Drink 1 cup of cool tea twice each day as needed.

✔ Sniff the Pounds Away

We all know that our sense of smell is the one most closely tied to our memories. But scents do a whole lot more than just carry our minds back to bygone days. They also stimulate all sorts of mental and physical functions. For instance, studies show that smelling strawberries before you

---

Your Strawberry Preparedness Plan

HEALTHFUL
HINT

Attention, home strawberry growers—or you folks who buy your berries at a pick-your-own berry farm! For those times when you're fresh out of fresh strawberries, keep a supply of strawberry-leaf mouthwash on hand. The leaves contain many of the same plaque- and germ-fighting chemicals that make the fruits so good for your teeth and gums. To make the brew, put 1 cup of fresh strawberry leaves into a heat-proof glass or ceramic bowl, and cover them with 1 cup of boiling water. Let it steep until the water has reached room temperature, strain it into another bowl, and mix in 2 teaspoons of either vodka or lemon juice (not both). Store the mixture in the fridge, and use it as you would any other mouthwash.

exercise causes you to burn more calories. So before you head off on your next power walk, or hit the treadmill at the gym, pull some berries out of the fridge, and take a good long whiff!

✔ Say "Ta-Ta" to Tartar

Strawberries contain chemicals that help prevent the buildup of tartar on your teeth, thereby fending off tooth decay and gum disease. You can put this healthy power to work in two ways:

1. Simply rub your teeth every few days with the cut face of a strawberry.

2. For a more thorough dental hygiene experience, mash a strawberry, dip your toothbrush in the pulp, and brush as you would with your regular toothpaste.

In either case, wait at least half an hour before you rinse—longer if possible—because the longer the berry juice remains on your teeth, the more effective it will be at removing tartar.

✔ Cool a Fever

Juice from freshly sieved strawberry pulp has a cooling and purifying effect that's just the ticket for reducing a fever. Simply chop a handful of berries, and whirl them in a blender with a little water. Then strain out the solids, and drink up. (Or serve the beverage to your resident patient.) Repeat frequently throughout the day until the thermometer registers a healthy 98.6°F.

A Berry Beautiful You

✤ Brightening Blackberry Facial Cleanser

To freshen and nourish your skin at the same time, mash two or three blackberries in a bowl, and mix in 2 tablespoons of plain yogurt and 1 teaspoon of distilled rose water (available in herb shops and health-food stores). Gently massage the mixture into your skin for 30 seconds. Rinse with cool water, and follow up with your usual moisturizer.

❖ Stain Your Lips

Lip stain is all the rage these days, and for good reason: Unlike lipstick, it stays on your lips all day long, and it won't smear off onto your clothes, your coffee cup—or your husband. You can buy commercial stains, of course, but it's a snap to make your own using either fresh or frozen berries. Just follow this easy-as-pie four-step procedure:

STEP 1. Gather your ingredients. You'll need 3 blackberries, 3 raspberries, ½ strawberry, and ½ teaspoon of olive oil.*

STEP 2. In a heat-proof bowl, microwave the berries until they're soft, then whirl them in a blender or food processor until smooth.

STEP 3. Strain the juice into a clean bowl, and stir in the olive oil.

STEP 4. Pour the stain into a glass jar with a tight-fitting lid. Store it in the refrigerator, where it will keep for about a month, or in the freezer for up to two months.

Apply the stain to your lips using a cotton swab or lip brush. To add shine, apply a clear lip gloss as needed.

* Adjust the type and quantities of berries to suit your color preference. For instance, for a pinker shade, use a whole strawberry, and cut back on the blackberries. To get a more intense, purplish hue, eliminate the strawberry, and add another blackberry.

POTENT POTION

CRANBERRY COMPLEXION COMPLEX

Cranberries are chock-full of ellagic acid, an antioxidant that fights the breakdown of collagen and elastin in your skin. What's more, according to a study in the journal, *Experimental Dermatology*, applying the acid topically helps prevent wrinkles caused by the sun's UVB rays. So whether you spend lots of time in the sun (for work or play), or you simply want to protect your skin as you stroll around town, this fabulous formula has you covered.

2 tbsp. of fresh or frozen cranberries
¼ cup of cornmeal
1 tbsp. of buttermilk
2 tsp. of honey

Crush the cranberries in a bowl, and blend in the other ingredients. Wash your face and neck as usual, then massage the paste into your still-damp skin for two to three minutes. Rinse with lukewarm water, and pat dry. Repeat once or twice a week.

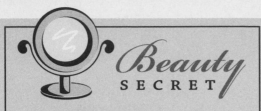

Beauty SECRET

CLEANSE, TONE, AND MOISTURIZE!

When it comes to time- and money-saving beauty treatments, this triple-threat mask is the berries. Mash 4 medium-size, ripe strawberries and puree them in a blender or food processor with 1 tablespoon each of heavy cream and organic honey. (You'll want to sneak a lick, but hold off! You can always make another batch for eating later.) Spread the mixture on your face and neck, keeping it away from your eyes. Wait 10 minutes, rinse with lukewarm water, and pat dry.

❖ Calling All Redheads!

Natural redheads, that is. Would you like to make your tresses shinier and the color more vibrant? If the answer is yes (duh . . .), then go soak your hair in 100 percent cranberry juice. Leave it on for two minutes, then wash it out with a mild shampoo and follow up with a gentle, rinse-out conditioner.

❖ Anti-Acne Mask

Zits don't stand a chance against this powerful, but gentle treatment: Mix equal parts of mashed red raspberries, uncooked oatmeal, and honey. Smear the paste onto your skin, wait 20 minutes, and rinse off. That's all there is to it!

❖ Serve Your Face Some Raspberries

You couldn't ask for a simpler—or healthier—way to smooth and soften your skin. Just mash a handful of ripe raspberries (black or red) in a bowl, and stir in enough cornstarch or potato starch to make a smooth paste. Apply it to your face, avoiding the area around your eyes. Leave it on for 10 to 20 minutes, and rinse with warm water.

❖ One Shine Booster Fits All

No matter what color your hair is, this little trick will make it gleam: Mix 8 mashed strawberries with 1 tablespoon of mayonnaise, and massage the mixture into your damp hair. Put on a shower cap, cover it with a warm towel, and go about your business for 15 minutes or so. When the time is up, rinse your hair thoroughly, then wash and condition as usual and get ready to shine!

✤ Sip Strawberry for Clear Skin

Strawberry juice is rich in alpha-hydroxy acid and vitamin C, both of which fight acne, eradicate dead skin cells, and help restore your skin's youthful appearance. The recommended dose for clearer, healthier skin: Drink ½ cup per day of 100 percent strawberry juice (available in health-food stores and most large supermarkets).

✤ See Spots Run

If you've got more freckles than you'd like to have, try this vanishing act. Cut a large fresh strawberry in two, and rub the cut side over your spots. Repeat the procedure every day or two until the speckles disappear, or at least become less noticeable.

✤ Re-energize Tired Feet

When a long day on your feet has left your dogs dog-tired, try this berry effective nighttime treat. In a blender or food processor, mix 8 strawberries, 2 tablespoons of olive oil, and 1 teaspoon of sea salt or kosher salt. Massage the paste into your feet, then rinse it off and dry your tootsies thoroughly before dropping into bed. By morning, you should be rarin' to go!

✤ Scrub Away Cellulite

Troubled by unsightly cellulite? Well, you're not alone. Now you could fork out big bucks for an anti-cellulite wrap at a fancy spa—or you could whip up a highly effective alternative for a tiny fraction of the cost. In a blender or food processor, blend 1 cup of strawberries with 1 tablespoon of ground coffee to make a paste. Massage the mixture vigorously into your skin using circular motions, then immediately rinse it off (there's no need to leave it on).

YOU DON'T SAY!

America's Most-Eaten Berry Award goes to the strawberry, hands down. California produces 90 percent of the strawberries that are grown in the United States—to the tune of more than 1 billion pounds of fruit per year—and if the average year's harvest was laid out berry to berry, it would circle the globe 15 times. Those figures are courtesy of the California Strawberry Commission, as is this finding from a recent national survey: Asked to describe the personalities of strawberry lovers, respondents wrote, "health-conscious, fun-loving, intelligent, and happy." Folks who did not care much for the fruits were labeled "weird, boring, stuffy—picky, fussy eaters who avoid healthy foods."

Best of the Rest

★ A Grape Way to Ease Arthritis Pain

Grape skins contain resveratrol, a natural compound that helps reduce inflammation caused by an injury or disease. A study published in the *Journal of Biological Chemistry* confirmed that eating 1 cup of either green or red grapes each day would increase your comfort level considerably. Drinking 100 percent purple grape juice (the recommended dose is one 8-ounce glass per day) does the trick, too.

★ Melons Beat Bloat

All kinds of melons contain a substance called cucurbocitrin, which increases the natural leakiness of tiny blood vessels in your kidneys. This makes your body able to process and eliminate more water. So the next time your monthly period—or simply a period of stress—makes you feel like an overfilled water balloon, dig into some tasty cantaloupe, honeydew, or watermelon.

★ Concord Conquers Cuts

When you have stubborn cuts that just don't want to close up—but they're not infected—100 percent Concord grape juice can come to your aid. How you use it depends on where the wound is:

ON YOUR HEEL. Because your heels see constant action, any cut down there seems to take forever to heal. Although this remedy won't close cuts up overnight, it is safe and effective. Every night

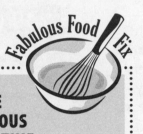

GREAT GRAPE AND MARVELOUS MELON SMOOTHIE

For a healthy perk-me-up on a hot summer day (or any other time), reach for this fast and easy recipe.

2 cups of cantaloupe or honey-dew melon, peeled and cubed

2 cups of seedless red or green grapes

⅔ cup of 100 percent white grape juice, chilled

4 ice cubes

Puree the first three ingredients in a blender or food processor on high speed. While the machine is running, add the ice cubes through the feed tube, one cube at a time, until the mixture is smooth and thick. Serve immediately.

YIELD: 3 CUPS

before bedtime, soak your foot for half an hour in a porcelain (not metal) bowl filled with enough Concord grape juice to cover the wound. Gently pat dry with a soft cotton cloth, but don't rinse off the grape juice, and don't get the area wet when bathing. Healing time varies, but it should be gone within three weeks.

ELSEWHERE ON YOUR BODY. Saturate a gauze pad in Concord grape juice, apply it to the wound, and fasten it in place with adhesive tape. Replace the dressing every day, but don't wash the affected area.

★ Eat Rhubarb for Regularity

Rhubarb is one of Mother Nature's yummiest—and most powerful—natural laxatives. It acts by stimulating mucus production in the large intestine to ease elimination, which typically occurs within 6 to 10 hours after you eat the fruit or drink the juice. So enjoy a big slice of strawberry-rhubarb pie. Or, if you prefer a more fluid remedy, puree 3 cups of raw rhubarb stalks and 1 cup of fresh or frozen strawberries in a blender or food processor. Mix in ¼ cup each of water and honey, then sip and go!

> **CAUTION** ⚠
>
> Whenever a medicinal potion or recipe calls for rhubarb, make sure you use only the stalks. The leaves contain large quantities of toxins called oxalates that can cause stomach irritation and kidney problems.

★ Rub Out Tooth Decay

Rhubarb is chock-full of calcium and potassium, both of which are potent tooth protectors. To put them to work guarding your choppers, crush a couple of fresh rhubarb stems to extract the juice, then dip a clean finger into the liquid, and rub your teeth with it every other day.

★ Peel Away Prickly Heat

Prickly heat (a.k.a. heat rash) is best known as a baby affliction, but it can strike people of any age—typically in very hot, humid climates. One excellent remedy: Rub the affected area with the inside of a watermelon rind. It'll help ditch the itch and discomfort in a hurry.

★ Grapes Turn Back the Clock

Well, not literally. But grapes *can* help minimize those tiny lines that Father Time leaves around your eyes and mouth. Just cut seedless green grapes in half, and squeeze the juice directly onto your little creases.

★ Condition Your Hair with Cantaloupe

Cube one-quarter of a small cantaloupe, and blend the chunks with slices from half a medium-size banana and 1 tablespoon each of olive oil and plain yogurt. Apply the mixture to your freshly washed hair, saturating the strands from roots to ends. Leave it on for 30 minutes or so, then rinse it off with cool water.

★ A Whole Bunch of Skin-Care Help

Who needs a lot of fancy cosmetics when you've got a bunch of grapes in the fridge? Just take a gander at the feats these fruits can perform:

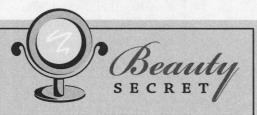

Beauty
S E C R E T

CANTALOUPE ANTI-AGING MASK

You can help hold back the sands of time with this simple recipe. Put 1 tablespoon of honey in a bowl, and microwave it until it's runny (rhyme intended!). Add ⅛ cup of mashed or pureed cantaloupe, and mix well. (If the texture is too liquid, stir in a little more honey.) Spread the mixture onto your cleansed face and neck, and leave it on for 15 to 20 minutes. Rinse it off with warm water, then rinse again with cool water to tighten your pores. Follow up with your usual moisturizer for picture-perfect results!

MAKE YOUR FACE GLOW. After washing with your normal cleanser, mash two or three grapes, dip your fingers into the fruit, and gently massage your skin. Rinse with luke-warm water.

RELIEVE ACNE AND OTHER SKIN IRRITATIONS. Peel some grapes (the number depends on how large an area you need to treat). Then place the skins, inner side down, on the afflicted area. Keep the peels on for 15 to 20 minutes, then rinse.

SOFTEN AGING SKIN. Mash three grapes with 3 tablespoons or so of aloe vera gel. Smooth the gel-paste mixture onto your face, leave it on for 20 minutes, and rinse it off.

TIGHTEN YOUR PORES. Mash two or three grapes and strain off the juice. Mix in 1 teaspoon of honey, and apply the paste to your face. Wait 20 minutes or so, then rinse.

Note: After any of these treatments, follow up by applying your usual moisturizer.

5

Carrots

Folks have been tapping into the health-giving, beautifying power of carrots since the days of ancient Greece. But it seems that every day we learn more about the truly astounding feats these tasty roots and their juices can perform—everything from softening your skin and moisturizing your hair to dramatically reducing your risk for cancer, stroke, and heart disease. In fact, Bugs Bunny's favorite snack now ranks high on nutritionists' superfood lists from coast to coast.

Put Carrots in Your Corner

✔ Eradicate an Earache
If you've got an ache that just won't quit, grate a large carrot, wrap the pulp in a piece of cheesecloth, and hold it against your ear for 15 minutes or so. The enzymes in the orange root will help draw out the infection that's causing the pain. Repeat every few hours until your misery is history.

✔ Douse Sore Throat Flames
When a sore throat strikes, grate a large carrot and spread it on a soft, clean cloth. Wrap the cloth around your throat (with the gratings against your skin, of course!), and cover it with a scarf to keep it in place. To make the poultice even more effective, you can top it with either an ice pack or a hot compress (the choice is yours).

✔ Can the Cancer Sticks

Want to quit smoking? Then try this time-tested trick: Whenever you get the urge to light up a cigarette, reach for a raw carrot instead. I'll bet gold bricks to bunny rabbits that before long, your nicotine cravings will cave in.

✔ Treat a Blocked Milk Duct

Attention, nursing mothers! If your breast is red and swollen because of a blocked milk duct, reach for a fresh carrot poultice. Grate a large carrot onto a piece of cheesecloth, fold the sides in to form an envelope, and moisten it. Place it on your sore breast all the way up to your armpit, and cover it with a hot-water bottle. Leave it in place for one hour. Apply a fresh poultice several times a day until the inflammation is gone. **Note:** If you also have a fever and flu-like symptoms, see your doctor immediately. You could have a serious infection.

Fabulous Food Fix

FRENCH CARROT SALAD

This simple, tasty salad is a classic in southern France, and for good reason: Besides tasting sweet and delicious, it delivers a full load of carrots' health-giving benefits to your lungs, liver, blood, and digestive system. Plus, the parsley boosts your kidney and adrenal functions, and the mint helps eliminate bad bacteria in your body.

1 lb. of carrots, grated
2 tbsp. of extra virgin olive oil
1 tbsp. of fresh-squeezed lemon juice
1 garlic clove, finely chopped (optional)
Pinch of sea salt
3 tbsp. of fresh Italian parsley, finely chopped
1 tbsp. of fresh mint, finely chopped

Toss the first five ingredients together, and sprinkle the parsley and mint on top. Then serve it up!

YIELD: 4 TO 6 SERVINGS

✔ Heal Bothersome Blisters

A blister is annoying enough at any stage, but when it's been punctured and becomes irritated, it's pure agony. So what do you do? Head to the kitchen, and grate a fresh carrot or two—that's what! Apply the gratings to the afflicted area, and cover it with a warm, moist washcloth. Leave the carrots and cloth in place for 20 to 30 minutes. **Note:** This remedy is also effective for clearing up weeping sores, skin ulcers, and cuts. But if the wound is already infected, get medical help ASAP.

✔ Say "So Long" to Sunburn

Carrots and their juice are packed with germ-killing chemicals that make them perfect for treating sunburn and other minor burns. To put that soothing power to work, first sponge the afflicted skin with ice water. Then dip a piece of gauze in 100 percent carrot juice, and squeeze it out so that it's wet, but not dripping. Put this dressing over the affected area, and secure it lightly with more gauze or lightweight fabric. Repeat several times a day until the pain and swelling are gone.

✔ Make Treatments Easier

When radiation or other cancer treatments make you too sick to eat, then it's time to juice a pile of carrots. The mild-tasting juice should sit easy in your queasy stomach—and even more importantly, you'll get a mega-dose of antioxidants, which you need to help neutralize the toxins from chemotherapy or radiation.

✔ Banish Bursitis Pain

When bursitis strikes, drink a 12-ounce glass of 100 percent carrot juice with breakfast and lunch until you feel relief. The nutrients in the juice will help break down the sediment residue in your bursae that causes the inflammation.

✔ Save Your Memories

Calling all ladies of, um, a certain age! During your childbearing years, your free-flowing supply of estrogen protects your memory by combating free-radical molecules that damage your brain cells. So what do you do when your body's estrogen levels wane during menopause? Feast on carrots and other veggies

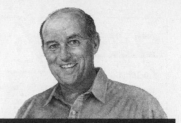

YOU DON'T SAY!

How many fish can you catch with a carrot? Apparently, quite a few—at least judging by the success of a company called Cellu-Comp that manufactures fishing rods from a substance called Curran®. The material is a carbon fiber that's derived largely from carrots. (*Curran* is the Scottish Gaelic word for "carrot.") Two Scottish scientists, David Hepworth and Eric Whale, created the substance at their company in Fife, and they made quite a splash in their debut at the American Sportfishing Association's 50th Annual Convention. Their surf fishing rod won the prize for Best Saltwater Rod, and its "brother," the E21 Carrot Stix rod, took top honors as Best in Show!

and fruits that are rich in natural antioxidants. You will soon find that you are better able to recall not only the names of your childhood pals—but also where you put those darn car keys last night!

✔ Improve Your Vision

No, it's not just an old wives' tale—or a joke about rabbits not wearing glasses. Carrots really can make your eyesight better. Simply making carrots a regular part of your diet will help keep your vision sharp. But to actually improve your faulty eyesight, do what country doctors have recommended for ages: Drink 5 to 6 ounces of 100 percent carrot juice twice a day for two weeks. You should see a definite improvement.

✔ Calm Your Frazzled Nerves

After a long, hectic day, relax with a carrot cocktail. Just mix equal parts of carrot and celery juice, and add honey to taste (plus a shot of Grand Marnier® if you'd like). Then sit back, relax, and drink up!

✔ Cure Baby's Diarrhea

A bout of diarrhea is miserable for an infant—and it's no bed of roses for his or her parents either! Fortunately, one of the most effective remedies is probably in your kitchen cupboard. What is it? Strained carrots. Just mix a jar of the baby food with a jar of water, and feed the mixture to the tiny tot until the runs have run their course.

✔ Ease Your Gas Worries

If you love beans, but you're not so fond of their infamous aftereffects, take an age-old tip from folks who live in the Appalachian Mountains: Whenever you cook your beans, toss a small whole carrot into the pot or baking dish. Somehow, the orange root reduces the beans' gas production, so you can eat your fill of the healthful legumes without fear of polluting the air around you.

✔ Develop a Drinking Habit . . .

For carrot juice, that is—preferably made in your own home juicer or bought fresh from the machine at your local juice bar. In many parts of the world, folks consider this golden treasure to be the "king of juices," and for good reason: Drinking an 8-ounce glass of carrot juice several times a week can work wonders for your health and well-being. Benefits include:

■ Balancing your blood sugar levels

■ Cleansing your liver

■ Decreasing the risk of jaundice in newborn infants

■ Fortifying your blood and helping prevent anemia

■ Guarding against the effects of secondhand smoke

■ Helping fend off asthma attacks and other respiratory ailments

■ Increasing the quantity and quality of a nursing mother's breast milk

■ Nourishing your skin

■ Preventing water retention

■ Strengthening your immune system

Note: Bottled 100 percent carrot juice offers the same health benefits, but the fresh version is much more potent.

✔ When There's No Baby On Board

Carrots can help cure diarrhea just as effectively for children and adults as they do for babies. In this case, cook a

POTENT POTION

TIP-TOP MOUTHWASH

If you grow your own carrots, or buy them at a farmers' market, don't toss the tops out—at least not all of them. Turn them into an effective mouthwash instead. Believe it or not, those frilly greens are chock-full of antiseptic compounds that kill germs and sweeten your breath.

3 cups of water
½ cup of chopped carrot tops

Bring the water to a boil, add the carrot tops, and simmer for 20 minutes. Remove the pan from the heat, and let it sit for another half hour. Strain, and store the potion in a glass container with a tight-fitting lid and keep it in the refrigerator. Then use it each morning to rinse and gargle as you would with any other mouthwash.

YIELD: APPROXIMATELY 2½ CUPS

few carrots until they're slightly soft, then mash or puree them with a little water or milk, and eat the mixture—or serve it to your patient—throughout the day.

HEALTHFUL HINT

Cook 'Em Crisp

Most folks think that to get the maximum health benefit from carrots, you should eat them raw. Not so! In fact, carrots are one of the few vegetables that release more of their important nutrients when they are either juiced or cooked whole (not sliced) until they are just tender-crisp. One example: A recent study at Newcastle University in England found that boiling carrots *before* slicing them increases their anti-cancer properties by 25 percent. Whatever you do, though, don't cook carrots longer than two to three minutes. If you overcook them (or any other vegetables), all their food value ends up in the cooking water.

Roots of Radiance

✤ Amazing Astringent

You won't find a homemade skin treatment that's any easier than this one: After cleaning your face each morning and evening, dip a cotton ball into 100 percent carrot juice, and wipe it over your face and neck. It'll remove any excess oil and cleanser residue and leave your skin positively glowing. **Note:** Before you use carrot juice or pulp on your face, test it on an inconspicuous spot to make sure it doesn't turn your skin slightly—but temporarily!—orange.

✤ Zap the Zits

Has acne got you (or your resident teenager) crawling up the walls? No problem! Just boil three carrots until they're soft, and mash them in a bowl. Mix ½ cup of the pulp with just enough dry milk to form a smooth paste. Apply it to your face, wait 20 minutes, and wash it off with lukewarm water. Repeat once a day until you've banished the blemishes.

✣ Detox Your Hair

Over time, shampoos, conditioners, and styling products build up in your hair, making it dull, drab, and hard to manage. This simple trick can fix that problem in a flash: Grate a medium-size carrot, and massage the gratings through your hair. Wait 15 minutes, then rinse out the carrot slaw. **Note:** Either perform this maneuver over your kitchen garbage disposal, or cover your sink drain with a piece of screen or old panty hose so that carrot pieces don't clog your plumbing.

✣ Hey, Carrot Top!

To intensify the color of your red tresses, grind up three medium-size carrots in a blender or food processor. Then mix the carrots in a bowl with about 2 tablespoons of honey and 3 tablespoons of plain yogurt, adjusting

---

POTENT POTION

ULTRA-HEALTHY HAIR CONDITIONER

This powerful but oh-so-gentle formula reduces dandruff, minimizes hair loss, helps preserve the natural elasticity of your hair—and makes it shine to beat the band!

1 large carrot, sliced
1 medium-size banana, sliced
⅓ cup of honey, warmed*
¼ cup of olive oil
Water

Boil the carrot slices in water until they're soft. Strain off the water, and puree the carrots and the banana in a blender or food processor until they're smooth, with no lumps. Pour the mixture into a bowl, stir in the honey and olive oil, and mix well. Massage the conditioner into your hair, coating it completely. (This is a messy procedure, so you may want to wear rubber gloves to make cleanup easier.) Cover your hair with a shower cap, and go about your business for at least 45 minutes, or up to eight hours for an extra-intensive treatment. Rinse thoroughly, and shampoo as usual.

* Warming the honey will make it easier to mix with the other ingredients.

the quantities as necessary to form a coarse paste. Shampoo as usual, and apply the carrot mixture to your hair. Keep it on for one to two minutes, and rinse. **Note:** To bring out any copper undertones in your hair, chop up ½ cup of cranberries along with the carrots.

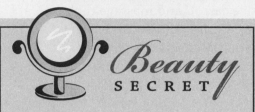

Beauty
S E C R E T

WHO IS THAT MASKED WOMAN?

Carrots are packed with vitamins and other nutrients that help increase blood circulation, which in turn fights the formation of wrinkles, enhances your skin's elasticity, and both repairs and tones its texture. To put this cosmetic powerhouse to work for you, slice three large carrots and boil them until they're soft. Mash them, and add 3 tablespoons of honey. Massage the mixture gently onto your face, using a circular motion, and leave it on for 20 minutes. Rinse with warm water, and pat dry.

✣ Strengthen Brittle Fingernails

If your nails are constantly breaking and peeling, then do yourself a big favor and start quaffing carrot juice. Replace your usual breakfast OJ with the other orange-colored juice several times a week, and before you know it, your nails will be beautiful and as tough as, well, nails.

✣ Brighten Your Smile

Munching on raw carrots is a dandy way to remove tooth stains—and it's a darn sight cheaper than those commercial whitening treatments. As an added bonus, carrots are one of Mother Nature's most effective breath sweeteners!

✣ Remove Warts

When one of the unsightly bumps appears, reach for a carrot. Grate it, and mix the shavings with 1 teaspoon or so of olive oil. Put the mixture on the wart, cover it with a soft cloth or bandage, and leave it on for 30 minutes or so. Repeat twice a day until the bump has vanished.

✣ We Have Liftoff!

When it comes to removing dirt, excess oil, and dead skin cells from your face, nothing beats a peel-off mask. If you do the job correctly, all of the gunk in your pores will adhere to the mask, and when you pull it off, your skin will be really deep-down clean. Here's the simple liftoff routine:

STEP 1. Gather your supplies. You'll need ½ cup of 100 percent carrot juice, ½ teaspoon of lemon juice, 1 teaspoon of unflavored gelatin, a bowl that's microwave safe, and a washcloth.

STEP 2. Mix the juices and gelatin in the bowl, and heat in the microwave until the gelatin dissolves. Stir well, and refrigerate for 20 to 30 minutes, or until the mixture thickens to a spreadable consistency. Don't let it get as firm as a gelatin salad!

STEP 3. Soak the washcloth in very warm water, and hold the cloth to your face for 15 minutes.

STEP 4. Smooth the gelatin mixture evenly over your freshly steamed skin. Wait until the mask has dried completely, then carefully peel it off.

STEP 5. Wash your face to remove any residue, and rinse with cold water to tighten your pores. Pat dry, and apply your usual moisturizer.

Best of the Rest

★ Beets Beat Constipation

When you wake up in the morning with your insides feeling as backed up as a freeway at rush hour, make your way into the kitchen. Scrub two small beets thoroughly, and eat them raw. (Either bite into them like apples, or dice them and eat them with a fork—it's your call.) Within 12 hours or so, "traffic" should be moving again.

★ Classic Help for Hemorrhoids

Remedies—for hemorrhoids or anything else—don't come much simpler than this old-time cure: Chop up a cabbage, lay the pieces on a towel, and sit on them for 30 minutes or so. And don't forget to take your pants off first!

★ Keep Your Cool

As you baseball historians know, the great Babe Ruth had his share of eccentricities, but at least one of them made a whole lot of sense: He stayed

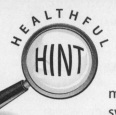

Cabbage Cures Ulcers

For centuries, folk-medicine gurus have sworn by cabbage and cabbage juice as top-notch ulcer remedies. Well, recently, numerous medical studies (including one at the Stanford University School of Medicine) have shown that drinking 8 ounces of 100 percent cabbage juice four times a day can heal both gastric and duodenal ulcers in anywhere from 2 to 10 days. Eating raw cabbage can perform the same miraculous feat. But if you'd rather not drink a quart of cabbage juice every day, you can substitute a wedge of raw cabbage, or about 1 cup of cabbage slices, for each 8-ounce cup of juice.

cool on the field and in the Yankees' non-air-conditioned dugout by wearing a cabbage leaf under his cap. He changed it for a fresh one every two innings. It still works—give it a try the next time you're puttering in the yard or sitting in the Little League bleachers on a hot summer day.

★ Leaves Relieve Menstrual Cramps

Ladies, if you're prone to pain every month, do yourself a favor: Before and during your period, eat plenty of raw cabbage, lettuce, and other leafy greens. Not only will their nutrients help relieve your cramps, but their diuretic power will also help reduce bloating.

★ Relax and Smell the Cucumbers

Rather, I should say smell the cucumbers and relax. Studies have shown that the scent of cukes helps you calm down during tense situations. The next time you're anticipating a stressful experience—say, a job interview or some medical tests—wash your hair with cucumber-scented shampoo (see "The Perfect Pair for Your Hair" on page 72) and/or put a dab of it on a hankie or a piece of cloth to take with you.

★ Lettuce Removes Rashes . . .

And sunburn, too! Whichever skin ailment you have, separate and clean the leaves of one small head of lettuce. Toss them into a pan of boiling water to cook for five minutes, then drain (saving the water). Let the leaves cool, then put them on your face and neck. Wait 5 to 10 minutes if you can—the leaves will be slippery! Pat your skin dry, without rinsing. Pour the reserved liquid into a jar with a tight-fitting lid, and store it in the refrigerator. Use it as a skin lotion as needed.

★ Soothe a Sour Stomach

When you've overindulged in tummy-troubling food, reach for this remarkable remedy: Grate a raw potato, and squeeze it through cheesecloth into a bowl. Mix 1 tablespoon of the juice with ½ cup of warm water. Drink the potion slowly, and before you know it, you'll be feeling right as rain!

★ Put Taters on the Tootsies

Got a young'un who's in bed with a fever? Tape a slice of raw potato on the bottom of each of the child's feet. Besides lowering his or her temperature, the unconventional footgear should give both of you some hearty chuckles—and, after all, laughter *is* the best medicine! **Note:** Just make sure the patient doesn't try to walk around in the slippery "slippers"!

★ Ease Your Allergy Miseries

Tomato juice does double duty as an allergy reliever—if you spike it with horseradish. Just grate a teaspoon or so of the tangy root into a tall glass of tomato juice, and drink up. It'll clear your inner airways from your nose right up through your sinuses.

Fabulous Food Fix

BAKED POTATOES HOT OFF THE GRILL

Believe it or not, the humble spud contains 60 different phytochemicals and vitamins that perform health and beauty feats ranging from boosting your immune system to supporting your skin structure. What's more, the potato is one of the few plants that contain compounds called kukoamines, which help lower blood pressure. So the next time you fire up your barbecue grill, put some tater power to work with this simple recipe.

6 medium russet potatoes, freshly baked
4 tbsp. of extra virgin olive oil
Salt and freshly ground black pepper to taste
12 small sprigs of fresh rosemary

Cut the potatoes in half lengthwise, and brush the cut sides with the olive oil. Season with the salt and pepper, and push a rosemary sprig into each spud half. Set the potatoes cut side down on the grill. Cook for about 10 minutes, until the potatoes are heated through and brown grill marks show on the surface (but don't let them blacken). Serve 'em hot and tasty.

YIELD: 6 SERVINGS

★ You Can't Beat Beet Blush

That is, if you're looking for a super-simple and ultra-healthy way to color your cheeks. Just cut a small red beet in half, and rub the cut side over your cheekbones until you get the shade you want. Then, for good measure, run a cotton swab over the beet's surface, and smooth the juice onto your lips to tint them rosy red.

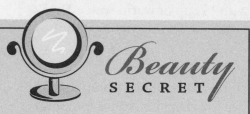

THE PERFECT PAIR FOR YOUR HAIR

Forget about those commercial two-in-one products that shampoo and condition your hair in one step! Instead, do it yourself by pureeing a peeled, diced cucumber and a peeled, sliced lemon in a blender or food processor. Strain out the seeds, wash your hair as usual with the dynamic duo, and rinse it out. The lemon cleans your tresses like nobody's business, while the cuke acts as a terrific conditioning agent.

★ A Tomato Tone-Up

Here's a nice 'n' easy way to tone oily or really acne-prone skin: Mash a medium-size tomato and spread it onto your face. Wait about 30 minutes, then rinse and pat dry. **Note:** Tomatoes are mildly acidic, so if your skin is sensitive, use yellow tomatoes, which are lower in acid than red varieties.

★ Brunettes, Take Note!

To put glistening highlights in your brown locks, boil a large, unpeeled baking potato in a quart of water, then dip a pastry brush in the liquid, and saturate your hair. (Be careful not to get the spud water in your eyes!) Wait for 30 minutes, then rinse with cool water. Repeat every two to three weeks to retain the "spudtacular" highlights.

★ Tomatoes Help Hair Care

The acids in tomatoes help balance the pH levels in your hair, thereby making your locks shinier and more manageable. To perform this balancing act, just mix 1 teaspoon of cornstarch with 1 cup of tomato juice, and comb the solution through your clean, wet hair. Leave it on for about 10 minutes, and rinse well.

6 Castor Oil

Back in our grandmothers' day, castor oil was the remedy of choice for everything from curing bronchitis and loosening up stubborn bowels to removing "liver spots" on faces and hands. Then came World War II, and in its aftermath, boatloads of commercial medicines and cosmetics arrived on the scene. The result? In most households, castor oil went the way of the dinosaurs. Well, modern medical researchers, doctors, and beauty-biz pros have recently "discovered" that Grandma was right after all: A big bottle of castor oil belongs in every medicine chest—and on every vanity table.

Cast Your Eyes on Wellness

✔ Heal Hangnails in a Hurry

When you've got a hangnail that's bound and determined to hang in there, reach for the castor oil. Rub a dab of it into the skin around the painful projection every night at bedtime. Before you know it, that hangnail will be history! **Note:** This same treatment also works to heal dry, cracked cuticles.

✔ Get Some Shut-Eye

Have trouble falling asleep at night? Just rub a little castor oil over your eyelids at bedtime. It'll help you relax deeply so that you can get a restful night's slumber without using any drugs.

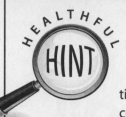

A Royal Flush

Once upon a time, castor oil was considered the King of Laxatives—so much so that lots of folks took it regularly just to keep things moving right along. The problem is that it's so strong, your system can become dependent on it if you use it for an extended period of time. So if you would like to use this classic remedy, it's okay to take 1 teaspoon of 100 percent pure castor oil in the morning (you'll probably want to mix it with fruit juice to disguise the bitter taste). You should then have a bowel movement within four hours or so. If not, continue the treatment once a day for two more days, but no longer! If your system isn't back to normal by then, call your doctor immediately. **Note:** If you are pregnant, don't take castor oil before speaking with your doctor; it is a strong stimulant that can bring on labor.

✔ Ease Irritated Eyes

All kinds of things, ranging from dust particles to cooking fumes and secondhand cigarette smoke, can make your peepers red and sore. To ease the discomfort, just put 2 drops of 100 percent pure castor oil in each eye. Repeat as needed once or twice a day until you get relief.

✔ Say "Bye-Bye," Styes

These painful bumps are actually infected oil glands on your eyelid—and the antibacterial properties of castor oil are just the ticket for clearing them up. Apply a very small drop of 100 percent pure castor oil directly onto the sty two or three times a day until the little sore has vanished.

✔ Can Canker Sores

Medical gurus tell us that canker sores are probably brought on by stress. Well, there's no "probably" about one thing: You can get rid of the annoying things by dabbing them with 100 percent pure castor oil frequently throughout the day until they're gone.

✔ Cast Off Corns

Castor oil's mighty moisturizing power makes it a perfect choice for softening up painful corns. Your action plan: Cover the bump with a commercial, non-medicated corn pad (the kind with a hole in the center to corral the oil). Then use a cotton swab to reach inside the hole and coat the corn with a thin layer of castor oil. Cover the pad with adhesive tape to keep the fluid in constant contact with the corn. Replace the dressing every day until the corn has disappeared.

✔ Treat Carpal Tunnel Syndrome

Has too much time spent pounding your computer keyboard left you with carpal tunnel syndrome? If so, here's good news: A castor oil compress can deliver relief directly to the site of the pain. Soak a soft cloth in the oil, and heat it in the microwave until it's warm, but not hot. Wrap it around your wrist, cover it with plastic wrap, and leave it in place for several hours—then stay away from the computer as much as you possibly can!

✔ Soothe and Heal Injured Muscles

Simply apply castor oil to the affected area, cover it with plastic wrap, and top it off with a heating pad set on low. The heat will help the oil penetrate your skin and act directly on your muscles to ease the pain and stiffness. Leave the pad on for 20 to 30 minutes, then wash the oil off with soap and water. Repeat the treatment several times a day as needed. **Note:** For all you runners, this routine works just as well to heal shin splints.

✔ A Sensational Sciatica Solution

Your sciatic nerve is your body's biggest nerve, and it can also produce one of its biggest pains. But—as unlikely as it may seem when that "fire" is shooting down your leg—you *can* relieve the discomfort. Just mix equal parts of castor oil, arnica oil, and St. John's wort oil, and gently massage the mixture onto the nerve track. Begin at your buttocks, and go down the back of your leg. If you have a disk problem, massage the oil into that area, too. Repeat as needed for soothing relief. **Note:** You can buy arnica oil and St. John's wort oil in health-food stores and herb shops, as well as from numerous websites.

✔ Preempt Plantar Warts

Unlike warts on your hands or face, which are merely unsightly, plantar warts can make

> **CAUTION** ⚠
>
> If you will be ingesting castor oil or using it in or around your eyes, ears, or mouth, make sure you use only 100 percent pure castor oil. If you're using it as a muscle rub or anywhere on your skin, look for cold-pressed or cold-processed oil (also safe to ingest). It is readily available in health-food stores and from numerous websites. Avoid any product that's labeled "refined" castor oil. Studies have shown that more than 95 percent of the compounds that give the oil its healing power are removed when the oil goes through the conventional refining process. And whatever you do, steer clear of any industrial-grade castor oil that you may see in hardware or home-improvement stores. It is processed in a way that makes it unsafe for either oral or topical use.

POTENT POTION

INFLAMED-EAR ELIXIR

When an ear infection strikes, reach for this gentle, but powerful remedy.

1 tbsp. of castor oil
1 tbsp. of milk

Heat (but don't boil!) the ingredients in a non-aluminum pan. Let the mixture cool to a comfortable temperature. Put 4 drops into your inflamed ear every hour, and plug the opening with cotton. **Note:** If your ear pain is severe and persistent, get medical attention pronto.

every step you take a painful experience. The nasty things start as little black dots on the soles of your feet—usually in clusters. The natural reaction is to simply scrape them off with a fingernail. But don't do it—you'll only make the infection spread. Instead, simply rub castor oil on the spots several times a day. Before you know it, they'll be gone with the wind.

✔ Stop the Ringing

Church bells and sleigh bells are one thing. But bells that ring . . . and ring . . . and ring in your ears are something else again—namely, tinnitus, and it can be the very dickens to get rid of. One remedy that has proven effective for many folks is castor oil. Just before bedtime each day, put 3 or 4 drops of 100 percent pure castor oil into each ear. Plug the openings with cotton, and keep it in place overnight. After a month or so, the ringing should have lessened considerably. Within another few months, there's a good chance it will be gone completely. If it isn't, see your doctor to make sure you don't have a more serious illness.

✔ Pack Away Your Problems

A castor oil pack is just what the doctor ordered for relieving inflammation and promoting internal healing anywhere on—or in—your body. To make this magic bullet, follow this four-step procedure:

STEP 1. Pour some castor oil into a bowl, and add a soft, clean cloth that's big enough to cover the problem area. (A towel or a piece of wool or cotton flannel is perfect.)

STEP 2. Lay the oil-soaked fabric on your bare skin, and add a sheet of plastic wrap over it. Make sure you've got complete coverage—believe me, you don't want castor oil stains on your clothes or sheets!

STEP 3. Top the plastic wrap with a heating pad set on low. Or, if you pre-fer, use an old-fashioned hot-water bottle wrapped in a towel. Make sure that the heating pad isn't set on high or that the water bottle is too hot. You want your heat source to be just comfortably warm.

STEP 4. Leave the pack in place for 20 to 60 minutes. Repeat as needed once or twice a day until you feel relief.

Between uses, tuck the pack into a plastic bag, and store it in the refrigera-tor. **Note:** If your problem hasn't cleared up within a week or two, see your doctor just to make sure your condition isn't more serious than you think.

Pick a Pack of Power

Physicians and naturopathic professionals routinely prescribe castor oil packs to treat a passel of problems (see "Pack Away Your Problems," at left, for the how-to). Here's a handful of the most common uses for this powerful remedy.

ANNOYING HEALTH PROBLEM	HOW TO SOLVE IT
Arthritis and bursitis pain	Cover the affected area, and leave the pack in place for 45 to 60 minutes, once a day.
Chest cold	Lay the pack on your chest, and lie down for about 60 minutes.
Constipation	Keep a tummy-sized pack on your abdomen for 20 minutes or so. That should be plenty of time to get the show on the road.
Endometriosis	Make a pack that's large enough to cover the area between your breast bone and your pubic bone. Then relax for 30 to 60 minutes.*
Tender breasts (caused by fluctuating hormones before menopause)	Lay a pack across your breasts, and leave it on for 60 minutes or so.

* To deliver long-term relief, this treatment is most effective if you use it when you are not menstruat-ing. You can also use it to reduce pain during your periods, but only if your cramping is not accompanied by heavy bleeding.

A Beauty-Kit Classic

✤ Soften Your Hands

Rough, dry skin is no match for this combo: Mix 1 teaspoon of castor oil with 1 drop of either lemon oil or peppermint oil (available in health-food stores and many large supermarkets). Massage the mixture into your hands or feet at bedtime, put on cotton gloves or socks, and leave them on overnight. Your skin will be silky smooth in no time at all!

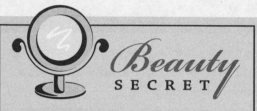

Beauty
S E C R E T

ALL EYES ON YOU

Eye makeup can be eye-catching all right, but removing it with commercial products can irritate the extra-tender skin around your peepers. On the other hand, this gentle combo will not only clean off the colors you've applied, but also soothe and moisten your skin. Simply mix 1 tablespoon each of 100 percent pure castor oil, olive oil, and canola oil in a glass jar with a tight-fitting lid. Then moisten a tissue or cotton ball with the oil as needed, and gently wipe away your eye shadow, eyeliner, or mascara.

✤ Eliminate Warts

There are more wart-removal remedies than you can shake a toad at, but this is one of the best: Mix 2 parts castor oil with 1 part baking soda to make a paste. Before you go to bed, apply the paste to the wart, and cover it with a bandage. In the morning, remove the bandage, and rinse off any paste residue. Repeat each night until the wart is gone. It will take anywhere from a few days to a few weeks to banish the unattractive bump, depending on the severity of the condition.

✤ Lighten Age and Sun Spots

Troubled by brown spots on your hands or face? You can lighten them with the dynamic duo of vitamin E and castor oil. Simply apply vitamin E oil directly to the spots once a day, then at night, rub on some castor oil. The marks will begin to fade in a few weeks.

✤ Fade Freckles Fast

Whether you got your unwanted skin spots from spending too much time in the sun, or they just run in your family—or a combination of both—this lovely lotion can produce a major vanishing act. To make it, follow this four-step routine:

STEP 1. Rinse four medium-size dandelion leaves thoroughly, and tear them into small pieces.

STEP 2. Mix the leaves with 5 tablespoons of castor oil in a glass or enamel pan.

STEP 3. Simmer the mixture, uncovered, over low heat for 10 minutes. Then turn off the heat, cover the pan, and let it steep for three hours.

STEP 4. Strain the potion into a bottle with a tight-fitting lid.

Every evening, massage a few drops of the oil into the freckled area, and leave it on overnight. Come morning, rinse it off with lukewarm water. You should start to see dramatic results within just a week or so.

✤ Thicken Your Lashes and Brows

If you'd like to have thicker, fuller eyelashes (and what woman wouldn't?), just rub a little 100 percent pure castor oil over the base of your lashes before bed each night. It will prevent thinning and promote rapid growth of the hair. To thicken your eyebrows—whether they've become naturally sparse over time, or you've plucked them more thoroughly than you'd intended to—wipe a little castor oil over your brow line each night.

✤ Condition Your Cuticles

Let castor oil and cocoa butter team up to keep your cuticles soft and beautiful. To make the conditioner, warm 4 tablespoons of cocoa butter over low heat until the butter liquefies. Stir in 4 table-

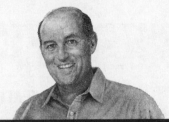

YOU DON'T SAY!

*C*astor oil comes from the seeds of the castor bean plant (*Ricinus communis*), and it's been a health and beauty staple since the days of ancient Egypt. Besides using the oil to soften their skin and speed up their inner workings, the Egyptians used it as a lubricant for sliding giant stone blocks over wooden rollers to their pyramid construction sites. Fast-forward 6,000 years to the 21st century, and you'll still find castor oil lubricating our means of transportation—namely, the engines of jet airplanes, trucks, and automobiles. In fact, castor oil is the prime ingredient in Castrol R® motor oil, which is specially designed for use in high-performance racing cars.

spoons of castor oil, and pour the mixture into a deep bowl. Let the potion cool to a comfortable temperature, then soak your fingertips and nails for 10 to 15 minutes. Rinse your fingers in warm water, and gently push back your cuticles. Store any leftover conditioner in a jar with a tight-fitting lid for up to three months at room temperature.

POTENT POTION

WINTER-WEATHER GUARD

Cold, dry, windy weather can damage your skin fast—besides making it itch like crazy. This lovely lotion acts like a suit of armor to protect your face and neck from Old Man Winter's ravages.

6 oz. of castor oil
2 oz. of water
2–4 drops of frankincense oil*
2–4 drops of lavender oil*

Mix the castor oil and water in a plastic bottle that has a screw-on cap with a lift-up spout.** Add the frankincense and lavender oils, and shake to blend the mixture. If it's too thick or too thin, add a little more water or castor oil, as needed. To use the potion, shake the bottle, pour a small amount of the oil into your hands, and spread it over your face and neck. **Note:** This formula is also a great way to protect children's skin from chapping and windburn before the tykes head out to play in the snow.

* Available in herb shops and health-food stores and from many websites.
** Available in the cosmetic or travel-supply section of drugstores and supermarkets.

❖ Minimize Scars

Applying castor oil to both accidental and surgical wounds can greatly reduce scarring and may even prevent it altogether. Gently wipe the oil into your skin periodically throughout the day as the wound heals. (Be sure to let the oil dry thoroughly before it touches any fabric.) The secret "weapon" is castor oil's ability to increase your body's quantity of T lymphocytes (a.k.a. white blood cells), which studies have shown to play an important role in skin healing.

✤ De-Line Your Face and Neck

Castor oil can help minimize the fine lines that appear in your skin as time marches on. Each night at bedtime, just dab a little 100 percent pure castor oil into the creases in your neck and around your eyes and mouth. Unfortunately, it won't halt the parade, but it will help to slow down its pace.

✤ Protect and Moisturize Dry Skin

Besides adding moisture, castor oil creates a protective barrier between your skin and the harsh environmental conditions of the sometimes not-so-great outdoors *and* indoors. To make this fabulous formula, simply mix ½ cup of castor oil with ⅔ cup of olive oil, and add 20 drops of your favorite essential oil. (Rose and geranium oils are both excellent for dry skin.) Use it as you would any other facial moisturizer.

Best of the Rest

★ Buddies Banish Back Pain . . .

With the help of eucalyptus oil. Put 20 drops or so of the aromatic oil in a cup, and heat it in the microwave for a few seconds. (It should feel comfortably warm to the touch—not hot.) Then have a friend or your spouse gently massage the oil onto the painful area of your back. After the hands-on healing session, you should feel a whole lot better!

★ Eucalyptus Conquers Coughs

Got a cough that just won't quit? Then rub the outside of your throat with eucalyptus oil. Besides getting rid of the built-up mucus, it'll help you relax enough to get some much-needed rest.

Come to Your Senses

HEALTHFUL HINT

When a head cold has your air passages so congested that your senses of taste and smell have all but vanished, try this trick: Sprinkle a few drops of eucalyptus oil on a cotton ball, and tuck it into a clean, empty pill bottle. Carry it around with you, and whenever you feel the need, remove the cap and take a few quick whiffs. You'll be tasting the wine and smelling the roses quick as a wink!

★ Relax, Cheer Up, and Charge!

Eucalyptus oil stimulates your nervous system in a way that calms you down, lifts your mood, and boosts your energy. To tap into this multipurpose powerhouse, simply mix 15 to 20 drops of eucalyptus oil per ounce of distilled water in a spray bottle, and mist yourself whenever you're feeling anxious, down, or stressed out.

POTENT POTION

SINUS-CLEARING BATH OIL

Whether the sinus-clogging culprit is a head cold or seasonal allergies, a soak in this soothing solution will help clear your airways—and relax your mind and body to boot!

8 drops of eucalyptus oil*
8 drops of peppermint oil*
8 drops of tea tree oil*

Put the three essential oils in a small bottle, screw the lid on tightly, and shake the bottle until the mixture is thoroughly blended. Then head to your bathroom and start filling the bathtub with water that's as hot as you can handle, pouring the oil under the spigot. Settle into the tub, and soak for at least 20 minutes, breathing deeply to inhale the wonderful (and wonderfully clearing) aroma.

* You can find these oils in health-food stores and herb shops.

★ Go Fishing for Psoriasis Relief

Recent studies have shown fish oil to be effective in healing psoriasis, and a combination of fish oil and avocado oil seems to be especially successful. That's because in addition to providing infection-fighting antioxidants, avocado oil quickly penetrates the psoriasis patches, so the fish oil can deliver its healing power. Put the dynamic duo to work for you with this three-step procedure:

STEP 1. Pour concentrated fish oil into one bowl and an equal amount of cold-pressed avocado oil into another bowl. (If you like, add a little lemon oil to the fish oil to improve its aroma.) Set the two containers close together, so you can reach them both quickly.

STEP 2. Using your very clean fingers, apply the avocado oil to the psoriasis lesions in gentle, circular motions. Immediately follow up with the fish oil, using the same easygoing, circular pattern. Work on one small area of skin at a time to maximize the synergy of the two oils.

STEP 3. Wait until the oils have dried thoroughly—at least 10 minutes—before you let clothing or other fabric touch your skin. Or, if you really need to scurry in a hurry, wait three to five minutes, then lightly pat the treated area with a damp cloth to remove any excess oil.

Note: Be sure to use cold-pressed avocado oil to ensure the maximum antioxidant content, and choose a concentrated fish oil for the highest levels of EPA and DHA omega-3 fatty acids. These are the magic bullets that deliver the results you want.

★ Give Bruises the Brush-Off

The next time you bang your shin—or any other part of your body—fetch some fish oil. It's a first-rate way to reduce inflammation in and under your skin. Take 1 to 2 tablespoons of 100 percent pure fish oil a day until the bruise is gone. (You can mix the oil with fruit juice to minimize the fishy taste.)

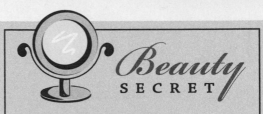

Beauty SECRET

FABULOUS FISHY SCAR REDUCER

*A combination of fish oil and vitamin E oil can greatly reduce the appearance of scars, and sometimes even make them vanish entirely. The process is simple: First, squeeze the contents of a fish oil capsule and a vitamin E capsule into a bowl, and mix thoroughly. Gently rub all of the liquid into the scarred area, and let it air-dry completely. Repeat the procedure once a day, or as often as you can, until the proud skin (as the old-timers called it) diminishes. **Note:** This same treatment works wonders for removing stretch marks caused by pregnancy or major weight loss.*

★ Nix Nail Fungus with Tea Tree Oil

There are few skin afflictions more annoying—or harder to get rid of—than a fingernail or toenail fungus. But it'll clear up fast if you paint your nails with tea tree oil three times a day. Also, keep your nails short and unpolished, and if the "victims" are your toes, go barefoot or wear open sandals as often as you can. This way, you'll maximize your nails' exposure to air, which encourages faster healing.

POTENT POTION

LOVELY LEG LOTION

Shaving and waxing can leave your legs bumpy, burned, irritated—and at prime risk for developing painful ingrown hairs. The healing power of tea tree oil in this recipe, along with the softening properties of lavender and thyme, can help minimize those nasty side effects.

1 bottle (8 to 10 oz.) of
   unscented body lotion
10 drops of tea tree oil*
5 drops of lavender oil*
5 drops of thyme oil*

Add the essential oils to the lotion, and shake the bottle well. Use the moisturizer daily to keep your legs (or any other part of your body) silky smooth and oh-so-soft to the touch.

* You can find these oils in health-food stores and herb shops.

★ Hair's to Eucalyptus

When it comes to healthy hair, eucalyptus oil is a triple-threat champ. It promotes hair growth, battles dandruff, and improves the elasticity of your locks (thereby leading to less breakage). Your job: Just add about 10 drops of the oil to a bottle of your regular shampoo, shake to mix, and wash your hair as usual.

★ Get Glowing

If your skin is looking dull and dry—or worse, chapped and flaking—reach for some eucalyptus oil. Add a few drops to a gentle, unscented face cream, and use it as you would any other moisturizer. Your complexion will have its healthy glow back in no time at all!

★ A Little Drop'll Do Ya

Looking for a really effective dandruff remedy? Well, look no further—this one's a dandy: Just add a few drops of either eucalyptus oil or tea tree oil to your usual shampoo, and use it each time you wash your hair. Your white-flake worries should be gone for good.

★ Banish Body Odor

Chronic body odor is generally caused by bacteria on your skin, so you need to boot out the bad bacteria to get rid of the unpleasant smell. Enter tea tree oil, which is a very potent antibacterial agent. Add several drops of the oil to your bathwater each day. Or, if you prefer showers to baths, mix 2 drops of tea tree oil per ounce of water in a spray bottle, and use it as a deodorant. But beware—it may sting a little on your freshly shaved underarms!

7 Cayenne Pepper

Cayenne pepper is a hot topic in health and beauty circles these days, and for good reason: Capsaicin, the ingredient that gives this—and all hot peppers—their firepower, also heats up your body's internal "machinery" like there's no tomorrow. Whether you add the ground pepper to food, take it in capsules, or mix it into creams and salves, cayenne can ease aches and pains, give you a glowing complexion, and even cure the common cold.

A Red-Hot Healer

✔ Stop a Toothache

Press just a few grains of ground cayenne pepper to your painful tooth and gum. Yes, I know that it will sting like the dickens at first—but only for a second or two. As soon as the "fire" goes out, your toothache should be gone.

✔ Warm Up Your Tootsies

If you're one of those people whose feet go into lockdown mode the minute you go outdoors in cold weather, this tip has your name written all over it: Before you pull on your boots or shoes, put on a pair of thin socks. Then grab a second, thicker pair, and sprinkle 1 teaspoon of ground cayenne pepper into each sock and pull 'em on over your stockinged feet. With a little pepper power, your dogs will stay toasty warm, even on the coldest winter day.

✔ Stay Cozy All Over

To rev up your circulation, thereby helping to keep your whole body warmer in cold weather, use either, or both, of these surefire remedies:

■ Drink about ¼ teaspoon of ground cayenne pepper in a glass of warm water once a day.

■ Stir 1 or 2 teaspoons of ground cayenne pepper into a tub of bathwater, and settle in for a nice hot soak. Just beware that the oils in the pepper will heat up the water, so run warm water to start with, and add more hot water from the tap if you need to.

Note: It goes without saying (I hope!) that these preventive measures are *not* substitutes for bundling up when you go outdoors!

✔ Fabulous Fever Reliever

It might seem odd that something as hot as cayenne pepper could reduce your body's temperature, but it does just that in this classic health helper. And making it is a simple three-step process:

STEP 1. Boil ½ teaspoon of ground cayenne pepper in 1 quart of water.

STEP 2. Let the potion cool until it's comfortably warm, but not hot.

STEP 3. Pour 1 cup of the "tea" into a bowl or measuring cup. Mix in ¼ cup of orange juice and 1 teaspoon of honey, and drink the potion slowly.

Store the remaining cayenne-water solution in the fridge, and drink the

---

POTENT POTION

SWEET AND SPICY SORE THROAT CURE

This two-timing gargle will make a sore throat scurry in a hurry!

⅛ tsp. of ground cayenne pepper
⅛ tsp. of ground ginger
8 oz. of hot water
Ice-cold pineapple juice

Mix the spices in the water. Pour the juice into a glass, and set it aside. First, gargle with a swig of the spicy mixture. Then follow up by gargling with the pineapple juice. Switch back and forth between the hot and cold liquids until both glasses are empty. Repeat the routine several times a day. The combination of hot and cold liquids will ease the burning sensation. And the dual action of the spices and bromelain (an enzyme in the pineapple) will loosen that irritating mucus in your throat.

remaining 3 cups throughout the day, heating it up each time, and adding the orange juice and honey to each cup. **Note:** You don't have to be running a fever to benefit from this bracing beverage. Anytime you drink it, you get a potent dose of cayenne's health- *and* beauty-enhancing power.

✔ Ease the Pain of Strains and Sprains

Whether you're a weekend warrior, or you just slipped on a patch of ice and twisted your ankle, cayenne pepper can come to your aid. Just mix a pinch of the fiery stuff in a cup or so of apple cider vinegar, dampen a cloth with the solution, put it on your sore body part, and leave it on for about five minutes. Repeat as often as necessary until the pain is gone and you're back to normal.

✔ Alleviate Arthritis Aches

Here's an ultra-simple way to ease the pain in your joints: Twice a day, mix ⅛ teaspoon of ground cayenne pepper in a glass of water or fruit juice, and drink up. The capsaicin in the pepper will block the debilitating pain. If you can't take the pepper's heat, get out of the kitchen, and head for the closest health-food store. Buy cayenne pepper capsules, and take two a day, as recommended, washed down with either water or fruit juice.

Conquer Carpal Tunnel

HEALTHFUL HINT

No one can deny that the computer age has given us many benefits, but it has also produced its share of unpleasant "side effects"—including carpal tunnel syndrome. If too much time at the keyboard has landed you with this painful affliction, reach for a jar of ground cayenne pepper. Mix 1 teaspoon of the red-hot powder into ¼ cup of skin lotion (any kind will do), and rub 1 teaspoon of the mixture—no more!—on the sore area. **Note:** Be careful not to get the steamy mixture on any broken skin or near your eyes, and wash your hands thoroughly after you've performed the procedure.

✔ Block Back Pain

Almost every adult on the planet gets a backache at one time or another. No matter what caused the problem, cayenne pepper liniment will send the pain packin' pronto. To make it, mix 2 tablespoons of ground cayenne pepper in 2 cups of boiling water. Reduce the heat, and simmer for 30 minutes. Remove the pan from the heat, and stir in 2 cups of rubbing alcohol. Let the potion cool, and store it at room temperature in a glass bottle with a tight-fitting lid. Then whenever you feel the need, rub the liniment into your sore back—or ask your spouse to do the honors. **Note:** With this or any other topical cayenne pepper remedy, test the potion on a small patch of skin first. And make sure you wash your hands thoroughly after applying it.

> **C A U T I O N** ⚠️
>
> Cayenne pepper is widely used to dissolve blood clots, but it also interacts with antacids, aspirin, and blood thinners. So if you take any of these medications on a regular basis, in either prescription or over-the-counter form, consult with your doctor before you dose yourself with any of these cayenne remedies.

✔ Protect Your Heart

In order to stay in good working order, your heart needs to receive a steady supply of blood. One of the best ways to ensure an ongoing flow of that life-giving fluid is to drink ⅛ teaspoon of ground cayenne pepper in a glass of water, herbal tea, or pure fruit juice every day.

✔ Mitigate Migraines

If you suffer from migraines, here's an old-time tip that could help end your agony: At the first sign of symptoms, dip a flat-ended toothpick into a jar of ground cayenne pepper, and sniff a teeny-tiny bit into each nostril. This remedy works for two reasons: Hot pepper contains both magnesium, which helps ward off migraines, and capsaicin, which blocks pain impulses from traveling to your brain. But remember to use only a few grains—even a midsize dash of pepper in your nose will deliver a very HOT surprise!

✔ Make Ulcers Say "Uncle"

For the most part, doctors advise ulcer sufferers to avoid spicy foods because they can further irritate your stomach's lining. But there is one major exception to this rule: cayenne pepper. Studies show that it can actually help heal ulcers and prevent them from forming in the first place. It works in three ways:

KILLS BACTERIA. Cayenne pepper kills harmful bacteria in your stomach—including *Helicobacter pylori,* which is the prime cause of ulcers.

REGULATES STOMACH SECRETIONS. The capsaicin in cayenne pepper not only acts as a natural pain reliever, but it can also stop your stomach from producing acid, which irritates ulcers. What's more, when you consume the fiery red powder, your stomach automatically produces more protective juices that may prevent the formation of new ulcers.

RELIEVES COMMON SIDE EFFECTS. This versatile spice can relieve heartburn, indigestion, and other gastrointestinal discomforts that often accompany an ulcer.

Note: If you're under medical care for an ulcer, consult with your doctor or naturopathic professional before you embark on a cayenne pepper treatment routine. And keep the doses small—too much pepper, especially in the beginning, may inflame your ulcers.

✔ Lower Your Stress Level

No matter what has you all hot and bothered, cayenne pepper can help reduce tension and give you a pleasant burst of energy to boot. Start by drinking ⅛ teaspoon of the ground pepper in 8 ounces of warm water once a day. Stick with that dosage until you've gotten used to its firepower, then increase the amount of pepper to ¼ teaspoon, then ½ teaspoon. Continue this "drinking habit" until you're feeling calmer.

✔ Control the Burn

Not everyone is accustomed to eating spicy foods, so be aware that when you first start drinking cayenne pepper in water, it *will* burn when you swallow it *and* when it comes out the other end. Over time, your body should adjust to the heat, but in the meantime, you can minimize the discomfort by

Fabulous Food Fix

FETTUCCINE SWEET AND HOT

This delicious dish serves up the health-giving power of cayenne and sweet bell peppers.

12 oz. of dry fettuccine
2 red bell peppers, thinly sliced
3 garlic cloves, minced
¾ tsp. of ground cayenne pepper
1 cup of reduced-fat sour cream
¾ cup of reduced-sodium chicken broth
¾ cup of grated Parmesan cheese
Salt and pepper to taste

Cook the fettuccine according to the package directions, and drain. Coat a large skillet with nonstick cooking spray, and sauté the peppers, garlic, and cayenne over medium heat for three to five minutes. Mix in the sour cream and chicken broth, and then simmer uncovered for five minutes. Remove the pan from the heat, and stir in the cheese. Toss the pasta with the sauce, and season with salt and pepper.

YIELD: 4 SERVINGS

taking your cayenne in capsule form. If you want the more direct impact of the ground pepper mixed in water, start with no more than ⅛ to ¼ teaspoon and work your way up to bigger doses if the situation calls for that. Also, keep a second glass of water, juice, or milk close at hand to dilute any burning feeling in your mouth.

POTENT POTION

SPICY SORE THROAT SYRUP

Cayenne pepper adds its therapeutic heat to this soothing remedy.

6 tbsp. of honey
3 tsp. of grated lemon peel
3 tsp. of horseradish
¾ tsp. of ground cayenne pepper

Combine all of the ingredients in a small bowl, and take 1 tablespoon every hour or so throughout the day. Mix up a fresh batch each morning, and you'll be warbling again in no time at all!

✔ Slow the Flow

Almost every woman of childbearing age knows that excessive menstrual flow is a major inconvenience—to put it mildly. Well, here's good news: Cayenne pepper can help regulate your profuse bleeding. Just mix ⅛ teaspoon of the ground pepper into a cup of warm water or your favorite herbal tea. Drink a "cuppa" as often as needed throughout the day until the raging stream has slowed to a healthy trickle. **Note:** If you're not sure whether your bleeding is due to extreme menstrual flow or hemorrhaging, don't take any chances—call your doctor pronto!

✔ Rub Away Bruises

The next time you have a run-in with your coffee table or any other body-bashing object, mix 1 part ground cayenne pepper with 5 parts petroleum jelly, and rub the ointment onto your bruise. Repeat the procedure every day or two until the black-and-blue patch vanishes.

✔ Nix a Nosebleed

Just about everyone gets a nosebleed now and then. The cause can be anything from allergies to a sinus infection, cold weather, or a bump on the schnozz. Regardless of what started the bleeding, you can stop it by drinking a glass of warm water with ⅛ teaspoon of ground cayenne pepper mixed into it. **Note:** If you have recurrent nosebleeds, it may signal an underlying ailment, so see your doctor. And if you're experiencing nasal hemorrhaging—blood flowing from both nostrils—hightail it to the nearest doctor or emergency room!

The Pepper Potential

✣ Slay Dragon Breath

Cayenne's firepower not only kills germs in your mouth, but also leaves your breath feeling spicy fresh. Just dilute 5 to 10 drops each of cayenne tincture and myrrh tincture (available in health-food stores) in half a glass of warm water, and use it as you would any other mouthwash.

✣ Conquer Cellulite

Besides revving up your circulation, cayenne pepper improves the efficiency of your lymphatic system, thereby allowing your body to eliminate toxins—including the ones that cause cellulite. Each time you consume

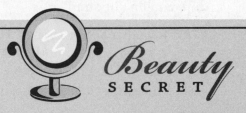

HAIR'S TO YOU!

*B*ecause cayenne pepper increases the blood flow to your scalp, it helps to make your hair fuller and glossier and promote its growth. So if you've got thinning hair, include more cayenne in your diet to assist in this process. For more direct action, mix 1 to 2 teaspoons of the ground pepper with enough olive oil to make a thick paste. Massage it thoroughly into your scalp and hair, cover it with a shower cap, and leave it on for 10 to 15 minutes. (Don't worry about burning your scalp; the olive oil will help neutralize the heat.) Then remove the cap, and follow up with your usual shampoo and conditioner. **Note:** To really intensify the effect, you can leave the paste in your hair overnight, with the shower cap on, of course!

Beauty SECRET

cayenne pepper, you help the detox process along, but here's a specific remedy that has proven effective: Squeeze the juice of one lemon into a glass, and add a pinch of ground cayenne pepper. Fill the balance of the glass with water, stir, and drink up. (You'll want to gulp this spicy-sour concoction down quickly.) Perform this routine three times a day, and within 30 days or so, you should begin to notice a difference.

✤ Fight Off Wrinkles . . .

And gradually make your skin more radiant. How? Just add more cayenne pepper to your diet, or drink it mixed in water, tea, or juice. It works its magic by stimulating blood flow, which in turn improves the softness and elasticity of your skin.

✤ Take Time for Tincture

One of the easiest ways to enjoy the beauty and health benefits of cayenne pepper is in tincture form. Just put a few drops of it in a glass of water or fruit juice, and drink up. You can buy cayenne pepper tincture in health-food stores, but don't waste your money; it's easy—and cheaper—to make your own supply. It does take a while to "cook," but the four-step procedure couldn't be simpler:

STEP 1. Gather your supplies. You'll need 2 cups of ground cayenne pepper; a 1-quart, wide-mouthed jar with a tight-fitting lid; 100-proof vodka; cheesecloth; a bowl or pitcher; a funnel; and small, dark-colored bottles with droppers (available in health-food stores and online).

STEP 2. Pour the ground pepper into the jar, and add the vodka to within ½ inch of the jar's top.

STEP 3. Fasten the lid tightly, and put the jar in a cool, dark place for six to eight weeks.

STEP 4. Strain the tincture through cheesecloth into a bowl or pitcher, then use the funnel to pour the tincture into the small bottles. Store them in a cool, dark place (like a closed kitchen cabinet that's not near the stove), where the tincture will keep indefinitely.

Note: If you'd rather not use alcohol in your tincture recipe, you can easily substitute either apple cider vinegar or glycerin (available in most drugstores) for the vodka. The tincture won't be quite as potent as the alcohol version, but it will still be effective.

Best of the Rest

★ Black Pepper Banishes Earwax

Earwax may not be a major health problem, but if you've got it, it sure is annoying. To send the wax on its way, warm 1 tablespoon of corn oil to a comfortable temperature, and sprinkle in a little ground black pepper. Dip a cotton ball into the mixture, and put the soaked blob in your ear. Wait five minutes, and remove the wax-covered cotton ball.

★ Relieve a Toothache

Why is it that toothaches always strike when you can't possibly see a dentist—like on a Saturday night or over a holiday weekend? When that happens to you, try this kooky-sounding—but highly effective—pain reliever. Cut a piece of brown paper grocery bag that's the size of your cheek. Soak the paper in apple cider vinegar, then sprinkle one side with ground black pepper. Put the peppered side against the outside of your face, over the aching tooth. Secure the paper with a bandage or two, and keep it there for at least an hour. Remove the dressing, and your pain should be gone.

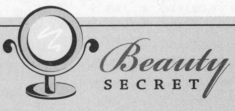

DE-WRINKLE, TONE, AND HEAL
Beauty SECRET

Cumin's antibacterial and hydrating powers team up to deliver a toner that heals blemishes and helps prevent wrinkles. To make it, bring 3 cups of water to a boil, toss in a handful of cumin seeds, reduce the heat, and steep for about three minutes. Strain out the solids, let the liquid cool to room temperature, and mix in a few drops of tea tree and lavender essential oils. Pour the potion into a dark-colored glass bottle with a tight-fitting lid, and store it in the refrigerator. Apply the toner to your face morning and evening after your normal cleansing routine. Then follow up with your usual moisturizer.

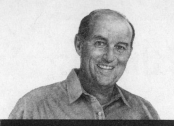

YOU DON'T SAY!

When it comes to spicy food, what one person considers steamy may be mild to others. But back in 1912, a pharmacist named Wilbur Scoville came up with a scale that objectively measures the heat in peppers and hot-pepper sauces. He called it the Scoville Organoleptic Test, and it's still used today. The scale begins at 0 Scoville Heat Units (SHUs) for pimento and bell peppers and goes up . . . and up. Habanero peppers top the scale at 200,000 to 300,000 SHUs. (The heat in any kind of pepper varies, depending on where and how it was grown, and when it was harvested.) As for hot sauces, the record holder is a brand called The Source, which measures a tongue-melting 7.1 million SHUs!

★ De-Gasify Your Beans

If you love beans, but could do without their all-too-common side effects, flavor them with ground coriander seed and ground cumin. These tasty spices help diminish legumes' gas production, so you'll have no worries about polluting the air.

★ Count on Cumin

The folks who study such things tell us that cumin is the second most popular spice in the world (black pepper ranks number one). We know it best for adding zing to tacos and other Mexican food, as well as Indian, Middle Eastern, and North African cuisines. But it also packs a powerful load of health benefits. It boosts your energy, fights the free radicals that cause cancer and other diseases, and improves your kidney and liver function. To make this superstar part of your health-care team, simply work it into your diet a few times a week. You'll find scads of scrumptious recipes on the Internet, in food magazines, and—of course—in ethnic cookbooks.

★ Hot Sauce Clobbers Cold Symptoms

You couldn't ask for a simpler solution than this one: Grab a bottle of hot-pepper sauce, and shake it well. (Any brand that suits your taste buds will do the trick.) Then put 10 to 20 drops into a glass of water, and drink up. Repeat the procedure three times a day until you're rarin' to go again.

★ A Hot Tip for Weight Loss

Recent studies have shown that adding just a few dashes of hot-pepper sauce to your daily diet not only reduces your levels of a hunger-causing hormone called ghrelin, but also raises your level of GLP-1, a compound that naturally suppresses your appetite. One of the tastiest ways to put this firepower to work: Add it to tomato juice.

★ Turmeric Trumps Heartburn

Turmeric is to Indian cuisine what salt and pepper are to basic American fare. But this exotic flavor enhancer is also a powerful digestive aid. It stimulates the flow of saliva, which both neutralizes acid and empowers your digestive juices. So before you eat something that typically gives you heartburn, jazz it up with ground turmeric. If the meal at hand does not lend itself to a hot, spicy additive, take two or three turmeric capsules (available in health-food stores) before you chow down for the same effect.

★ Spicy Help for Body and Mind

Curcumin, the active ingredient in turmeric, is one of the most powerful, naturally occurring anti-inflammatory substances ever identified—and therefore, it's one of the most potent weapons in the fight against chronic diseases. What's more, turmeric has also been shown to have strong anti-cancer properties and to reduce the buildup of plaque in the brain that causes Alzheimer's disease and cognitive decline. Your R_x for good health: Simply add ground turmeric to your favorite soups, stews, and other foods as often as you can—as they say, the more, the merrier!

★ Treat Your Face to Turmeric

In India, turmeric is renowned for its power to soften, cleanse, soothe, and clear up any type of skin. This mask is especially effective for dry skin: Mix 2 teaspoons of flour and 1 teaspoon of

Fabulous Food Fix

SPICY CHICKPEA DIP

The mixture of tangy spices in this scrumptious dip gives you a load of health and beauty benefits. Serve it with raw veggies and pita chips at your next party or poker game.

2 cans (15-oz. each) of chickpeas, rinsed and drained
2 tbsp. of lemon juice
3 garlic cloves, chopped
1 tsp. of cumin seeds
¼ tsp. of hot paprika
⅛ tsp. of ground cayenne pepper
2 tbsp. of olive oil
Salt and pepper to taste

Combine the first six ingredients in a food processor until they become finely chopped. With the machine running, add the olive oil in a steady stream, and process until the mixture is smooth. Spoon the dip into a shallow bowl, and season with the salt and pepper. Serve at room temperature.

YIELD: ABOUT 3 CUPS

ground turmeric in a bowl, make a well in the center, and add 1 teaspoon of honey to it. Mix until you have a smooth orange paste. Wash your face, then smooth the concoction onto your skin, and leave it on for 10 to 15 minutes. Wash the mask off with warm water, then splash your face with cool water, and pat dry. **Note:** Although turmeric will not stain your skin, it *does* stain fabric, so wear old clothes and use old towels for this project!

★ Exfoliating Pepper Scrub

Troubled by rough skin on your elbows, knees, or feet? Don't fret— smoother skin is as close as your kitchen. Mix a handful each of coarsely ground black pepper and salt with just enough plain yogurt to hold them together. Massage the mixture into your "alligator" skin, then rinse it away with lukewarm water.

★ Double-Duty Coriander Mask

To soothe your skin and lighten dark spots at the same time, puree a peeled, chopped cucumber in a blender or food processor, and mix in enough ground coriander to make a paste. Apply it to your face, leaving it on for 20 minutes. Then rinse with warm water, and follow up with your usual moisturizer.

POTENT POTION

ACNE-ERASING TONER

If you've got oily or combination skin that's prone to inflammation and blemishes, this toner is just the ticket.

¾ cup of water
1 tbsp. of whole black peppercorns
1 sprig of fresh rosemary
2 tbsp. of apple cider vinegar

Bring the water to a boil, and add the peppercorns and rosemary. Continue boiling until half the water has evaporated, then remove the pan from the heat, and let it cool to room temperature. Strain the liquid into a glass bottle with a tight-fitting lid, add the vinegar, and store it at room temperature. Then each evening, after washing your face, smooth the toner onto your skin with a cotton pad. End of story.

---

8 Chamomile

It's probably safe to say that chamomile is the very first herb that most of us ever heard of—when our mothers lulled us to sleep with Beatrix Potter's *The Tale of Peter Rabbit*. But Mrs. Rabbit was far from the first loving mama to cure her youngster's ills with chamomile tea. The first recorded use of the herb dates back to ancient Egypt, and over the centuries, it's been used for just about every health and beauty purpose under the sun. As the Germans like to say, chamomile is *alles zutraut*, which means "capable of anything."

A Health-Care Classic

✔ Soothe Sore Eyes

Chamomile has potent anti-inflammatory powers that make it a perfect choice for reducing redness, puffiness, and irritation around your eyes. Simply steep two chamomile tea bags in 1 cup of freshly boiled water for three minutes. Remove them from the water, and tuck them into the fridge to cool for about five minutes. Then lie down, and put a bag over each eye. Relax for 15 minutes or so, and jeepers creepers—your peepers should be back to normal.

✔ When You've Picked Your Poison . . .

Rather, when your poison has picked you—and it came from poison ivy, poison oak, or poison sumac—chamomile can clear up the itchy, burning rash. Just steep 2 tablespoons of dried chamomile in 2 cups of boiling water for about 10 minutes. Let the tea cool to a comfortable temperature, then soak a clean washcloth in it. Lay the cloth gently on your afflicted skin, and leave it on for 15 minutes or so. Repeat as often as needed until your rash has healed.

HEALTHFUL HINT
Classic Chamomile Tea

No matter how you intend to use it, the basic recipe for chamomile tea is the same: For each serving, pour 1 cup of freshly boiled water over one chamomile tea bag or 1 to 2 teaspoons of dried chamomile (or more if you prefer a stronger brew). Cover the pot or cup to keep the herb's volatile oils from dissipating, and steep for three to five minutes. Remove the tea bag, or strain out the herbs. Add honey or lemon if you like, and drink up.

✔ Peter's Mother Knew Best

Chamomile tea is just what the doctor ordered for curing a stomachache. (The recommended dose for humans is 3 or 4 cups a day until you feel chipper enough to romp through a garden again.) But this versatile beverage can also perform a boatload of other health-giving feats, like these, for instance:

ALLEVIATE MENSTRUAL CRAMPS. At the first twinge of monthly discomfort, start sipping chamomile tea throughout the day until your cramps are gone.

CLEAR UP STRESS-RELATED HIVES. If your itchy, red blotches just happen to arrive during a period of anxiety or emotional turmoil, there's a good chance that stress is the culprit. So before you try any over-the-counter antihistamines, treat yourself to a few cups of nerve-calming chamomile tea every day. It may just make your spots disappear right before your eyes.

CURB CARPAL TUNNEL SYNDROME. Drink several cups of chamomile tea each day until your wrist feels better—and cut back on your keyboard time as much as possible!

ENCOURAGE PICKY EATERS. If you've got a youngster who frequently turns up his or her nose at what is on their plate, don't get caught up in endless rounds of mealtime meltdowns. Instead, make a cup of chamomile tea, and add just a pinch of ground ginger to it. Give the tyke 1 teaspoon of the warm brew half an hour before each meal. That should stimulate the child's appetite enough to appreciate any cuisine.

RELIEVE INDIGESTION. Drink 1 cup of chamomile tea after each meal until you're feeling better. Or if you have a chronically sensitive digestive system—and you know that you have no serious underlying medical condition—make a post-meal "cuppa" part of your regular routine.

SACK SAD SYMPTOMS. In addition to feeling gloomy and tired, people with seasonal affective disorder (SAD) tend to experience intense cravings for carbohydrates. One effective antidote: Whenever a carb craving strikes, drink a cup of chamomile tea. It'll divert your attention from food and give you a much-needed energy boost at the same time.

✔ Hic- Hic- Hiccup No More

Hiccups may not pose a serious health threat, but they sure are annoying! Here's one way to stop them: Put a drop of chamomile essential oil in a brown paper bag, hold it over your nose and mouth, and breathe in deeply. Bingo—end of problem!

POTENT POTION

TEA TIMES TWO

An herbal infusion is simply an extra-strong tea that's ideal for topical use—although you can also drink it, provided the herbs are edible and you prefer your tea on the strong side. This recipe makes 1 cup of brew, but you can double, triple, or even quadruple the recipe if you need more for a particular use (like soaking your feet), or if you simply want to keep a supply on hand.

2 heaping tbsp. of dried chamomile
8 oz. of fresh spring water

Put the herbs in a ceramic or glass mug, jar, or pitcher, and pour just-boiled spring water over them. Cover, and let the mixture steep for 10 to 15 minutes. Strain, and pour it into a clean container. Let the brew cool before you use it on your skin, but drink it at whatever temperature suits your fancy. Either use the infusion right away, or store it in the refrigerator, where it will keep well for about five days.

✔ Let's Ear It for Chamomile

When you've got an earache from you know where, put a tablespoon or so of dried chamomile in a bowl, and pour in just enough hot (not boiling!) water to moisten the herbs. Spread them on one-half of a piece of moistened cheesecloth or other soft, clean fabric that's a little more than twice the size of your ear. Fold the sides of the material over to form an envelope. Then put the poultice over your painful ear for 15 minutes or so. **Note:** If you don't have the dried herb on hand, substitute a couple of chamomile tea bags.

CAUTION ⚠

Chamomile is one of our most effective herbal health and beauty herbs, but there are a couple of things you need to be aware of. First, it contains coumarin, which reacts with blood-thinning drugs. So if you are taking any of those meds, consult with your doctor before you consume chamomile in any oral form. Second, because chamomile is a member of the ragweed family, you should use this herb with caution if you suffer from pollen allergies. It won't cause you any long-term harm, but it may trigger some sneezing, or wheezing, or even contact dermatitis.

✔ Towel Off a Sore Throat

It seems that everybody and his uncle has a favorite sore throat cure. Well, this is one of mine: Make a quart of strong chamomile infusion (just quadruple the recipe for Tea Times Two on page 99), and strain it into another pan. Let the brew cool just enough so you can handle it, then soak a clean towel in the solution. Wring it out, and wrap it snugly around your neck. As soon as the towel cools off, warm up the tea, remoisten the towel, and reapply it to your throat. The chamomile will help draw out the pain, and the heat will ease the tension that's built up in your throat muscles. Repeat the procedure as needed until you feel better. (It shouldn't take more than one or two additional dips.)

✔ Prevent Gingivitis

If your dentist has told you that you're at risk for gingivitis—or if you've already been treated for the disease and you want to keep your gums in good health—this preventive potion can help: Put 2 teaspoons of dried chamomile in 1 cup of boiling water, and let it steep for 10 minutes or so. Drink a cup after every meal, and let the herb do what it does best: kill germs and reduce your risk of developing (or redeveloping) the dreaded gum disease.

✔ Pull Out a Toothache

The same hot chamomile compress that relieves a sore throat can also draw out the pain of a toothache. In this case, saturate a clean washcloth in a strong chamomile infusion, wring it out, and press it against the part of your face that's outside the aching tooth. As soon as the cloth cools off, resoak and reapply it. Your pain should be gone before you need to reheat the brew.

✔ Chopper-Calming Mouthwash

Here's a quick (and tasty) way to ease denture pain: Drop 1 teaspoon of dried chamomile into 1 cup of hot water, and steep for 10 to 20 minutes. Strain out the herb, and when the tea has cooled down, take a mouthful, swish it around for 30 seconds or so, and spit it out. Repeat the procedure until you've used up all of the brew.

✔ Sponge Off Sunburn

Cool the burn with a mild chamomile tea (one tea bag or 1 teaspoon of dried chamomile per cup of freshly boiled water). Let the brew cool, then gently sponge it onto the affected areas.

Fabulous Food Fix

CHAMOMILE ICE

This granita (as our Italian friends call it) makes a delicious and healthful treat at any time, but it's especially useful for relaxing you—or your youngsters—on a hot summer night when you just can't get to sleep.

2½ cups of water
4 chamomile tea bags or ¼ cup of dried chamomile
¼ cup of fresh-squeezed lemon juice (or to taste)
¼ cup of honey (or to taste)

Boil the water in a saucepan, remove it from the heat, and add the tea bags or dried herb. Steep for 5 to 10 minutes. Strain the tea into a bowl, add the lemon juice and honey, and stir to mix thoroughly. Pour the mixture into a 2-inch-deep, freezer-proof dish or roasting pan, and freeze for six to eight hours, stirring occasionally with a fork. Just before serving, put the pan in the refrigerator for five minutes, then mix again with a spoon or fork to make ice crystals. Spoon the ice into cups, and garnish each one with a lemon slice and a crisp, thin cookie.

YIELD: 4 TO 6 SERVINGS

POTENT POTION

FABULOUS FLU BATH

In addition to clearing your stuffed-up nasal passages and soothing your aches and pains, a nice long soak in bathwater spiked with this herbal combo will help you get a good night's sleep. And that's exactly what you need when your body is wracked with the flu!

1 tsp. of dried chamomile
1 tsp. of dried lavender
1 tsp. of dried rosemary
1 tsp. of ground cinnamon
1 tsp. of ground ginger

Put all of the ingredients in a jar with a tight-fitting lid, and shake it until the herbs are thoroughly blended. Add 1 teaspoon of the mixture to a panty hose toe or a coffee filter, and close it tightly with a twist tie. Toss the pouch into a tub of hot water, and let it steep for 10 minutes or so. Then sink into the fragrant brew, and soak your troubles away!

✔ Defeat Athlete's Foot

There are a lot of antifungal remedies for athlete's foot, but many of them sting like the dickens. If you'd prefer a kinder, gentler remedy, rinse your feet in a chamomile infusion in the morning, at night, and after each shower at your health club. Then dry your feet (especially between your toes) thoroughly.

✔ Soften Corns and Calluses

A chamomile footbath is just what the doctor ordered for softening up these annoying—and often painful—tootsie terrors. Just fill a tub or basin with enough chamomile infusion to cover your feet (see Tea Times Two on page 99), then sit back in a comfortable chair and soak your dogs. Repeat as needed until the corns or calluses are gone.

✔ Tame Your Ticker

Almost everyone experiences heart palpitations (a.k.a. *arrhythmia*) at one time or another. That's because, no matter how healthy you are, the electrical impulses that power your heart are not absolutely perfect. If you've received a clean bill of health from your doctor and still your heart starts thumping, or seems to skip a beat or two, try this old-time trick to calm it down: Make 2 cups of strong chamomile tea, and while it's brewing, shred three or four cabbage leaves and steam them. Combine the tea and the leaves in a bowl, and sip the soup. It won't be the tastiest dish you've ever had, but it should tune up your ticker in a hurry. **Note:** If your palpitations persist, or if they're accompanied by chest pain, dizziness, or fainting spells, seek immediate medical help!

✔ Belly-Rub Your Stress Away

Feeling so stressed out you could climb the walls? An abdominal massage can help you release emotional stress and nervous tension, both of which (especially for women) are often held in the belly. Just add 4 to 6 drops of chamomile essential oil (available in health-food stores) to 1 tablespoon of massage oil. Then, using gentle pressure, smooth the oil over your abdomen. Begin at your belly button and, making small circles with your fingertips, massage in a clockwise direction in gradually bigger circles.

✔ Relieve Rosacea Flare-Ups

As you know, if you suffer from rosacea, there is no cure for this chronic acne-like condition. But with regular treatment from a dermatologist and your Johnny-on-the-spot response to facial flushing—the trigger mechanism for a full-fledged attack—it can be controlled. To make a fast-response weapon, toss a handful of dried chamomile into 3 cups of boiling water, remove it from the heat, and steep for 10 minutes. Strain the brew into a container with a tight-fitting lid, and stash it in the fridge. Then whenever the need arises, dip a soft cotton cloth in the cold solution, and apply it to the affected area until you feel relief.

✔ Healing Hemorrhoids: A Teutonic Tip

An old German folk remedy calls on a chamomile bath to reduce the pain and itching of hemorrhoids. To make the potion, toss a handful of dried

Fabulous Food Fix

BACK PAIN PANACEA

Even if it's not the result of a serious condition, back pain can be so crippling that it can ruin your entire day. Relieve the agony with this terrific tea that's tailor-made for those times when your schedule needs to keep running smoothly.

1 part dried chamomile flowers
1 part dried peppermint leaves
1 part grated fresh ginger
1 cup of water

Mix all of the ingredients together, and add 1 teaspoon of the mixture to 1 cup of just-boiled water. Cover, and steep for 10 minutes. Store any remaining herbal blend in a container with a tight-fitting lid. Drink 1 cup of the tea three or four times a day to ease your pain and keep your plans on track.

chamomile in 2 quarts of freshly boiled water, and steep until the brew is comfortably warm to the touch. Pour it into a tub that's big enough for you to sit in, and soak your posterior for 15 minutes. Perform this routine two or three times a day (if your schedule permits) until you're feeling better. If multiple bottom baths aren't feasible on a daily basis, you can ease your discomfort by applying the tea to your hemorrhoids with a cotton ball after each bowel movement.

Chamomile Comeliness

✤ Invite Your Face to Tea

A chamomile infusion (see Tea Times Two on page 99) can work the same wonders for your skin that chamomile tea does for the inside of your body. Use it as either a stand-alone treatment, or as a skin prep before one of the facial masks found throughout this book. In either case, just dab the potion onto your face with a cotton pad, and let it air-dry. It will reduce inflammation as well as soothe and cleanse your skin. **Note:** Anytime you make enough tea or infusion for more than one treatment, store the extra supply in the refrigerator, where it will keep for about five days.

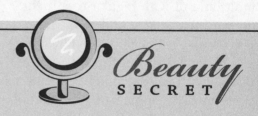

CHAMOMILE SHAMPOO

This delightful DIY shampoo is as gentle on your budget as it is on your hair. To make it, steep four chamomile tea bags in 1½ cups of boiled (not boiling!) water for 10 minutes. Remove the tea bags, add 4 tablespoons of pure soap flakes, and let the mixture stand until the soap softens, stirring occasionally.

Beauty SECRET

Pour in 1½ tablespoons of glycerin, and stir to blend. Pour the liquid into a plastic bottle with a pop-up spout (a clean shampoo or conditioner bottle is perfect). Keep it in a coolish place, and use as you would any other shampoo.

POTENT POTION

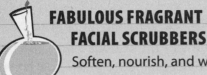

FABULOUS FRAGRANT FACIAL SCRUBBERS

Soften, nourish, and wash your face at the same time with these gentle, aromatic (single-use) cleansing bags.

3 bars of mild, unscented facial soap, grated
1½ cups of dried chamomile flowers
1 cup of dry oats
½ cup of dried sage leaves

Toss all of the ingredients together in a bowl until they're thoroughly blended. Put 1 tablespoon of the mixture in the middle of a 4-inch square of doubled cheesecloth. Bring the corners up to form a pouch, twist them, and tie the "handle" with a string. Wet both the bag and your face, then using a circular motion, gently scrub your skin with the bag. Rinse with lukewarm water, pat dry, and follow up with your normal moisturizer. **Note:** You can either store the remaining mixture in a jar with a tight-fitting lid (away from light and heat), or make up a supply of scrub bags in advance and keep them in a tightly closed container.

YIELD: ENOUGH FOR ABOUT 13 SCRUB BAGS

✤ Fair and Shinier

Here's a simple and gentle way to put glistening highlights in your blonde or light brown tresses: Add 4 tablespoons of dried chamomile to 2 cups of just-boiled water, let it steep for two hours, and strain out the solids. Shampoo and rinse as usual, then massage the herbal potion through your hair. **Note:** If you perform this procedure over a plastic basin, you can save the solution and use it for two or three more shampoos.

✤ Ramp Up the Lights

To intensify the blonde highlights in your hair, combine 3 cups of brewed (and cooled) chamomile tea with 1 cup of lemon juice. Pour the liquid over damp hair, then head outdoors. Sit in the sun for an hour or so, rinse your hair thoroughly, and follow up with a good conditioner. Repeat the process until your hair reaches the desired shade.

✤ A Mayo Mask-arade

Facial masks don't come any easier—or any more skin-friendly—than this one. Just mix 5 drops of chamomile essential oil into ½ cup of full-fat mayonnaise. Smooth the mixture over your face and neck, and leave it on for 15 to 20 minutes. Rinse with warm water, and follow up with your usual toner and moisturizer. **Note:** Don't even think about using low-fat or "light" mayonnaise for this mask. It's the eggs and oil in the full-fat version that soothe, soften, and condition your skin.

✤ Full Steam Ahead!

An herbal steam treatment opens your facial pores, flushes out ingrained dirt, and enriches your blood with skin-renewing oxygen. Many herbs, herb combos—and even fruits and vegetables—can be effective facial sauna partners. But chamomile's calming, antibacterial, and anti-inflammatory properties make it one of the best choices for all types of skin.

No matter what ingredients you use, the steaming routine is a simple five-step process:

STEP 1. Tie your hair back out of the way, then clean and rinse your face thoroughly.

STEP 2. Bring a big potful of water to a boil, and add about ⅓ cup of fresh or dried chamomile, or a few drops of chamomile essential oil. Boil for one to two minutes, then remove the pan from the heat, cover, and let the brew steep for five minutes or so.

STEP 3. Set the pot on a counter or tabletop (using a towel or place mat to protect the surface), and remove the lid. Position your face over the water, and cover your head with a large clean towel, letting the sides drape over the pot like a tent to capture the steam.

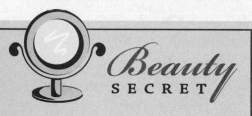

Beauty S E C R E T

CHAMOMILE MILK SOAK

When you're in the mood for an ultra-indulgent—and ultra-skin-softening—bath, steep five chamomile tea bags in a bowl of just-boiled water for 20 to 30 minutes. Remove the tea bags from the solution, and wring them out into the bowl. Dissolve 2 tablespoons of honey in the brew, then add 1 cup of dry milk, and mix well. Add the mixture to a tub of water, then settle in and enjoy!

STEP 4. Keep your eyes closed and hold your face at least 10 to 12 inches away from the water. Relax, and enjoy the fragrant steam for five to seven minutes—no longer! If at any time you feel dizzy or overheated, stop immediately.

STEP 5. When you're finished, splash your face with cool water, pat dry, and apply your regular moisturizer.

A weekly steam treatment is fine for normal, oily, or combination complexions, but limit it to once a month if you have dry or mature skin.

✤ A Variation on the Steam Theme

If leaning over a pot of steaming water is not your cup of tea, soak several clean washcloths in hot chamomile-infused water, and wring them out. Then sit down, lean your head against a chair back or other support, and put the cloths over your face. Relax for five minutes or so, redipping the cloths in the water if necessary to keep them hot. When time's up, rinse your face with cool water, pat dry, and moisturize as usual.

Fabulous Food Fix

SKIN-SOOTHING CHAMOMILE SMOOTHIE

Soften and detox your skin from the inside out with this tasty—and very healthful—drink.

½ cup of milk
1 apple, peeled, cored, and diced
¼ cantaloupe, peeled and cubed
2 tbsp. of plain yogurt
1 tbsp. of fresh or 1 tsp. of dried chamomile flowers

Put all of the ingredients into a blender or food processor, and puree until smooth. Pour the beverage into a tall glass and enjoy!

✤ Tea and Oats Treatment

In this super-simple facial, chamomile teams up with the protein and minerals in oatmeal to leave your skin beautifully soft, supple, and healthy. To make the mask, mix ½ cup of strong chamomile infusion with ¼ cup of uncooked oatmeal, and let the mixture thicken for a few minutes. Apply it to your face and neck, relax for 15 to 20 minutes, then rinse, tone, and moisturize as usual. Just make sure that you set a plastic basin or shallow pan in the sink before you rinse—otherwise, you'll wind up with an oatmeal-clogged drain! **Note:** Both this and the chamomile-mayo mask (see "A Mayo Mask-arade," at left) are gentle enough to use on your delicate eye area, but be careful not to get the stuff *in* your eyes.

✿ Tub-Time Treats

At the end of a long, hard day (or even a short, easy one) there's no better way to relax than settling into a soothing chamomile bath. You can simply pour a cup of chamomile infusion into a tub of hot water, but it's a snap to jazz up your routine with one of these homemade treasures:

BATH OIL. Mix 3 parts castor oil with 1 part chamomile essential oil, and pour 1 teaspoon of the mixture into the tub.

BUBBLE BATH. Mix 1 cup of mild, unscented dishwashing liquid with ¼ cup of glycerin, 1 teaspoon of sugar, and ⅜ teaspoon of chamomile essential oil. Use 2 to 3 tablespoons of the potion per bath.

FIZZING BATH SALTS. Combine ½ cup of baking soda, ¼ cup each of citric acid (available in health-food stores and online) and cornstarch, and ¾ teaspoon of chamomile essential oil. Mix thoroughly to distribute the oil evenly through the dry ingredients. Just before you get into the tub, sprinkle 2 tablespoons of the salts over the water.

Whichever bath treat you choose to use, store the leftover mixture in a container with a tight-fitting lid.

Best of the Rest

★ Angelica Conquers Constipation

When your internal "plumbing" ceases to function, don't reach for an over-the-counter laxative. Instead, hightail it down to your local health-food store or herb shop and pick up a bottle of angelica tincture (or order it for overnight delivery from a reputable herbal website). Drink 20 to 30 drops mixed in 1 cup of water three times a day until things are moving along normally again.

★ An Angelic Headache Remedy

As soon as that familiar devilish throbbing starts, mix ½ teaspoon of angelica tincture in ¾ cup of hot water, and drink it down. Not only will it ease the pain in your head, but it will also lift your spirits—and maybe a case of the blahs that caused your headache in the first place.

★ Kitty Knows Best

Catnip tea is famous for its ability to do everything from reducing fevers to relieving nausea and nasal allergy symptoms—and, of course, to help you relax and get a good night's sleep. But catnip can also provide those same benefits in other forms, and it's delicious to boot. So give yourself a healthful treat by cutting up fresh leaves and tossing them into salads, or adding dried leaves to soups or stews. They're also great simply sprinkled over meats.

Fabulous Food Fix

CARMELITE WATER

Eau de Carmes was first made in Paris in the early 17th century by Carmelite nuns. They used it to treat anxiety and headaches as well as to "comfort the heart and driveth away melancholy and sadness." It works and tastes just as good today as it did in the 1600s.

3 tbsp. of angelica leaves, roots, and/or stalks*
3 tbsp. of lemon balm leaves*
2 cups of unflavored vodka

Put the herbs in a large jar with a lid, pour the vodka over them, fasten the lid tightly, and shake to mix the ingredients thoroughly. Leave the jar in a warm place for three weeks, shaking it once a day. Strain the mixture into a sterilized bottle with a tight-fitting lid, and store it in a cool place, where it will keep indefinitely. Then whenever your head is throbbing—or you simply want to enjoy a relaxing after-dinner beverage—pour a little into a cordial glass, and toast to good health and good times!

* Either fresh or dried.

YIELD: 16 (1-OUNCE) SERVINGS

★ A Gentle Dental Helper

Catnip leaves, straight from the plant, can relieve sore gums or aching teeth fast. Just pop a leaf into your mouth, and hold it against the painful area until the hurt goes away—which should be almost faster than you can say "Here, kitty, kitty!"

★ Comfrey Comforts Sprains

Sprained ligaments are no bed of roses. But a stroll (or hobble) into an herb garden—or the produce section of a health-food store—can speed up

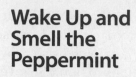

Wake Up and Smell the Peppermint

Why? Because sniffing the mint in any form, whether it's fresh or dried leaves, extract, essential oil—or even candy or chewing gum—can do a couple of things for you:

INCREASE YOUR ENERGY LEVEL. The aroma of peppermint works directly on your sensory nerves to increase alertness and get-up-and-go power.

HELP YOU LOSE WEIGHT. In a study by the Smell & Taste Treatment and Research Foundation, 3,193 volunteers who regularly sniffed the scent of peppermint, green apples, or bananas lost an average of 30 pounds in six months.

the recovery process. Just blanch two to four comfrey leaves, and put them over your sprained body part. Cover the leaves with an elastic bandage, and go about your business. Renew the dressing every day, and you'll be back in the running before you know it.

★ Please Pass the Mint

No matter where you're from, a headache is a major pain in the, um, head. In two far-flung places, old folk remedies use mint as a surefire cure for the throbbing:

■ In Mexico, folks say to paste or (in more modern times) *tape* a fresh mint leaf on the part of your head where the ache is most severe, and leave it there until the pain is gone.

■ Our English friends juice their mint leaves and use the fluid as eardrops (yes, you read that right). To try this trick, liquefy a few mint leaves in a blender or food processor, and mix in enough water so the fluid will flow easily through a medicine (a.k.a. eye) dropper. Put a few drops into each ear, and before you know it, your headache should be history.

★ Drink to Cold Relief

Say good-bye to cold symptoms with this tasty beverage: Mix ¼ teaspoon of peppermint extract and 2 teaspoons of sugar in ½ cup or so of hot water. Drink the potion as needed throughout the day to calm your cough, loosen congestion, and relieve that achy-all-over feeling.

★ Angel Breath

Looking for a way to sweeten your breath without using a commercial mouthwash that's full of alcohol and chemicals? Look no further! Just put

3 tablespoons of angelica seeds in a teapot or other heat-proof container, and pour 2 cups of boiling water on top. Cover, and steep until the brew cools to room temperature. Strain it into a glass bottle with a tight-fitting lid, and use the solution as you would any other mouthwash.

★ Comforting Comfrey Mist

For a soothing, nourishing facial treat, give this triple-play tea a try: Make 1 cup each of comfrey, chamomile, and rose hip infusions, and let each one steep for one hour (see Tea Times Two on page 99). Mix the trio in a spray bottle, and refrigerate the solution for at least 10 minutes. Just before cleansing, lightly mist your face with the potion, and let it air-dry. Store in the fridge between uses, and it'll stay fresh for about five days.

★ Mighty Minty Face Mask

Clay and mint perform a perfect balancing act for oily skin. Just mix 1 tablespoon of finely chopped fresh mint leaves with 2 tablespoons of cosmetic-grade clay (available in health-food stores and online) with enough water to make a smooth, but thick paste. Spread it gently onto your clean face and neck, avoiding the eye area, then lie down and relax for 20 minutes. Wash the mask off with warm water, splash your face with cold water to close your pores, and pat dry. Follow up with moisturizer.

★ Defeat Dandruff

When white flakes are falling on your shoulders so hard that you feel like you're in the final scene of *White Christmas*, boil 1 cup of apple cider vinegar, 1 cup of water, and ¼ cup of fresh mint leaves for three minutes or so. Strain out the solids, and pour the solution into an airtight container. Wait until it cools, then gently massage the potion into your scalp, and let it air-dry. Do not shampoo or rinse your hair for at least 12 hours. Repeat as needed.

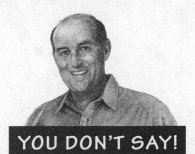

YOU DON'T SAY!

For generations, Americans have been growing and using mint as a flavorful ingredient in things like digestive remedies, toothpaste, and other dental hygiene products, and—of course—in chewing gum, candy, and ice cream. But to the ancient Romans, mint was far more than a healthful and refreshing taste treat. For one thing, they believed that eating mint increased a person's intelligence. Furthermore, the scent of mint was said to keep people from losing their temper. For that reason, whenever the royal Roman ambassadors went anywhere on official business, they always carried mint sprigs in their pockets ...just in case!

9

Cinnamon

You'd be hard-pressed to find a healer—homemade or otherwise—with a more impressive past than cinnamon. In the book of Exodus, God instructs Moses to include it in his holy anointing oil. The Chinese wrote about its medicinal prowess as early as 2800 BC, and the ancient Egyptians considered it more precious than gold. Fast forward to the 21st century, and more than ever, you'll find health and beauty gurus singing the praises of cinnamon for its ability to prevent and cure diseases, boost your brainpower, soften your skin—and a whole lot more!

Dr. Cinnamon Is In

✔ Alleviate Athlete's Foot

Fight the foul fungus with a cinnamon footbath. Bring 4 cups of water to a boil in a medium saucepan, and add 10 broken cinnamon sticks. Reduce the heat to low, and simmer for five minutes. Remove the pan from the stove, cover, and steep for another 45 minutes. Pour the brew into a basin, and soak your feet for 30 minutes. Repeat daily until the fungus has fled.

✔ Clear Up Yeast Infections

The same cinnamon brew that cures athlete's foot can also get rid of the notorious vaginal infection *Candida albicans*. Make the potion as described above, and when it's cooled to lukewarm, use it as a vaginal douche.

✔ Dodge Diabetes

It's no secret that type 2 diabetes is rapidly reaching epidemic proportions across our country. But here's good news: Numerous studies show that adding ½ to 1 teaspoon of ground cinnamon to your diet every day could be enough to help control your blood sugar levels and avoid this dreaded disease. That's because it can improve the ability of your body's cells to recognize and respond to insulin—a process that goes haywire in diabetics. **Note:** If you already have either type 1 or type 2 diabetes, consult your doctor before you start dosing yourself with cinnamon—or anything else!

✔ A Spicy Sprinkle

Protecting you against diabetes isn't cinnamon's only health-care service. Research shows that consuming just ½ to 1 teaspoon of the tasty ground spice each day can lower your LDL (bad) cholesterol, lessen your risk for chronic diseases, and may reduce the growth of leukemia and lymphoma cancer cells.

It's a snap to get your daily dose of cinnamon. Just sprinkle it on cereal, toast, or English muffins; add it to coffee or tea; stir it into yogurt or applesauce; or blend it into a healthful drink like the Banana-Walnut Smoothie (at right).

✔ Cure Your Cold

Sore throats, coughs, and stuffy noses are no match for cinnamon! To put its power to work, pour 1 cup of water into a saucepan, add a cinnamon stick, bring the mixture to a boil, and continue to boil for two minutes. Remove the cinnamon stick, and use the freshly boiled water to brew a cup of your favorite tea. **Note:** If your cold symptoms last longer than a week, consult your doctor.

Fabulous Food Fix

BANANA-WALNUT SMOOTHIE

In addition to providing you with a healthy helping of disease-fighting cinnamon, this delicious drink serves up a major load of vitamins, minerals, and protein. Whip it up and take it along as an on-the-go breakfast, or multiply the recipe and serve it to your youngsters as a nutritious after-school snack.

**1½ cups of milk
1 banana, peeled and sliced
¼ cup of chopped walnuts
2 tbsp. of honey
½ tsp. of ground cinnamon**

Put all of the ingredients in a blender, puree until smooth, and drink up.

YIELD: 1 SERVING

✔ Fend Off the Flu

If there's anything better than a remedy for the flu, it's a magic bullet for preventing it. This is one of the best: As soon as possible after you've been exposed to someone with the flu, start taking 5 drops of cinnamon oil in 1 tablespoon of water three times a day. Just to play it safe, continue this routine for the duration of flu season.

POTENT POTION

SPICY FLU FIGHTER

The next time you start coming down with a cold or flu, show those germs the door with this powerful (and quite pleasant) potion.

3–4 whole cloves

1 cinnamon stick

2 cups of water

2 shots of whiskey

1½ tbsp. of blackstrap molasses

2 tsp. of lemon juice

Put the cloves, cinnamon stick, and water in a saucepan, and bring the mixture to a boil over medium heat. Let it boil for three minutes or so. Remove the pan from the stove, and mix in the whiskey, molasses, and lemon juice. Cover the pan, and let it sit for about 20 minutes. Drink ½ cup of the toddy every three to four hours (warm it up each time). Before you know it, you'll be back in full swing again!

YIELD: ABOUT 5 DOSES

✔ Suck Your Cravings Away

Whether the objects of your desire are cigarettes or sweet treats, cinnamon can help conquer your cravings. Whenever you feel an overwhelming need to light up or pig out, reach for a cinnamon stick, and suck on it (or brew a cup of cinnamon tea and sip it slowly) until the feeling passes. Eventually, you should be able to kick your habit.

✔ Mitigate Menstrual Problems

Some women routinely suffer from menstrual cramps and/or heavy bleeding. But even those who generally breeze through their monthly periods can have these woes every now and then. Cinnamon can help on both counts—here's how:

CRAMPS. Cinnamon's potent anti-inflammatory and anti-spasmodic compounds are highly effective at relieving menstrual pain. As soon as the cramps strike, drink cinnamon tea as needed several times a day, or sprinkle ground cinnamon on your morning toast or cereal.

HEAVY BLEEDING. If you usually experience heavy flows, drink a cup or two of cinnamon tea the day before you expect your period to start and continue as needed for the duration.

✔ Conquer Cold-Weather Woes

The natural warming power of cinnamon can help relieve a couple of problems caused by low-digit temperatures:

HEADACHES. When a heavy dose of frigid air makes your head hurt like there's no tomorrow, mix 2 to 3 teaspoons of ground cinnamon with just enough water to make a fine paste. Smooth it onto your temples and forehead, and you should feel almost-instant relief.

COLD FEET. Warm up your chilly toes with this spicy brew: Mix ½ teaspoon of ground cinnamon into 8 ounces of hot water, and let it steep for 15 minutes. Drink this beverage three times a day, and it's all but guaranteed that your "hind paws" will be better able to tolerate the chilly temperatures.

✔ Ease Indigestion

If you suffer from heartburn or indigestion after meals, cinnamon can help ease the discomfort. Simply drink a freshly brewed cup of cinnamon tea after every meal. If you don't get relief after a few days and your indigestion persists, make an appointment to see your doctor.

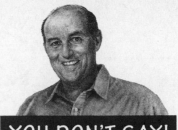

YOU DON'T SAY!

If you think clever marketing campaigns are modern concepts, think again. Back in the fifth century BC, Greek merchants bought cinnamon from Arab traders and sold it in Europe. To drive up the price of their product, the traders devised a tall tale about how hard the stuff was to get. They claimed that cinnamon birds flew to an unknown land, collected cinnamon bark, and carried it back to build their nests. The traders said they used large chunks of meat to lure the birds away from their homes. The story goes that when the birds took the heavy load back to their nests, they fell to the ground, where workers scrambled to pick up the pricey cinnamon pieces.

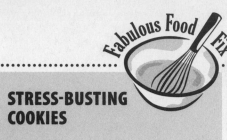

STRESS-BUSTING COOKIES

The intense cinnamon scent of these taste-tempting treats delivers major aromatherapy that will lower your anxiety and ramp up your brainpower. That's in addition to providing ample supplies of cinnamon's other health-giving benefits.

2 sticks of butter, softened
2¼ tsp. of ground cinnamon
½ tsp. of baking soda
½ tsp. of sea salt
1 cup of blackstrap molasses
¼ cup of dark honey
¼ cup of brown sugar
2 large eggs
½ cup of plain yogurt
4 cups of all-purpose flour

In a large mixing bowl, combine the first four ingredients. Gradually add the molasses, honey, and sugar. Then beat in the eggs, and stir in the yogurt and flour. Drop rounded teaspoonfuls of dough 2 inches apart onto cookie sheets, and bake at 400°F for 12 minutes, or until the cookies are lightly browned at the edges.

YIELD: ABOUT 4 DOZEN COOKIES

✔ Stop the Runs

When it comes to curing diarrhea, cinnamon is a world-class champ. How you put it to work is your call. Here's a trio of tried-and-true prescriptions:

■ Mix 2 pinches of ground cinnamon per cup of warm milk, and sip it slowly. Drink as much of the beverage as possible throughout the day. This is an old—and delicious—Pennsylvania Dutch folk remedy that's especially helpful to children.

■ Add 1 teaspoon of ground cinnamon and 1 teaspoon of sugar to 1 cup of hot water. Stir, let it cool to room temperature, and gulp it down as quickly as you can. One or two doses should get your inner workings back to normal.

■ In a saucepan, bring 2 cups of water to a boil, and add ¼ teaspoon of ground cinnamon and ⅛ teaspoon of cayenne pepper. Reduce the heat, simmer for 20 minutes, then remove the pan from the burner. When the liquid is cool enough to drink, start sipping ¼ cup of the brew every 30 minutes or so until the runs have run their course.

✔ Drive More Safely

If you're like most folks I know, a traffic-clogged, rush-hour commute can send your stress level soaring off the charts. Besides being unhealthy, it puts you at high risk for causing an accident. But, believe it or not, cinnamon can make you feel more at ease—and therefore safer—behind the wheel. In a recent study, participants reported that chewing cinnamon-flavored gum during simulated rush-hour scenarios significantly decreased their frustration, increased their alertness, and made the ride seem shorter. Not a gum chewer? Not to worry: You can achieve the same safety improvement by hanging a cinnamon-scented air freshener in your car. Now that's what I call a no-brainer!

✔ Maximize Your Memory

Numerous studies indicate that in addition to making you feel calmer and more relaxed, inhaling the aroma of cinnamon in any form can enhance your overall brain function and improve both your long- and short-term memory. So what are you waiting for? Cook up a cinnamon-rich recipe (see Stress-Busting Cookies, at left), toss broken cinnamon sticks into your favorite potpourri, or simply dab a spot of cinnamon extract onto a few lightbulbs around your house. (Just make sure the bulbs are turned off and completely cool to the touch before you anoint them!)

Ease Arthritis Pain

HEALTHFUL HINT

Thanks to its potent anti-inflammatory power, cinnamon has been shown to be remarkably effective at relieving joint pain and stiffness. The recommended dose (according to a study at the University of Copenhagen in Denmark) is ½ teaspoon of ground cinnamon mixed with 1 tablespoon of honey every morning before breakfast. Arthritis sufferers who swallowed this tasty medicine faithfully reported noticeable relief within the first week. And by the end of the first month, they were walking with no pain whatsoever.

Spice Up Your Looks

♣ Sweeten Your Breath

Eliminating halitosis isn't exactly a matter of life and death, but stinky breath sure has killed many a relationship—both social and professional. To maintain your standing among your friends, romantic partners, and colleagues, suck on a cinnamon stick every once in a while to keep your breath naturally clean and fresh.

✤ Sweeten Your Breath, Take 2

If you prefer your breath fresheners in liquid form, mix ½ teaspoon of tincture of cinnamon (available in health-food stores and online) in a glass of warm water, and use it as you would any other mouthwash. Besides eliminating odors caused by recently eaten food, the cinnamon will kill any germs that could lead to gum disease or tooth decay.

> **CAUTION** ⚠
>
> Cinnamon can irritate sensitive skin, so before you use any topical remedy—for either health or beauty purposes—always apply a dab of the mixture to a small patch of your skin. Wait for 10 minutes before proceeding, just to make sure you have no adverse reaction.

✤ Banish Blemishes

There are scads of ways to clear up pimples, but cinnamon's antibacterial and antifungal properties make it one of the most effective remedies of all. The process is simple: Mix 1½ teaspoons of ground cinnamon with 1 tablespoon of honey to make a paste. Smooth a thin layer over your face, and leave it on for 15 minutes. Then rinse it off with lukewarm water, and follow up with your usual toner and moisturizer. Repeat the procedure three times a week until your face is blemish-free. Depending on the severity of the problem, it could take up to several months.

✤ A Triple Play for Oily Skin

Balance, moisturize, and stimulate your complexion with this fabulous facial mask: Warm 2 tablespoons of organic honey in a small, heat-proof bowl, and set it in hot water just until the honey liquefies. Then add 1 teaspoon of fresh lemon juice, ¼ teaspoon of cinnamon, and ¼ teaspoon of nutmeg, and mix to form a smooth paste. Gently apply it to your clean face and neck, avoiding the eye area. Wait 15 minutes, then rinse it off with alternate splashes of cold and warm water, ending with cold. Pat your face dry, and follow up with your usual moisturizer.

✤ Soothe Stressed-Out Skin

As we all know, emotional stress can take a toll on your body—and, as your body's biggest organ, your skin is no exception. This DIY facial not only calms your complexion, but also reduces swelling and redness and sloughs off dead skin cells. To make the mask, mix 1 teaspoon of cinnamon and 1 teaspoon of nutmeg in 2 tablespoons of warm honey to form a thick paste. Apply it to your face and wait 30 minutes or so. Then wash it off with warm water, scrubbing gently in circular motions to exfoliate your skin.

✤ Make a Better Bronzer

Commercial cheekbone bronzers (a.k.a. blushers) can cost a pretty penny. Plus, you never know what chemicals you might be putting on your face. So here's a better idea: Put a few teaspoons of cornstarch into a bowl, and mix in pinches of ground cinnamon, cocoa, and nutmeg until you get the shade you like. Pour the final product into a small tin or empty makeup case (available in some drugstores and on many DIY cosmetic websites), and apply it with a makeup brush.

Prefer a firmer bronzer? Then just substitute cinnamon essential oil for the ground cinnamon. Stir to make a thick paste, scrape it into a container, and refrigerate until it hardens.

✤ Get a Safer Tan

When you want a sporty, bronzed-all-over look for a special event, don't rush off to a tanning salon. Instead, just add ground cinnamon to enough of your favorite skin lotion to cover whatever parts of your body you want to tan. Besides being safer than lying in a tanning booth—or baking in the

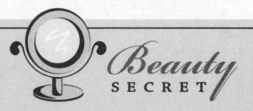

GET A GLOW ON

Cinnamon revs up your blood circulation, thereby giving your skin a healthy radiance—and energizing your whole body to boot. Plus, the spice's antibacterial and antifungal compounds help keep acne at bay. This body scrub can deliver those benefits every day. To make it, mix 1 cup of raw sugar (available in health-food stores) with ¼ cup of walnut oil and ½ teaspoon of ground cinnamon. Spoon the mixture into a clean, plastic container with a tight-fitting lid, and keep it in the shower. Every time you bathe, massage a few tablespoons of the scrub all over your wet body (using circular motions), then rinse thoroughly.

Beauty SECRET

POTENT POTION

WARMING WINTER BATH SOAK

Cold winter days call for indoor pampering to keep yourself warm and your skin smooth. This relaxing bath blend does the trick nicely. (It also makes a great Christmas present for all the ladies on your gift list!)

1 cup of baking soda
1 cup of dry milk
3 tbsp. of cornstarch
2 tbsp. of cream of tartar
1½ tbsp. of ground cinnamon

Mix all of the ingredients in a plastic container with a tight-fitting lid. At bath time, shake the container to make sure the contents are thoroughly blended, and pour about ½ cup of the mixture into a tub of water. Then settle in for a good soak, and think nothing but warm thoughts!

YIELD: ABOUT 4 USES

sun for hours on end—this tan won't turn into dry, flaky skin. Simply rinse it off in the shower when you get home. Just make sure you let the lotion dry thoroughly before you put your clothes on, and don't get your skin wet until you're ready to de-tan yourself! (It's best to skip this "tanning" technique if you're going to have even a remote chance of breaking a sweat; if you do, your tan will unfortunately slide off.)

✤ Extra-Luscious Lip Balm

To moisten and protect dry, chapped lips, and enjoy the delicious taste of cinnamon at the same time, mix 2 teaspoons of coconut oil, 2 teaspoons of honey, and ¼ teaspoon of cinnamon oil or extract in a small bowl. Scrape the mixture into a small container with a tight-fitting lid, and use it as you would any other lip balm.

✤ Calling All Guys . . .

Or gals who'd like to whip up this spicy aftershave for the men in their lives. In addition to smelling delectable, the potion helps stop bleeding from razor nicks. Plus, it couldn't be easier to make. Just fill a jar with dried bay leaves (a 1-quart canning jar is perfect). Add two cinnamon sticks, broken into pieces, and 1 tablespoon of cloves. Pour in enough dark rum to cover the herbs, and let the mixture steep for two to three weeks. Be sure to shake the jar daily. Strain out the solids, pour the liquid into a glass bottle with a tight-fitting cap, and then use it as you would any aftershave.

Best of the Rest

★ Aniseed: A New Mother's Ally

If you're a nursing mother, or know someone who is, here's something to remember: Tea made from aniseed increases the flow of breast milk. To make this helpful brew, just put about 7 teaspoons of aniseed in a pan with 1 quart of water, and bring it to a boil. Reduce the heat to low, simmer until the water has reduced to about 3 cups, and strain out the seeds. Then once or twice a day, drink two cups of the potion, sweetened to taste with honey if you like. **Note:** This tea also relieves indigestion.

★ Cloves Nix Nicotine

If you think you've tried every stop-smoking ploy under the sun, and you're still reaching for the cancer sticks, give this old-time trick a try: Always keep a whole clove in your mouth. Suck on one for a couple of hours, then toss it out and put in a fresh one. The cloves neutralize the taste of nicotine in your mouth, which (according to the experts) is a major reason a smoker always feels the need for another cigarette.

★ Fast Help for Kitchen Cuts

Yikes! You were slicing a tomato for sandwiches, got distracted for a second, and sliced into your finger instead. Well, at least it happened in the right place at the right time! Reach for the ground cloves, and pour a thin layer over your cut. It'll stop the pain and help prevent infection.

Multipurpose Ginger Rub

HEALTHFUL HINT

This versatile formula clears up coughs and chest congestion *and* delivers fast relief to sore muscles and stiff, achy joints. Just before bedtime, mix 1 teaspoon each of ground ginger and dry mustard with 2 tablespoons of olive oil. Rub a dab on your inner arm, and wait 10 minutes. If your skin shows no sign of irritation, smooth the rest of the mixture onto the troubled area until you feel a warm, tingling sensation. Put on an old T-shirt, or cover your bed with a soft cotton cloth to protect your sheets from the oil. Then hop into bed and get a good night's rest. In the morning, wash off the residue with soap and water. Repeat as often as necessary.

POTENT POTION

ANISEED SYRUP

As unlikely as it may seem, this simple concoction can solve two of life's more annoying problems: It can silence a hacking cough and (are you ready for this?) improve your memory.

1 qt. of water
7 tsp. of aniseed
4 tsp. of glycerin
4 tsp. of honey

Bring the water to a boil, and add the aniseed. Reduce the heat to low, and simmer until the water is reduced to about 3 cups. Strain out the seeds, and while the brew is still warm, stir in the glycerin and honey. Pour the syrup into a jar with a tight-fitting lid. For cough relief, take 2 teaspoons every few hours until your hacking stops. To give the old gray cells a boost, take 2 tablespoons three times a day as long as you feel the need.

YIELD: ABOUT 24 DOSES

★ Ginger Mitigates Migraines

If you're a migraine sufferer, chances are you're always looking for new ways to conquer the pain and nausea those dreadful headaches bring on. Well, here's a cure that a lot of folks swear by: As soon as you feel the first hint of a coming attack, mix about ¼ teaspoon of ground ginger in a glass of water, and drink up.

★ Make Medical Tests Easier

The worst part about having colonoscopies, stomach X-rays, and many other medical tests isn't the procedures themselves—it's the foul-tasting liquid they make you drink beforehand. Fortunately, there's a simple way to improve the flavor: Just add a teaspoon of vanilla extract to the stuff. It'll go down a whole lot easier!

★ Scrub Your Skin with Ginger

For a body scrub that will exfoliate your skin and make you feel energized all over, start by smashing 4 tablespoons of warm, cooked rice with the back of a spoon. Then stir in 4 tablespoons of ground ginger and enough water to make a paste. Using a circular motion, rub the mixture into your damp skin, and rinse it off with warm water. That's all there is to it!

★ Quick Breath Freshener

It never fails: You're rushing out the door to work or a meeting, and you realize that your breath smells, shall we say, less than soda-pop sweet. Quick—reach into your spice cupboard, and grab a jar of either aniseed or whole cloves. Pop a pinch of aniseed or a few cloves into your mouth, and chew them on your way out. You *and* your colleagues will be glad you did!

★ All's Well with Allspice

When you have a little more time to spare, here's an easy and tasty way to sweeten your breath: Just dissolve 1 tablespoon of ground allspice in 1 cup of hot water, let it cool to a comfortable temperature, and use it as you would any other mouthwash.

★ Nutmeg Negates Acne Scars

The real agony of acne is not the annoying red zits, but the scarring and skin discoloration that they often leave behind. One removal remedy that has proven effective for lots of folks is ½ teaspoon or so of ground nutmeg mixed with just enough honey to make a paste (about ¼ teaspoon should do the trick). After washing your face, apply the mixture to the marks, leave it on for 30 to 45 minutes, and rinse it off with warm water. Repeat the procedure up to three times a day. Unfortunately (full disclosure), your scars may never

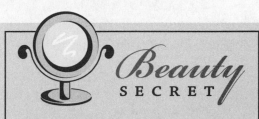

Beauty SECRET

VERY VANILLA FOAMING BATH BLEND

If you're a fan of vanilla ice cream and vanilla milk shakes, then you'll love this softening, relaxing tub-time treat: Mix 1 tablespoon of pure vanilla extract (not artificial!) with 1 cup of almond oil and ½ cup each of honey and mild liquid soap in a glass jar with a tight-fitting lid. To use the formula, shake the jar gently to remix the contents, and pour ¼ cup under running bathwater. Settle back, and dream of an old-time soda fountain.

POTENT POTION

SUGAR AND SPICE SCRUB

When you buy a commercial body scrub, there's no telling what chemicals might be in it. But this one's so safe, you could eat it!

1 cup of brown sugar
1 cup of white sugar
¾ cup of almond or coconut oil
2 tsp. of cinnamon
2 tsp. of ground ginger
2 tsp. of nutmeg

Mix all of the ingredients together in a bowl, and transfer the mixture to a plastic container with a tight-fitting lid. At bath or shower time, scoop out a small handful of the blend, and massage it all over your damp body. Then rinse with warm water.

YIELD: ABOUT 1¾ CUPS

disappear entirely, but over time, they will become less distinct, and your skin tone will even out.

★ Serve Yourself a Spicy Steam Facial

To get your skin deep-down clean and free of airborne toxins, cleanse your face thoroughly, then add ⅓ cup of whole cloves, ⅓ cup of aniseed, and 3 to 5 drops of peppermint essential oil to 4 cups of boiling water. Boil for two minutes, remove the pan from the heat, cover, and steep for five minutes. Then steam your face following the procedure described in "Full Steam Ahead!" on page 106.

★ Summerize Your Feet

Before sandal season comes around, get your feet looking their best with a bedtime foot scrub made from ¼ cup of brown sugar, ⅛ cup of almond oil, and 3 drops of ginger essential oil. Mix the ingredients thoroughly, spread the mixture generously onto your feet, and let it penetrate for three to four minutes. Then massage it into your skin, pull on a pair of old cotton socks, and hit the sack. When you wake up, your tootsies should be the toast of the town!

CHAPTER

10

Epsom Salts

So what makes Epsom salts such a hotshot healer? In a word: magnesium. This element is essential for maintaining crucial bodily functions such as muscle control, electrical impulses, energy production, tissue healing, and the elimination of harmful toxins. But because of modern commercial farming methods and less than ideal eating habits, most of us don't get enough magnesium in our daily diets. Enter Epsom salts, which delivers a potent dose of magnesium that can be absorbed through your skin—thereby giving you a super-simple solution for staying in—or getting back into—your peak of good health and good looks.

The Magic of Magnesium

✔ Remove a Stubborn Splinter

Having trouble getting a splinter out of your finger? Pour 2 tablespoons of Epsom salts into 1 cup of warm water, and soak your sore digit in the solution. It'll draw the invading fragment right out. **Note:** This trick is especially effective for removing tiny slivers that are stuck under your fingernails.

✔ Blast Blisters

Sweaty feet and blisters tend to go hand in hand (or should I say, foot in foot?). To get rid of both of those annoyances, try this old-time trick: Dissolve about 1 cup of Epsom salts in a basin of warm water, and give your tootsies a five-minute soak. Then dry 'em thoroughly. Repeat the procedure every week or so as needed for the freshest feet in town!

✔ Soothe Summertime Ailments

When you're living it up outdoors in the good old summertime, trouble can strike like lightning in the form of insect bites and stings, poison-plant rashes, and sunburn. Fortunately, Epsom salts can make the livin' easy again—fast. You have a trio of treatment choices, depending on what part of your body is under attack.

APPLY A LOTION. Dissolve 1 teaspoon of Epsom salts in 1 cup of hot water, and chill it in the refrigerator for 20 minutes or so. Clean the affected area and pat dry, then gently dab the solution onto your irritated skin.

MAKE A COMPRESS. Mix 2 tablespoons of Epsom salts per cup of cold water in a bowl. Soak a clean cotton washcloth in the mixture, and hold it against your skin until you feel relief.

TAKE A BATH. Pour 2 cups of Epsom salts under the spigot as you fill the tub, then settle in and soak for 20 minutes. **Note:** If you have an oversized tub, use 4 cups of salts.

> ### HEALTHFUL HINT
>
> ### Provide Dental First Aid
>
> Epsom salts is just what the dentist ordered for relieving a toothache or pain and swelling at the site of a tooth extraction. In either case, your treatment plan is the same: Mix 1 teaspoon of Epsom salts in 8 ounces of warm water, swish a mouthful of the solution for about 30 seconds, then spit it out. Repeat the procedure until you've emptied the whole glass. Just make sure you don't swallow any of the potion, or you could be in for a very unpleasant surprise (see "Move Things Along," at right)!

✔ Move Things Along

Epsom salts is one of Mother Nature's most effective laxatives. All you need to do is mix 1 to 2 teaspoons of salts in an 8-ounce glass of water to get relief. Stir in enough lemon juice to make the potion drinkable, then toss it back. (It's best to drink this on an empty stomach.) And don't stray too far from a bathroom because in anywhere from 30 minutes to six hours, your inner plumbing should spring into action. If it hasn't responded by then or shortly thereafter, it's time to give your doctor a call.

✔ Treat Cuts and Scratches

The magnesium in Epsom salts quickly reduces inflammation, which makes it especially useful for treating minor scratches, scrapes, and cuts. The simple process: Dissolve ½ cup of Epsom salts in 1 quart of water that's as warm as your comfort range allows. Wash your cut with soap and warm water, then soak the affected body part in the solution for 6 to 10 minutes. Dry the cut with a clean towel, and cover the site with a bandage. Repeat several times a day until your "owie" has healed.

✔ Heal Deeper Wounds

Clear up deep cuts and puncture wounds with this surefire routine: Dissolve 1 part Epsom salts in 8 parts hot water (it should take no more than 10 to 15 seconds). Then either submerge the wound in the solution or, if that's not possible, soak a clean washcloth in the liquid and press it against the site. Soak your injury, or keep the compress in place for 10 minutes—no longer, or you'll risk drying out the wound. Repeat the process three times a day until you're all better. **Note:** If you don't see continuous improvement, or if there is any sign of infection, see a doctor ASAP.

✔ Ease Trigeminal Neuralgia Pain

This agonizing condition occurs when a vein or artery compresses the trigeminal nerve on the side of the face. Unfortunately, there is no cure—at least none that's been discovered so far. But Epsom salts can help reduce the excruciating pain that strikes from out of nowhere. Just mix equal parts of Epsom salts and water that's as hot as you can stand. Dip a clean towel in the solution, wring out the water, and lay the towel at the base of your neck, which is where the trigeminal nerve originates. Keep the compress in place until it cools down, then repeat as needed until you feel relief.

✔ Good Health Over Easy

When it comes to overall good health, an Epsom salts bath is the closest thing you'll ever find to an all-purpose magic bullet. That's because the

> **CAUTION** ⚠
>
> While magnesium is essential for good health, it is possible to give yourself an accidental overdose, especially if you are taking any medications that contain the chemical. If you're pregnant (or think you might be) or nursing, or if you're under medical care for any chronic health condition—especially high blood pressure, heart disease, or diabetes—consult with your doctor before you use Epsom salts in any form.

POTENT POTION

BACK-IN-BALANCE BATH

Muscle aches, fatigue, spasms, and cramps—as well as mental and emotional burnout—can all be signals that your internal electrolytes are out of balance. To get back to normal, reach for this recipe.

2 cups of Epsom salts
2 cups of kosher or sea salt
2 tbsp. of potassium crystals*

Pour the salts and crystals into a tub of hot water, and soak your troubles away.

* Available in health-food stores and the health-food sections of many supermarkets.

magnesium in the salts is absorbed through your skin to benefit every part of your body. The pleasant R_x for maximum benefit: Three times a week, pour 2 cups of Epsom salts into a tub of warm water, and soak for 20 minutes. If you like, add ½ cup of your favorite bath oil. But don't use soap of any kind—it will interfere with the action of the salts. Besides improving your blood circulation, lowering your stress level, and relieving general aches and pains, this powerful soak can help alleviate a boatload of other health conditions, including these:

- Arthritis
- Bruises
- Gout
- Hives
- Kidney stones
- Sciatica

✔ Fight Fibromyalgia

The cruel irony of fibromyalgia is that it makes you so tired and achy that you can barely move. Unfortunately, inactivity leads to poor sleep, which in turn makes your muscles ache even more. You become so trapped in a pain-fatigue-pain loop that you may stop moving altogether. Well, here's one way to break free: Before bedtime, prime your body for a deep, restful sleep by soaking for 15 minutes or so in a tub laced with ½ cup of Epsom salts. Stick with this routine as long as necessary until you're regularly sleeping through the night.

✔ Relieve Ingrown Toenails

A warm Epsom salts footbath is a classic remedy for ingrown toenails, but recent studies show that alternating hot and cold soaks may provide faster relief. Your action plan: Soak your foot for three minutes in a solution of Epsom salts and hot water (100°F to 110°F) and then for 30 seconds in cold water with no Epsom salts added to it. Perform this routine at least three times a day, and your ingrown nail should soon grow out.

✔ Soften Psoriasis Scales

With the help of Epsom salts, saying good-bye to psoriasis lesions on your hands or feet is a simple three-step process:

STEP 1. Just before bedtime, soak for 15 to 20 minutes in a bath laced with about 2 cups of Epsom salts.

STEP 2. Pat your itchy skin areas dry, and massage them with warm peanut oil (do not substitute any other kind).

STEP 3. Cover the oil with a paste made from baking soda and castor oil, then pull on clean white cotton gloves and/ or socks, and hop into bed.

Repeat every few days as needed, and your scales should soon sail away. **Note:** Do not use this remedy if you are allergic to peanuts.

✔ Boomeritis: First Response

So many baby boomers are injuring themselves trying to get back into shape at the gym, overdoing it on the tennis court, or launching an impromptu game of hoops with their grandkids, that *boomeritis* has become an emergency room byword. Fortunately, a concentrated Epsom salts bath

HEALTHFUL HINT

Bathe and Breathe Acute Bronchitis Away

There's no mistaking a case of acute bronchitis: You have a deep, window-rattling cough that sounds like a barking seal and brings up gobs of mucus; your muscles ache head to toe from nonstop hacking; you have a slight fever—and your voice sounds as hoarse as Marlon Brando's. What to do about it? Climb into a steaming tub laced with 1 cup or so of Epsom salts, plus 2 drops each of eucalyptus, thyme, and rosemary oils. The steam will increase the flow of nasal mucus; the molecules from the oils will dilate your internal airways, thereby easing your breathing; and the mega-dose of magnesium in the Epsom salts (absorbed through your skin) will relax your stressed-out bronchi. Of course, if your bronchitis lasts more than a week with no letup, see your doctor right away to rule out (or head off) pneumonia.

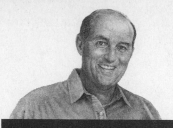

Epsom salts has been around since before the dawn of recorded history (it's a naturally occurring element with the scientific moniker of magnesium sulfate heptahydrate). But it didn't burst onto the health-care stage until the very dry summer of 1618, when a farmer named Henry Wicker was tending his cattle on Epsom Common in Surrey, England. One day, just before heading home with his herd, he noticed a trickle of water in a hollow hoofprint, and he dug a square hole around it. The next morning, the hole was running over with cool, clear water. The cows—as thirsty as they were—refused to drink it, but Henry tried it himself and quickly discovered its laxative effects. He set about promoting the water as medicine, and before long, folks were flocking to Epsom to partake of the foul-tasting, but health-giving fluid.

can relieve the pain of almost any sports injury. Add 1 to 2 pounds of salts to a tub of warm water, and soak those aches and pains away.

✔ Stop Back Spasms

If there's anything worse than a plain old backache, it's muscle spasms that make you feel as though you're being stabbed in the back—over and over again. Give that "knife" the heave-ho with this simple routine: Pour 2 cups of Epsom salts in a tub full of hot water, ease yourself in, and have a good soak. You'll start to feel relief almost instantly. Afterward, lie down for 30 minutes or so with an ice pack on your back.

✔ Treat Sprains

Whether your ligament injury is mild, moderate, or severe, Epsom salts can play an important role in your treatment plan by reducing inflammation and promoting the formation of joint proteins. For optimum results, soak your affected body part in a solution made from 2 cups of Epsom salts per gallon of water.

✔ Banish Bunion Pain

Unfortunately, you can't rub bunions away, but you can make the pain go away—fast. Just stir 1 to 2 cups of Epsom salts into about 3 cups of simmering water, then add just enough cool water to make the temperature comfortable. Pour the solution into a basin, and soak your feet for 20 minutes or so. You'll be ready to go out and dance the night away, or take Rover for a stroll around the block.

✔ Rub Away Corns and Calluses

These painful and annoying bumps are no match for this simple—but highly effective—routine: Pour ½ cup of Epsom salts into a basin of warm water, and soak your feet for 20 minutes or so. Then use a pumice stone to gently rub away the softened layers of skin. Dry your feet, then add 2 drops of peppermint essential oil to a handful of shea butter or cocoa butter, and rub it into your feet thoroughly to lock in the moisture. **Note:** Whatever you do, don't ever try to shave or cut corns or calluses; you could easily cause an infection.

✔ Give Shingles a Shove

If you had chicken pox as a kid, your body is still harboring the herpes zoster virus that caused it—and it could come back to haunt you in the form of painful, blistery shingles. For those of you who get a case of the shingles, help lessen the pain by making a paste of Epsom salts and water, and smooth it directly on your affected skin. Repeat the process as often as possible until your flare-up fades away.

✔ Reduce Rheumatism Miseries

There are lots of folks who can tell that a weather change is on the way because their toes, or maybe their knees or elbows, ache. But who wants to be a famous weather prognosticator at the price of painful, swollen joints? One of the most effective ways to relieve the swelling and discomfort of occasional bouts of rheumatism is to relax for 20 minutes or so in a warm bath with 2 cups of Epsom salts, 1 cup of sea salt, and 1 cup of baking soda mixed into the water. To soak your foot or elbow in a basin, or to make enough solution for a compress, use the same dry ingredients in the same proportions, but just use 1 or 2 tablespoons of the mixture per gallon of water. Store any extra in an airtight container.

POTENT POTION

PEPPERMINT FOOT SOAK

After a long day on your feet, there's nothing like a refreshing footbath to put you back in the swing of things.

¼ cup of Epsom salts
¼ cup of sea salt
4 drops of liquid menthol*
4 drops of peppermint essential oil
Water

In a foot-size basin, mix the first four ingredients with just enough very warm water to cover your feet. Then settle back in a comfortable chair and relax. Before you know it, your aches and tiredness will be an unpleasant memory.

* Available in health-food stores and pharmacies.

Epsom Elegance

❖ Wash That Oil Right Out of Your Hair

Mix 1 cup of Epsom salts and 1 cup of lemon juice in 1 gallon of water, and let it sit for 24 hours. Pour the solution onto your dry hair, wait 20 minutes, then shampoo as usual. The excess oil will exit, without leaving your scalp overly dry. **Note:** This same formula works equally well to remove hair spray buildup.

❖ Add Volume to Your Hair

Don't worry—this trick won't make you look like a country music star with a hairdo the size of a hot-air balloon! Rather, it will simply add healthy fullness and bounce to your hair. Here's what you need to do: In a pan, mix equal parts of Epsom salts and a high-quality deep conditioner. Heat the mixture until it's warm, work it through your tresses, and leave it on for 20 minutes or so. Then rinse with warm water.

❖ Easy Epsom Face Scrub

It's always smart to give your face an extra-thorough cleaning at night to remove not only your makeup, but also all of the airborne gunk that your skin absorbs during the day. The good news is that you don't have to run

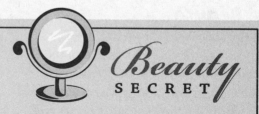

DETOXIFYING FACIAL MASK

Soften your skin and draw out impurities with this quick and easy formula: Mix 1 tablespoon each of Epsom salts, honey, and olive oil. (If you have oily skin, add a few drops of fresh lemon juice.)

Beauty SECRET

Smooth the mixture onto your face and neck, leave it on for 5 to 10 minutes, then rinse it off with warm water. Follow up with your usual moisturizer.

out and buy a special intensive cleaner. Just mix ½ teaspoon of Epsom salts with your regular cleansing cream. Massage it into your skin, and rinse with cold water. Follow up with your usual toner and moisturizer, and hit the road to dreamland.

✤ Banish Blackheads

Why is it that blackheads always seem to appear on your face just when you've got a special event coming up? Well, don't fret. Help is as close as your bathroom medicine chest. Mix 1 teaspoon of Epsom salts and 3 drops of iodine in ½ cup of boiling water. Let the mixture cool just enough so that you can stick your finger in it, then dab it onto each blackhead with a cotton ball, and let the solution dry. Repeat the procedure three or four times, reheating the solution if necessary. Gently remove the blackhead using a clean washcloth, and apply rubbing alcohol to the area.

✤ Exfoliate Your Skin

Long before fancy exfoliators came on the scene, women used plain old Epsom salts to remove dead skin cells and deep-down dirt from head to toe. It works as well now as it did then, and the process couldn't be simpler: Stand in the shower or bathtub, wet your skin, and then massage it with handfuls of the salts, starting with your feet and working up to your neck. When you're finished, rinse the stuff off and pat your skin dry.

POTENT POTION

FLOWERY BATH CRYSTALS

Mix up a batch of this beautiful blend to soak your troubles away. While you're at it, multiply the recipe and make extra "servings" to give as birthday or Christmas presents.

½ cup of Epsom salts
½ cup of sea salt
½ cup of fresh chamomile, lavender, or rosebuds
¼ cup of baking soda
15 drops of fragrance oil (any kind you like to match or complement the flowers' fragrance)
Food coloring (optional)

Blend the salts, flowers, and baking soda in a blender or food processor. Let the mixture sit for half an hour or so to dry a little, then add the oil and food coloring. Pour the blend into lidded glass jars. At bath time, add a heaping ½ cup of the mixture to the water.

YIELD: ABOUT 1½ CUPS

✤ Smooth Your Feet

When summer sandal season is on the way, make sure your feet are ready for action with this simple salt rub: Moisten a handful of Epsom salts with a small amount of olive oil. Then scrub your feet until the salts have dissolved and the oil has softened your skin. Rinse with lukewarm water.

✤ Deodorize Your Feet

No matter what the season, foot odor is no fun for anyone. To send the smell on its way, mix ½ cup of Epsom salts in a foot basin filled with warm water, and soak your dogs for 10 minutes. Repeat daily.

✤ Bath Salts Over Easy

Luxurious bath treats don't come any easier than this formula: Mix 1 cup each of Epsom salts, sea salt, or kosher salt and baking soda, and store the blend in an airtight container. To use it, add about 2 tablespoons of the mixture to your bathwater. For an aromatic bath, add a few drops of your favorite essential oil as the tub fills.

A Bath-Enhancing Menu

There are dozens of oils that can add aromatherapy power to an Epsom salts bath, but here's a baker's half-dozen of excellent—and readily available—choices.

HERBAL OIL	WHAT IT DOES FOR YOU
Chamomile	Soothes and relaxes
Cinnamon	Energizes and stimulates
Eucalyptus	Clears internal airways; great to use during cold and flu season
Geranium	Helps balance mind and body
Grapefruit	Lifts spirits
Lavender	Relaxes and rejuvenates; pairs well with chamomile in a nighttime bath
Peppermint	Cools and refreshes

Best of the Rest

★ Heal Insect Bites and Stings

There are plenty of DIY formulas that stop the pain and itch of bites and stings, but these are two of the simplest and most effective ways to control inflammation and ease the pain:

■ Dissolve two effervescent antacid tablets in a glass of water. Then moisten a soft cloth with the solution, and hold it on the bite for 20 minutes.

■ Wet the site, and rub an un-coated aspirin tablet over it.

Whichever remedy you choose, if the culprit was a bee, remove the stinger before you proceed.

★ A Fizzy Way to Quit Smoking

Trying to break the nasty nicotine habit? Great! As long as you're not on a low-sodium diet and don't have ulcers, drink a glass of water with two effervescent antacid tablets dissolved in it at each meal to help curb your cravings.

A Bedtime Boon for Blood Pressure

HEALTHFUL HINT

In a recent study, participants who took aspirin each night for three months registered a 5.4-point drop in their systolic blood pressure. But those who took the same dosage every morning saw no change at all. Don't start dosing yourself, but if your doctor has already prescribed aspirin to lower your blood pressure, ask whether you would be better served by taking it at night.

★ Milk of Magnesia Moves Mountains

Well, not *mountains* exactly, but it can relieve a trio of highly annoying health problems, namely these:

CANKER SORES. Coat each painful bump with milk of magnesia. Its alkalinity will counteract the acidic conditions in which the canker-producing bacteria thrive.

SKIN RASHES. Use a cotton pad to apply a generous layer of milk of magnesia over the affected skin. It will neutralize the acids that cause rashes and will also act as a natural disinfectant to prevent the problem from spreading. Best of all, milk of magnesia is gentle and safe to use even on infants suffering from heat or diaper rash.

SUNBURN. At bedtime, gently cover the burned area with a light layer of milk of magnesia. Let it dry, then hit the sack. Come morning, wash it off with cool water. Presto—end of pain!

Note: Although milk of magnesia can't cause any long-term harm, it can irritate skin that is allergic to either magnesium or zinc. So play it safe: Do a patch test on an elbow before using it on a larger area.

★ Aspirin Axes Corns and Calluses

This old-time remedy still works like a charm: Mash five uncoated aspirin tablets with equal parts of water and lemon juice (just enough to make a thick paste), and apply it to the annoying C-spot. Wrap the area in a warm towel, put a plastic bag over your foot, and leave it on for 10 minutes or so. Take off the wrappings, and scrub the bump away with a pumice stone.

★ Better Shaving with Aspirin

Ladies, to keep your bikini line free of ingrown hairs and razor bumps, apply shaving gel, leave it on for a few minutes, and shave with a wet razor. Then spritz the area with water in which you've dissolved two aspirin tablets and a drop of glycerin, which will reduce redness and swelling.

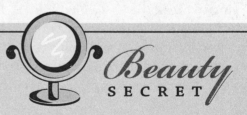

BID ADIEU TO DANDRUFF

You can pay a pretty penny for some of those fancy dandruff shampoos, but for my money, this easy treatment beats 'em all, hands down. Just mash five uncoated aspirin tablets, and put them in a bottle with 1 cup of cider vinegar and ⅓ cup of witch hazel. Cap the bottle and shake it thoroughly to mix the ingredients. Shampoo as usual, then comb the solution through your hair. Wait 10 minutes, rinse with warm water, and wave good-bye to white-flake woes.

POTENT POTION

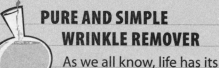

PURE AND SIMPLE WRINKLE REMOVER

As we all know, life has its little ups and downs. After a while, the accompanying smiles and frowns begin to leave their mark. Well, don't run out and pay megabucks for fancy cosmetics or painful Botox® treatments. Instead, erase those lines with this time-tested formula.

Mild soap

Warm water

Milk of magnesia

¼ cup of extra virgin olive oil

Witch hazel, refrigerated for 30 minutes or so

Wash your face with the soap and water, pat dry, and wait 10 minutes. Using a cotton pad, spread a thin layer of milk of magnesia on your face (making sure to keep it away from your eyes!), and let it dry completely. Apply a second layer of milk of magnesia; this will dissolve the first one. Wipe it all off with a warm, damp washcloth. Next, heat the olive oil in a small pan over low heat until it's just lukewarm. Apply it to your face with a cotton pad, leave it on for five minutes, and wipe it off with the witch hazel. Repeat this procedure twice a week. Within a couple of weeks, you'll be looking considerably better and less, um, experienced.

★ Aspirin Gets A+ for Facial Care

The salicylic acid in aspirin increases dead-cell exfoliation, which in turn helps minimize skin discoloration, fine lines, and wrinkles. To put this power to work for you, crush four uncoated aspirin tablets, and mix them with 1 teaspoon of freshly squeezed lemon juice. Stir until the aspirin dissolves and forms a paste. Then smooth it evenly over your face, using cotton pads (and avoiding the eye area!). Leave it on for 10 minutes, then remove it using a cotton pad saturated in a solution of baking soda and water. Follow up with your usual moisturizer. **Note:** You may feel a slight sting when you remove the mask, but don't worry—this is normal.

11

Garlic

It's no coincidence that folks in garlic-loving territory (like the Mediterranean region) tend to live longer and have fewer chronic health problems than those of us who don't partake of the pungent bulb on a regular basis. Study after study has shown that routinely incorporating garlic into your diet can be a magic bullet for health and longevity. In fact, eating as few as one or two cloves a day can help boost your immune system, control blood sugar, and reduce your risk of developing heart disease, cancer, and more—the list goes on and on. Plus, the same properties that make garlic such a powerful health partner also make it a must-have in your beauty-care arsenal.

The Goodness of Garlic

✔ Beat High Blood Pressure

Here's an old folk remedy that can't be beat for reducing your blood pressure: Soak ½ pound of peeled garlic cloves in 1 quart of brandy for two weeks, shaking the mixture a few times a day. Then strain it, pour it into bottles with tight-fitting stoppers, and drink up to 20 drops a day.

✔ Triumph Over Toothaches

This is far from the tastiest way to ease the pain of a toothache, but it is one of the quickest: Peel a garlic clove, crush it, and apply it directly to the gum above or below the affected tooth. Then hold it in place until the ache subsides. The relief should last long enough for you to get to a dentist's office—where, no doubt, the receptionist will promptly hand you a glassful of mouthwash!

✔ Can the Corns

You say painful corns are driving you nuts? No problem! Just slice off a sliver of peeled garlic that's the same size as the corn, put it on top of the blasted bump, and secure it with a bandage. Replace the mini-poultice every day until the corn drops off.

✔ Wave Bye-Bye to Boils

There's no getting around it: Boils hurt like the dickens. But garlic can make the pain vanish. Simply mash a peeled clove, apply it to the boil, and secure it in place with a bandage. The garlic will draw out the infection and send the pain packing pronto!

✔ Oily Pain Relievers

The potent antibiotic properties of garlic make this simple oil a natural choice for curing a couple of common ailments. To make the oil, peel and slice one garlic clove, add it to about 2 tablespoons of extra virgin olive oil, and heat it on the stove for a minute or two. Strain it, let it cool to lukewarm, and then use it to treat either of these annoying afflictions:

SORE THROAT. Rub the oil onto the front and sides of your neck, and breathe deeply. The volatile compounds will be absorbed right through your skin to the source of the pain. (You may need to multiply the quantities of garlic and olive oil, but stick to the same proportions.)

EARACHE. Put a few drops of the oil into your ear, using a medicine (a.k.a. eye) dropper. But if your pain is severe, or if it persists for more than two days, see your doctor. **Note:** Never heat garlic in the microwave because nuking destroys the bulb's health-giving properties.

✔ Fend Off a Cold

If you act fast, garlic can help you keep the nasty germs at bay. The minute you feel any symptoms of a cold coming on, start eating a whole clove every couple of hours. You won't win any popularity contests around the office, but you may avoid a lot of uncomfortable days and nights!

✔ When You Already Have a Head Cold . . .

Reach for one of these time-tested remedies:

■ Several times a day, crush a garlic clove, put your nose up close to it, and inhale deeply. You might not like what you're smelling—but neither will the cold germs!

■ Keep a whole, peeled garlic clove in your mouth, between your teeth and cheek. Don't chew the clove, but gently bite into it every once in a while to release a little garlic juice. Replace the clove with a fresh one every three to four hours.

Fabulous Food Fix

A GEM OF A GERM-BUSTING BREW

Plain old garlic tea can knock your cold or flu bug out of the ballpark, and with just a little tweaking, you can turn that tonic into a truly tasty beverage.

**3 or 4 garlic cloves,
    peeled and grated***
Boiled water
**1 tsp. of concentrated chicken
    or vegetable stock****
1 sprig of fresh rosemary

Let the grated garlic sit for 10 to 15 minutes, so the allicin (the compound that gives garlic its germ-chasing power) can develop its full potency.

Then put the gratings into a warmed mug, and fill it with the boiled water. Stir in the stock, and add the rosemary sprig. When the brew has cooled enough to drink, start sipping. Drink one or two cups a day until you're all better. Depending on the severity of your bug, that could be anywhere from less than 24 hours to several days.

* The more finely you grate or chop garlic, the more beneficial compounds will be released.

** Such as Better Than Bouillon®. You can also substitute a bouillon cube or 1 teaspoon of powdered bouillon.

■ Crush six peeled garlic cloves, and mix them into ½ cup of vegetable shortening. Spread the mixture on the soles of your feet, and cover them with a warm towel or flannel cloth. Then put plastic wrap under your feet to protect your bedding or, if you're sitting up, your carpet or footstool. Repeat the procedure every five hours until your cold is gone. **Note:** Be forewarned that even though you apply the garlic to your feet, the odor will still come out on your breath!

✔ Desperate Measures

When congestion is backing up into your ears, try this potent (some would say "desperate") treatment. Spread ½ teaspoon of prepared horseradish or mustard on three or four slices of garlic, and eat them. Wash the concoction down with a cup of peppermint tea. You should feel relief almost immediately.

✔ Find Your Voice

Lots of things, from a bad cold to too much vocal enthusiasm at the local ballpark, can cause laryngitis. There are plenty of ways to cure it, too, but this Amish remedy is one of the best—provided you have no social engagements on your calendar: Slice a peeled garlic clove down the middle, and tuck a half into each side of your mouth. Then suck on the slices as you would lozenges.

✔ The Milky Way to Cure Sciatica

Sciatica is not only as painful as all get out, but it can also be the very dickens to get rid of. Lots of folks have had remarkable success with garlic milk. To make it, mince two cloves of peeled garlic, put them in about ½ cup of milk, and drink it down without chewing the garlic. Take a dose each morning and evening, and within a week, you should feel much better. In two weeks or so, there's a good chance your pain will be gone entirely. **Note:** By not chewing the garlic, you'll avoid having the odor on your breath.

C A U T I O N ⚠

Even the healthiest substances can be harmful under certain circumstances, and garlic is no exception. Whether you intend to cook with it, eat it fresh, or take supplements in the form of tablets, capsules, or extracts, keep these pointers in mind:

■ If you're taking any kind of medication, in either prescription or over-the-counter form, be sure to consult your doctor before you dose yourself with any garlic remedy.

■ Avoid garlic entirely if you have a bleeding ulcer or any bleeding disorder.

■ Remember: It is possible to get too much of a good thing. So if you start to experience indigestion or stomach irritation, ease off on your intake until you find your comfort level.

POTENT POTION

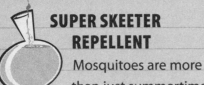

SUPER SKEETER REPELLENT

Mosquitoes are more than just summertime nuisances. They can also transmit deadly diseases like West Nile virus, yellow fever, and encephalitis. Fortunately, the aroma of garlic makes the villains scurry in a hurry—after all, they really *are* little vampires!

3 garlic cloves, peeled and
** minced**
1 oz. of mineral oil
1 tsp. of fresh-squeezed
** lemon juice**
2 cups of water

Put the garlic and oil into a container with a tight-fitting lid, and let it sit for 24 hours. Strain out the solids, and mix the garlic-scented oil with the lemon juice and water. Pour the potion into a spray bottle, and give yourself a good spritz before you head out.

YIELD: 2 CUPS

✔ When to Say "Whoa!"

Eating garlic can become too much of a good thing when you start to sweat out the scent. Stinky breath is manageable by gargling and chewing minty gum, but if you find that people start putting distance between themselves and you, you're probably exuding garlic from every pore and it's time to cut back.

✔ Alleviate Asthma Attacks

The potent garlic and milk duo mentioned in "The Milky Way to Cure Sciatica" (see page 141) can also minimize the discomfort of asthma. This formula, however, is a little different from the one for relieving sciatica. As soon as you feel an asthma attack coming on, peel and chop 10 garlic cloves, and add them to ¼ cup of milk. Heat the moo juice to boiling on the stove, then strain out the garlic. Let the milky "tea" cool to a comfortable temperature, and drink it down. If this potent potion doesn't stop the attack in its tracks, it should at least decrease the severity.

✔ Longer-Term Asthma Relief

Taking garlic syrup consistently may just help you ward off asthma symptoms. Here's your five-step game plan:

STEP 1. Separate and peel the cloves of three garlic bulbs.

STEP 2. Put them in a non-aluminum pan with 2 cups of water. Simmer until the garlic cloves are soft and there is about 1 cup of water left in the pan.

STEP 3. Using a slotted spoon, transfer the garlic to a jar with a tight-fitting lid.

STEP 4. Add 1 cup of apple cider vinegar* and ¼ cup of raw, organic honey to the water in the pan, and boil the mixture until it's syrupy.

STEP 5. Pour the syrup over the garlic in the jar, put the lid on, and let it sit overnight, or for at least eight hours.

Every morning, on an empty stomach, swallow one or two of the garlic cloves along with 1 teaspoon of the syrup.

* For medicinal and beauty purposes, always use raw, unfiltered apple cider vinegar (available in health-food stores and in the health-food sections of most supermarkets) rather than the clear, filtered kind that's on the shelves in the main grocery aisle.

Make a Lovely Liniment

HEALTHFUL HINT

If you suffer from rheumatism—or you just want to be prepared for treating muscle aches and sprains—this healing potion belongs in your medicine chest. Put 1 cup of high-quality, extra virgin olive oil into a glass jar with a tight-fitting lid. Peel and crush four garlic cloves, and add them to the oil. Cover the jar, and leave it in a warm place for a full week. Strain the oil into a clean bottle with a lid, and store it in a cool, dark spot. Then once or twice a day, massage a teaspoon or two of the oil onto your achin' body parts.

✔ Chase Athlete's Foot Away

You don't have to be a jock to get athlete's foot—and you don't have to be a doc to make the fungus flee. Just go at it with this simple (but odiferous) remedy: Steep half a dozen garlic cloves in a basin of hot water for an hour. Then soak your feet in the "tea" for 20 minutes once a day until the problem is gone.

✔ Tougher Stuff

When the athlete's foot fungus takes a more aggressive approach, reach for even stronger medicine. Crush six garlic cloves, put them in a jar with a tight-fitting lid, and add enough olive oil to cover them by half an inch or so. Put the lid on, shake the jar, and let the mixture fsit in a dark place for a few days. Then shake it again, and apply the oil to your clean, dry feet using a soft brush or cotton pad. Just one word of caution: This potent

A Garlic Shopper's Guide

There's nothing complicated about buying garlic: Simply look for plump, firm bulbs with tightly closed cloves. Whatever you do, steer clear of prepackaged garlic; it's all but guaranteed to be on its way downhill. To get the greatest health and beauty benefits—and the best flavor—you want the freshest stuff you can find. Then, when you get your garlic home, store it in a cool, dark place (but not in the refrigerator). Unbroken bulbs should last for up to eight weeks. Individual cloves, with their skin intact, can stay fresh for as long as 10 days.

stuff can burn sensitive skin, so use it with care, and don't get it on open cuts or sores.

Note: If you have diabetes, check with your doctor before you use any garlic athlete's foot remedy.

✔ Send Poison-Plant Rashes Packing

Garlic is just what the doctor ordered for easing the itch and redness of poison ivy, oak, or sumac. Simply boil four peeled, chopped garlic cloves in 1 cup of water. Remove it from the heat, let it cool to room temperature, and apply the liquid to your affected skin with a soft, clean cloth.

✔ Soothe Jock Itch

Like athlete's foot, jock itch is caused by a fungus, and it *does* tend to afflict its namesake victims. (It can spread rampantly in gyms and health clubs where the towels are washed with water that's not quite hot enough to kill the fungi.) Your best offense: Mash several peeled garlic cloves, and mix them with just enough olive oil to make a paste. Rub it onto your affected skin several times a day until the itching, burning, and redness are gone.

✔ Warm Up!

Attention, snowbelt dwellers! You know those days when you get so cold outdoors that after you come inside, you just can't stop shivering, even though the room is toasty warm? The next time that happens, try this old-time warmer-upper: Peel and grate two garlic cloves, and mix the pulp with a pinch of cayenne pepper. Divide the mixture into two portions, wrap each half in a piece of muslin, or old, clean panty hose, and fold it over to form a mini-envelope. Then put one of them behind each of your heels, where the backs of your shoes will hold them in place. You should feel warm all over within minutes.

✔ Conquer Constipation

Sluggish bowels have been plaguing mankind since the beginning of time. Hippocrates, the father of medicine who lived in Greece from 460 to 377 BC, had a surefire cure: garlic, and plenty of it. Unfortunately, Dr. H. didn't specify an exact quantity—at least none that we know of—but modern natural-health gurus recommend eating one or two minced garlic cloves a day, mixed in milk or plain yogurt, until your internal machinery is back in business again.

Fabulous Food Fix

GARLICKY BROCCOLINI

Here's an ultra-simple—and ultra-tasty—way to get your daily dose of dynamic, disease-busting garlic and the antioxidant power of broccolini.

1½ lbs. of fresh broccolini*
1 tbsp. of extra virgin olive oil
4 or 5 garlic cloves, minced
Coarse sea salt (optional)
Freshly ground pepper (optional)

Lightly steam the broccolini for one to two minutes until it's just crisp-tender. Put the olive oil and garlic in a skillet, and cook for two to three minutes over medium heat. Add the broccolini, and sauté for one more minute. Season the broccolini with the salt and pepper if desired, and serve it up.

* Or substitute frozen broccoli florets.

YIELD: 4 SERVINGS

✔ Trying to Become a Dad?

A great many things can cause male infertility, but in a full 90 percent of cases, the culprit is simply low sperm count. So if you and your wife just can't seem to conceive—and your doctors have ruled out medical reasons—give garlic a try. It's been proven highly effective at increasing sperm quantities by improving blood flow to the male sex organs. Just adding two cloves of garlic to your daily diet could take you a long way toward the first time you hear a tiny voice say "Daddy."

✔ Cure a Vaginal Yeast Infection

Simply making garlic a part of your daily diet can restore the natural pH balance in your vagina, thereby fighting the overgrowth of bacteria that cause yeast infections. If you'd prefer a faster and more direct approach, peel a garlic clove, and wrap it in a piece of sterile cotton gauze. Insert the little package you know where, as you would a tampon. Leave it in place for 24 hours, then replace it with a fresh one. Repeat the procedure until the infection is gone. **Note:** If the problem isn't resolved after two weeks, or if your irritation worsens at any point, see your doctor.

✔ Clear Up Varicose Veins

Surgery and drugs can clear up varicose veins, but garlic can help, too. Studies show that eating as little as one clove of fresh garlic each day will keep your blood moving through your vessels, thereby preventing clots, helping to alleviate the discomfort, and making your legs look more attractive.

✔ Undo Ulcers

Although garlic is a big no-no for anyone with a bleeding ulcer, it is a highly effective way to help relieve mild ulcers and prevent new ones from forming. That's because garlic's antibacterial properties fight the *H. pylori* bacterium that causes these annoying (and painful) stomach sores. The recommended dose is two small, crushed cloves a day, in whatever form you care to take them.

✔ Say "Get Out, Gout!"

This old-time gout remedy comes straight from Russia, where they eat a lot of garlic: Twice a day, drink a glass of 100 percent cherry juice with two cloves of minced garlic in it. Be sure not to chew the garlic—that way, it won't wind up on your breath.

✔ Ah—There's the Rub!

Cold sores are caused by viruses, and ringworm is a fungal infection, but the same simple garlic treatment can heal both of these nasty nuisances. Simply slice a clove in two, and rub the cut surface over the affected skin area.

✔ Toss Off Tinnitus

Tinnitus is almost never a serious health condition, but it is one of the most annoying afflictions under the sun. But never fear—here's a surefire cure. Put six large, peeled garlic cloves in a blender with 1 cup of cold-pressed, extra virgin olive oil, and blend until the garlic is finely minced. Pour the mixture into a sterile glass jar, put the lid on, and refrigerate it for seven days. Strain out the solids, and pour the liquid into several sterilized eyedropper bottles. Then each night at bedtime, pour a small amount of the oil into a bowl, wait a few minutes for the chill to wear off, and put 3 drops into each ear. Plug the openings with cotton balls, leave them in overnight, and remove them in the morning. Within two weeks, your bells should stop ringing. **Note:** To sterilize the jar, lid, and eyedropper bottles, simply place them in a large pot of boiling water for a few minutes, and let them air-dry before you add the oil. Also, always keep the oil in the refrigerator, where it will last up to a month.

Pretty and Pungent

✤ Spot-Treat Pimples

It never fails: Just when you've got a major social or business event on your calendar, a pimple pops up from out of nowhere. Not to worry! Just peel a fresh garlic clove, slice it in two, and rub one of the cut sides onto your blemish. The redness and swelling should vanish within a day or so.

✤ Make an Anti-Acne Mask

To treat more widespread acne, peel and mash five garlic cloves, and mix them with 1 tablespoon of raw, organic honey. Spread the mixture over the affected areas of your face, and leave it on for 10 minutes or so. Then rinse it off with lukewarm water, pat dry, and apply your normal toner and moisturizer. **Note:** The mask may sting a little when you first apply it, but don't worry—that feeling is normal and should vanish within a minute or two.

✤ Purify Your Pores

Garlic and tomatoes are a culinary match made in heaven. Their combined antiseptic properties also form a dynamic duo that can clear out

POTENT POTION

GARLIC-STRAWBERRY FACIAL SCRUB

This treatment gives any complexion a healthy glow. Thanks to the antiseptic action of garlic, it's also a special boon for oily or acne-prone skin.

2 tbsp. of boiled distilled water

1 small garlic clove, peeled and crushed

3 strawberries, mashed

2 tbsp. of ground oatmeal*

1 tbsp. of cornmeal

1 tsp. of plain yogurt

2 drops of tea tree oil

Pour the boiled water over the garlic, and let it steep for 30 minutes. Then strain out the solids, and mix the liquid with the rest of the ingredients. Scrub your face with the mixture, leave it on for 10 minutes or so, and rinse with lukewarm water. Pat your skin dry, and follow up with your usual toner and a light moisturizer.

* A coffee grinder, food processor, or blender will do the job nicely.

embedded makeup, environmental toxins, and everyday dirt that clogs your skin. Your action plan: Mash a peeled garlic clove and a medium-size tomato, and mix them together. Spread a thin layer of the mixture onto your face, and leave it on for 20 minutes or so. Then rinse it off with lukewarm water. Splash your face with cold water to seal your pores, and follow up with your usual moisturizer.

✤ Say Good-Bye to Warts

Of all the wart-removal methods out there, this may be the simplest (and it's certainly the cheapest!): Just before you go to bed, cut the tip off a fresh garlic clove, and rub the cut side directly onto the wart for a few seconds. Repeat the procedure each night until the ugly bump vanishes.

✤ Fortify Your Fingernails

Whether you're troubled by peeling, splitting fingernails all year round, or only during cold winter weather, this remarkable remedy can solve your problem: Add a finely minced garlic clove to a bottle of nail polish (either clear or your favorite shade), and let it sit for a few days. Then simply paint it onto your nails in the usual way. Once the polish has dried completely, remove any garlic odor by washing your hands with freshly squeezed lemon juice. Repeat the procedure once a week, and your nails will stay strong and healthy.

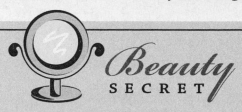

GARLIC BREATH, BE GONE!

*A*lthough garlic is one of the most powerful tools in your health and beauty arsenal, we all know that eating it leaves you with breath that would make a dragon keel over. The good news is that you have a number of effective options for sweetening the air around you. Like these, for instance:

■ *Chew a stick of gum (any flavor will do).*

■ *Drink a cup of mint tea.*

■ *Eat a sprig of fresh parsley or a tablespoon or so of the dried version.*

■ *Munch on a few coffee beans.*

■ *Sip a glass of milk.*

■ *Suck on a lemon wedge.*

The not-so-good news is that the aroma spewing out of your mouth is not just coming from your tongue—the odor of garlic actually gets into your lungs, and it can stay there for as long as 12 hours. So whichever breath-freshening method(s) you choose to use (and depending on how much garlic you've consumed), you may need to repeat the procedure every few hours.

✤ Scalp Salvation on the Double

Whether you're suffering from dandruff or shedding hair, a simple garlic treatment can solve your problem. Just pulverize two peeled garlic cloves in a food processor, and massage the mush into your scalp using small, circular motions. Wait 60 minutes, then massage 2 tablespoons of olive oil into your scalp. Cover your head with a shower cap, and leave it on for at least six hours. Wash with a gentle shampoo, and follow up with conditioner.

✤ Put Your Hair Back in the Black

Just about all of us develop gray hair over time, but the color change is most obvious in folks whose hair is naturally black. Here's an easy—and inexpensive—way to cover up the intruding gray strands:

STEP 1. Gather up peels from three or four garlic bulbs. (Ideally, save the peels from the garlic you normally use in your kitchen; otherwise, peel the

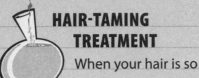

POTENT POTION

HAIR-TAMING TREATMENT

When your hair is so dry that it feels like it's about to split all the way up the shafts, replace the moisture with this sweet and pungent potion.

2 tbsp. of garlic oil*
1 tsp. of honey
1 egg yolk

Mix the oil and honey, then beat in the egg yolk. Rub the mixture into your hair one small section at a time. Cover your head with a shower cap or a plastic bag, and wait 30 minutes. Rinse thoroughly, and shampoo as usual.

* Available in health-food stores.

cloves, and use the cloves immediately, or preserve them in sherry or brandy for later use.)

STEP 2. Heat the peels in a frying pan over low heat until they're thoroughly dry and black.

STEP 3. Grind the blackened peels into a fine powder, using a coffee grinder, food processor, or a mortar and pestle.

STEP 4. Mix the grindings with enough olive oil to reach a consistency that's slightly thicker than shampoo (about the same thickness as commercial hair dye). Pour the potion into a stoppered glass bottle, and store it in a dark place for a week or so.

STEP 5. After a week, work the dye into your wet hair just before bedtime. Then cover your head with a shower cap, and hit the sack. Come morning, rinse your hair, and shampoo as usual. **Note:** The longer the dye stays on your head, the deeper it will penetrate into your hair shafts—and the longer the color will remain. Repeat the treatment when the color begins to fade, which is generally after three to four weeks.

Best of the Rest

★ Root for More Energy

Gingerroot, that is. It's an old Japanese remedy for boosting your energy level by revving up your circulation, and it comes on like gangbusters. Just add 1 cup of minced fresh ginger to 2 quarts of warm water, and soak your feet until they're a rosy shade of red. Then dry your "paws" thoroughly, and go out and conquer the world—or at least take a nice long walk.

★ Speed Up Sluggish Bowels

When your internal plumbing slows down, there are plenty of over-the-counter laxatives that can get things moving again. But if you prefer a less invasive approach, whip up a gentle gingery poultice. Here's what you need to do: Put 2 gallons of water in a pot, and bring it to a boil. Tuck 4½ tablespoons of grated fresh ginger into a cheese-cloth bag, dunk it in the water, and remove the pot from the heat. Let the pouch steep until the water reaches a comfortable (but still warm) tempera-ture. Then dip a clean towel into the brew, and lay it over your abdomen until the compress cools.

Repeat the process four more times, reheating the water and applying a fresh compress each time. You'll find that things will soon be moving along again.

★ Don't Horse Around with Arthritis

Make the pain gallop away with this ter-rific trick: Boil ½ cup of milk, and mix 3 tablespoons of grated horseradish into it. Pour the mixture onto a piece of cheesecloth, and lay it on your aching joint. By the time the poultice cools off, you should feel like hopping on your pony and headin' on down the trail!

★ Clear Your Sinuses

Are clogged sinuses driving you to drink (or merely increasing your con-sumption)? If so, take 1 teaspoon of

Fabulous Food Fix

HORSERADISH DETOX DIP

Horseradish is one of the most potent sources of glucosinolates—compounds that increase your liver's ability to detoxify carcino-gens. Not only does that action help lessen your risk of developing cancer, but studies show that it may suppress the growth of existing tumors. The recommended dose is as little as ¼ teaspoon a day, either freshly ground or bottled. And this tangy dip is an easy way to meet your quota.

1 cup of plain nonfat Greek yogurt
½ cup of fresh dill, chopped
3 tbsp. of horseradish (freshly grated or bottled)
½ tsp. of salt (optional)

Mix all of the ingredients in a bowl, and serve the dip with crackers, pita chips, or raw veggies.

YIELD: ABOUT 1 CUP

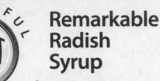

Remarkable Radish Syrup

If you or anyone in your family comes down with a cough or sore throat, make up a batch of this old-time Irish cure. (I learned it eons ago from a landlady who hailed from County Cork.) The recipe couldn't be simpler: Just cut six or eight radishes into thin slices, spread them out on a plate, and sprinkle them with a tablespoon or so of sugar. Cover them loosely with wax paper or aluminum foil, and let them sit overnight. In the morning, you'll find the slices swimming in a rich syrup. Drain it off into a glass bottle or jar with a tight-fitting lid, and take a teaspoonful whenever you feel the need.

grated fresh horseradish daily—or as needed—until your symptoms subside. Just how do you take this fiery stuff? Any way you like! It works wonders whether you spread it on a sandwich, mix it in tomato juice, or eat it straight from the spoon. After you're breathing freely again, a few teaspoons a month should help prevent future clogging.

★ Stimulate Your Water Flow

When you're having trouble urinating, belly up to the bar (or your kitchen counter) and grate ½ cup of horseradish. Add it to a pan with ½ cup of beer, and bring it to a boil. Let it boil for a minute or two, then remove it from the heat. When it's cool enough to drink, sip it down. Repeat two more times during the day, and the spigot should soon be functioning fine again.

★ R Is for Radish and Radiance

To look at a humble red radish, you'd never take it for a hotshot beauty helper, but it is. In fact, it makes a highly effective cleanser that gives your face a glorious glow. Just pop a couple of radishes into a blender, and whip them into a fine paste. Smooth it onto your face and neck, and leave it on for 20 minutes or so. Rinse with cold water, pat your skin dry, and apply your usual moisturizer. That's all there is to it!

★ Top o' the Morning Toner

Mix up a batch of this gingery potion, and use it each morning to get your day off to a rousing start. Bring 8 ounces of water to a boil, add three slices of fresh ginger, then reduce the heat to low and simmer for 15 minutes. Let the tea cool, strain out the ginger, and mix 2 ounces of the tea with

1 ounce each of witch hazel and aloe vera juice (available in health-food stores and online). Pour the mixture into a glass bottle with a tight-fitting cap, and store it in the refrigerator. Each morning, dampen a cotton pad with the cool potion, and smooth it over your freshly washed face. Apply your usual moisturizer, and you're ready to face the day.

★ Make Dark Spots Get Outta Dodge

Looking for a way to make freckles and age spots giddyup and go? Deputize horseradish and vinegar. Finely grate a 4-inch piece of fresh horseradish, and mix the pieces with ¼ cup of apple cider vinegar in a clean jar with a tight-fitting lid. Let the mixture sit for two weeks, shaking the jar daily. Strain the liquid into a second jar, and store it in the refrigerator. Then three times a day, rub the potion into your problem areas using a cotton ball or swab. You should start to see results within a month or so.

★ Say "So Long" to Cellulite

Ginger is famous as one of Mother Nature's most powerful cellulite reducers. When you mix it with sugar, olive oil, and lemon zest, you get a body scrub that will warm you up, wake you up, soften your skin—and reduce the appearance of cellulite. Just mix 2 teaspoons of freshly grated, peeled ginger with ½ cup of granulated sugar, ¼ cup of olive oil, and the zest of one lemon (preferably organic). In the shower or bath, gather up handfuls of the mixture, and scrub your body lightly. Rinse well, and enjoy your rejuvenated skin!

POTENT POTION

STIMULATING GINGER HAIR CLEANSER

The dynamic duo of ginger and green tea will recharge your skin cells, rev up your scalp circulation, and even soothe any irritation or inflammation you might have.

8 oz. of water
2 slices of fresh ginger
(¼ inch or so thick)
2 tbsp. of green-tea leaves
2 tbsp. of liquid castile soap

Bring the water to a boil, add the ginger and tea, and steep for 20 minutes. Let the mixture cool, then strain out the solids, and pour the liquid into a clean shampoo bottle. Add the soap, and mix thoroughly. Pour the entire amount of potion over your hair, and massage it into your scalp. Rinse well, apply your normal conditioner, and style your hair as usual.

12 Honey

Talk about old-time healers! Prehistoric rock paintings suggest that people were keeping honeybees as early as 13,000 BC (yes, you read that right). The ancient Greeks and Romans were particularly skilled beekeepers and highly adept at using "the nectar of the gods" for both medicinal and cosmetic purposes. And when the first English settlers arrived on our shores in the 17th century, they brought their beehives with them. The rest, as they say, is history. Every day, it seems, health and beauty experts find more ways to use honey to make us feel *and* look better.

Here's to Honey!

✔ Soothe Acid Indigestion

When you've overindulged at the dinner table, take 1 to 3 teaspoons of honey for instant indigestion relief. To ease a chronic problem, take 1 tablespoon each night at bedtime, on an empty stomach, until you feel better. **Note:** If your discomfort continues for more than a week, or if you experience other symptoms, call your doctor.

✔ *Arrivederci,* Arthritis

Bid good-bye to arthritis pain with this classic—and highly effective—treatment: Each morning and evening, take 1 teaspoon of honey mixed with 1 teaspoon of apple cider vinegar. That's all there is to it!

✔ Take the Sting Out

It has always seemed a bit ironic to me that an insect that delivers such searing pain can also produce one of the best antidotes to its sting. The solution? Just smooth a dab of honey on the spot (after removing the stinger, of course), and the pain and itch will vanish.

✔ Heal Cuts and Scrapes Fast

After you wash a wound, spread honey over it. Because honey is hygroscopic (that is, it absorbs water), it deprives infection-causing microorganisms of the moisture they need to survive. It also forms a natural bandage that helps your "owie" heal faster. Perhaps best of all (especially if the wounded warrior is a child), honey won't sting the way some antiseptics can.

✔ Treat Minor Burns

Serious burns demand immediate medical attention. But for treating common kitchen burns, like brief encounters with hot pans or ultra-hot coffee, honey is a first-class first responder. Here's how to get relief:

BURNED SKIN. Rinse the affected skin with cold water or apply a cold compress for a minute or so. Gently pat the area dry, then spread honey over the burn. It will ease the pain and help speed up the healing process.

BURNED THROAT. Swallow a tablespoon of honey. It'll coat and cool your tender tissue like nobody's business. If your throat pain lingers, repeat the dosage once or twice more over a few hours, and you'll soon be swallowing smoothly.

POTENT POTION

SOOTHING SUNBURN BATH

For those occasions when too much sun leaves you (or your resident youngster) looking like a boiled lobster, relieve the burn with this gentle tub-time healer.

1 cup of vegetable oil
½ cup of honey
½ cup of mild liquid soap
1 tbsp. of pure vanilla extract (not artificial)

Mix all of the ingredients together, pour the mixture into a bottle with a tight-fitting stopper, and store it at room temperature. At bath time, shake the bottle, then pour ¼ cup of the potion under running water, slip in, and say "Ahhh."

YIELD: 2 CUPS

✔ Head Off a Hangover

If you're going to a party or an after-work happy hour with your office buddies, take a tip from the experts at the National Headache Foundation: Before you start drinking, eat a piece of toast or a few crackers slathered with a generous layer of honey. It helps break down the by-products of alcohol in your bloodstream that make you feel so awful. **Note:** If you don't remember to take your preventive "medicine" before you start to imbibe, take it as soon as possible after the party's over. You'll still avoid most, if not all, of the typical morning-after miseries.

✔ Cure a Hangover

When a night on the town lays you low the morning after, forget the hair of the dog; take the juice of the bee instead. Eat 1 teaspoon of honey every hour until you feel better, which will be a lot sooner than you probably think possible! How you take your sweet medicine is up to you: It'll put you back in the land of the living whether you lick it straight from the spoon, stir it into milk or tea, spread it on toast or English muffins, or mix it with yogurt.

✔ Foil a Migraine

Fast action can often stop a migraine in its tracks. The minute you feel the early warning signs, eat a tablespoon of honey. If your headache isn't gone within 30 minutes, take another tablespoon of honey, and chase it down with three glasses of water. That should be all she wrote!

HEALTHFUL HINT

Choose the Right Stuff

To get the health and beauty benefits of honey, always use the pure, raw (a.k.a. unprocessed) kind, not the brands you find next to the peanut butter and jelly in most supermarkets. The common commercial types of honey have been put through a heating and filtering process that kills off the health-giving enzymes and nutrients. So while these sweet treats may taste fine, they aren't worth beans for treating ailments or improving your looks. Fortunately, the good stuff is easy to come by: You can find it in health-food stores, at farmers' markets, in the organic/natural-food sections of most major supermarkets, and (of course) on scads of websites. **Note:** Studies have shown that dark-colored honey, like that made from buckwheat and blueberry pollen, contains more antioxidants than lighter types and therefore offers the most protection against debilitating diseases.

✔ Sleep Tight

Sleepless nights are no fun—and they're not good for your health either. So if you find yourself tossing and turning when you should be cuttin' some z's, try this time-tested remedy: At bedtime, mix 1 teaspoon of honey in warm milk or lukewarm water, and drink it down. In no time flat, you should drift off to dreamland.

✔ Fight Fatigue

Yes, honey helps you get a good night's sleep (see "Sleep Tight," above), but it also does the trick when you need a quick energy boost to make it through your workout or other strenuous exercise. Simply take 1 table-spoon of honey washed down with 8 ounces of water. Studies have shown that it delivers just as big a jolt of get-up-and-go power as the glucose used in energy bars and fancy sports gels, at a much lower price!

✔ Bounce Back Fast

After your workout, have another spoonful of honey. It'll help your muscles recuperate quickly by replacing the carbohydrates your body burned during your exercise routine.

Fabulous Food Fix

GET-UP-AND-GO HONEY BARS

The next time you venture out on a hike, a day of cross-country skiing, or simply a long day at the office, tuck some of these power-packed energy bars into your backpack or briefcase. They also make terrific after-school snacks!

⅓ **cup of honey**
¼ **cup of butter, melted**
3 **egg whites**
1 **tsp. of cinnamon**
½ **tsp. of almond extract**
3 **cups of low-fat granola**
¾ **cup of dried cherries**
½ **cup of almonds, coarsely chopped**

Whisk together the first five ingredients, then stir in the granola, cherries, and almonds. Spoon the mixture into a greased 9- by 9-inch baking pan. Using a piece of wax paper, firmly press the batter in place. Bake at 350°F for 20 to 25 minutes, or until lightly browned. Remove from the oven, cool completely, and slice into bars. Store them in a covered container at room temperature.

YIELD: 12 BARS

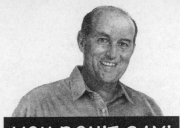

✔ Drop Some Weight

Trying to shed a few pounds? Well, forget about elaborate diets or expensive weight-loss products. Instead, half an hour before each meal, mix 2 teaspoons of honey in a glass of water, and drink it down. It'll naturally suppress your appetite so you won't be as tempted to overeat.

✔ Speak Easier

We've all been there: You open your mouth to speak, but nothing comes out. Well, don't force the issue. Even a whisper puts undue stress on your vocal cords and could lead to further complications. So just send your voice on vacation for a few days. In the meantime, throughout the day, sip this time-honored singers' remedy: 2 teaspoons of honey and 1 teaspoon of fresh-squeezed lemon juice mixed in a glass of hot water. **Note:** If your voice hasn't returned to normal after three days or so, or if you experience other symptoms, see your doctor.

✔ Speak Up!

We've all been here, too: You're all set to give a major speech, ace a big job interview, or maybe pop that crucial question, and bingo! Your mouth goes dry, and you can barely muster up a mumble. Your instinct may say, "Down a cold beverage." Well, don't do it! It will moisten your mouth, all right, but it'll also tighten up your already-tense throat muscles. Instead, mix 1 tablespoon of honey in ½ cup of warm water. Gargle with the mixture, and swish it around in your mouth for three to five minutes. Then rinse your mouth with clear water to cut the sweetness. The honey will increase the secretion of saliva, thereby relieving the dryness and making it easier for you to utter your important words.

✔ Hack No More

To relieve a cough, mix a full cup of honey with ½ cup of olive oil and 4 tablespoons of fresh-squeezed lemon juice. Heat the mixture on low for five minutes, then stir vigorously for two minutes. Pour the potion into a jar with a tight-fitting lid and keep it at room temperature. Take 1 teaspoon every two hours as needed. Before you know it, your hacking will be history! **Note:** If you prefer to take your medicine straight, sip 1 teaspoon of honey at bedtime, and let it trickle down your throat.

✔ Stop a Bronchial Cough

If you're prone to bronchitis during the winter months (as many folks who live in cool, damp climates are), this potent syrup is just what the doctor ordered. Mix up a batch or two, and keep it close at hand. Here's what to do: Put 6 tablespoons of honey in a clean bottle with a tight-fitting lid, and add 3 drops of oil of anise and 3 drops of oil of fennel (both available in health-food stores and from websites). Store it at room temperature, and take 1 teaspoon of the syrup whenever you start to feel the wheezing coming on.

✔ All Allergies Are Local

Well, not *all*, but hay fever sure is! When seasonal allergies have you sneezing up a storm, hightail it to your nearest farmers' market, farm stand, or independently owned health-food store. Buy a jar of locally produced, raw honey, and start taking 1 tablespoon a day in whatever form(s) you like. Your immune system will become accustomed to the neighborhood pollen contained in the honey, and your body will stop kicking up such a fuss. You may not feel 100 percent better, but it's highly likely that you'll be a lot more comfortable.

Fabulous Food Fix

A HONEY OF A HOT TODDY

When cold and flu season rolls around, keep this curative recipe close at hand.

1 tbsp. of honey
½ cup of hot water
3 tbsp. of brandy*
3-inch by ½-inch strip of
    lemon peel
1 cinnamon stick

Stir the honey and water in a toddy glass until the honey dissolves, and pour in the brandy. Twist the lemon peel over the edge of the glass, then add it to the drink. Stir with the cinnamon stick, and drink to your good health!

* Or substitute bourbon or scotch.

✔ Plan Ahead for Sneeze-Free Days

Next year, two to three months before allergy season starts, begin taking 1 to 3 teaspoons of locally produced honey a day. By the time the pollen starts flying, your immune system will have built up enough resistance that your symptoms should be greatly lessened, if not eliminated entirely.

✔ Clear Up Cold Sores

Cold sores (a.k.a. fever blisters) are caused by the herpes virus. Although they have no direct relation to either colds or fevers, they do hurt like crazy. Never fear, honey can help relieve the pain. Mix 3 tablespoons of the "bee juice" with 1 tablespoon of unfiltered apple cider vinegar, and store it in a jar with a tight-fitting lid. Then dab the mixture onto your sore(s) in the morning, in the late afternoon, and just before bedtime.

✔ Fix Your Internal Plumbing

When Mother Nature doesn't call, or when she just won't get off the "line," reach for a jar of honey. It can solve both of those (usually) minor, but annoying problems. Here's what to do:

CONSTIPATION. Mix a tablespoon or two of honey in a glass of warm water, and drink it down. Things should start moving along within 24 hours. If they don't, you can take another dose.

DIARRHEA. Drink 10 ounces of water with 3 teaspoons of honey mixed into it. It'll kill the bacteria that cause diarrhea and also soothe your stomach and relieve that cramped feeling that generally accompanies a case of the runs.

Note: Whichever condition you're dealing with, if it persists for more than a few days, or if you have other symptoms, call your doctor.

CAUTION !

Although honey supplies heaping helpings of health benefits, it should *never* be given to babies under one year of age. That's because honey contains the spores of *Clostridium botulinum*, which causes infant botulism. While adults and children can digest the spores with no harm at all, the human gastrointestinal tract is not fully operational until an infant reaches 12 months of age. And to play it extra safe, consult with your doctor before you give honey to a child under the age of two.

✔ Banish Bursitis Pain

Whether it goes by the name of housemaid's knee, tennis elbow, or (my personal favorite) weaver's bottom, a case of bursitis is a royal pain in the body part. There are plenty of topical remedies that can ease your discomfort. But here's a simple routine that works from the inside to help reduce the inflammation in your bursae, strengthen your joints, and boost your immune system. One hour before breakfast, drink a 12-ounce glass of water with 2 tablespoons of honey, ½ cup of apple cider vinegar, and 1 teaspoon of cayenne pepper mixed into it. Repeat each morning until your joints are jumpin' again.

Sweet and Wonderful

❖ Make Your Teeth Glow

To get your pearly whites whiter without the high cost of a trip to the dentist, brush them with a mixture of 1 tablespoon of honey and 1 tablespoon of activated charcoal (available in pharmacies and health-food stores). **Note:** Do not confuse activated charcoal with the kind that's made for barbecue grills!

❖ Lighten Skin Spots

Natural-beauty pros have more spot-removal remedies than Howdy Doody has freckles, but this is one of the simplest and gentlest: Once a day, mix 1 teaspoon of honey with 1 teaspoon of plain yogurt. Apply the mixture to the problem areas, and let it dry. Then wait another 30 minutes, and wash it off. Besides bleaching the marks, it will soften your skin.

❖ Bye-Bye, Blackheads

Here's a sweet way to banish blackheads: Just heat about ⅛ cup of honey until it's lukewarm, and dab it onto the blemishes. Let it sit for a couple of minutes, wash it off with warm water, and rinse with cool water. Pat your skin dry with a soft towel, and follow up with your usual moisturizer.

❖ Get a Shine On

With a little help from honey, you can turn your normal conditioner into a hair-care dynamo that will make your tresses softer, silkier, and shinier. Simply mix ¾ cup of your usual conditioner with ¼ cup of honey, and work it through your hair. Leave it on for 10 to 15 minutes, then shampoo.

POTENT POTION

ALL-OVER HONEY AND HERB SCRUB

You could go to one of the fanciest spas in the country to have this sweet, softening scrub massaged into your face and body—and pay triple-digit dollars for the privilege. Or you could step into your kitchen and whip up the simple recipe yourself.

2 tbsp. of honey

1 tbsp. of extra virgin olive oil

3 tbsp. of sugar

2 tsp. of fresh basil, finely chopped

2 tsp. of fresh mint, finely chopped

3–4 drops of lavender essential oil*

Warm up the honey, and stir in the olive oil. Add the remaining ingredients, and mix thoroughly. Step into the bath or shower, and massage the potion all over your body and face. Rinse with warm water, and pat dry. Then go out and buy yourself a special treat or dinner with all the money you've saved!

* Or substitute your favorite aroma.

❖ Send Crow's Feet Flying

The crinkles at the corners of your eyes are the natural result of years of smiling and squinting. If you view them as blemishes, rather than souvenirs of a well-lived life, you could opt for expensive (and painful) Botox® treatments. Or you could do what beauty-conscious women have been doing since the days of ancient Egypt: Smooth honey over your face, and leave it on for 20 minutes or so. Then rinse it off with warm water, and pat dry. Not only will it lessen the appearance of wrinkles, but it'll also deliver deep-down moisture to your skin and leave your face feeling dewy soft.

❖ If It Was Good Enough for Cleopatra . . .

It's good enough for you. The beautiful Egyptian queen claimed that she owed her good looks in large part to her baths of milk and honey. But don't just take her word for it, try it yourself. Pour 1 to 2 cups of whole milk and ½ cup of honey under warm water as it flows from the spigot. Swish the water around with your hand to mix the ingredients, and settle in. Close your eyes, relax, and think lovely thoughts for 20 minutes or so. Then step out, pat dry, and apply your usual moisturizer. **Note:** To get the maximum softening and exfoliating effects, lightly brush your skin in circular motions with a dry brush or loofah before you get into the tub.

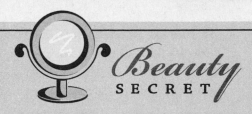

ANTI-AGING MASK

Let's face it: Nothing can make you look 25 (or even 40) forever. But this mask has been known to keep women's skin looking soft, smooth, and firm well into their senior years. The magic formula: Mix 1 tablespoon of honey, 2 table-spoons of heavy cream, and the contents of one vitamin E capsule until the mixture has a smooth,

creamy consistency. Spread it onto your face and neck, and leave it in place for 15 to 20 minutes. Then rinse it off with lukewarm water, and pat dry. Repeat once a week or so, and before long, your friends will be demanding to know where you've found the Fountain of Youth!

✤ Soften Up Your Birthday Suit

Dry skin can result from cold weather, frequent bathing, too much sun exposure, or chemicals that leach the natural oils from your skin. But whatever caused your dryness, a milk-and-honey massage can help you replace the lost moisture fast. Just mix equal parts of whole milk and honey. Starting at your feet, massage the lotion into your thirsty skin. Then step into the shower and rinse yourself off. **Note:** Don't even think of using reduced-fat milk for this or any other skin-softening routine. This job demands the heavy-hitting power of full-strength moo juice.

Best of the Rest

★ Fight Cancer with Chocolate

Studies show that compounds called polyphenols slow the growth of cancer cells. And 1 ounce of dark chocolate contains almost as many polyphenols as a cup of green tea does and twice as many as a glass of red wine does (two widely touted sources of the compounds). Remember—the operative word is *dark*. So look for chocolate that consists of more than 70 percent cocoa.

★ Have Some Molasses, Baby

Nobody knows what causes colic in babies, but fortunately for harried parents (as well as suffering infants), the problem usually diminishes within a few months. In the meantime, molasses can calm the turbulence. Just mix 2 teaspoons of it with ¼ cup of warm water in a baby bottle, and give it to the youngster to suck on. It will soothe the tyke's stomach in a flash—thereby delivering instant gratification to the victim and everyone else in the household. **Note:** Unlike honey, molasses is perfectly safe for babies of any age.

★ Gelatin Stops the Runs

This plumbing-repair tip works for anyone, but it's an especially appealing way to cure a child's case of diarrhea. Mix a 3-ounce package of fruit-flavored gelatin according to the package directions, let it set just until it's soft, and give it to your young patient. That should help halt the flow. **Note:** If the problem persists, or if other symptoms are present, call your doctor.

★ Fade Varicose Veins

Troubled by painful varicose veins? Lighten them up by taking 2 to 3 teaspoons of blackstrap molasses daily. It will improve your circulation, thus opening up the channels and clearing the discoloration. **Note:** If you don't have varicose veins yet, but they run in your family, there's a good chance you can head trouble off at the pass by making molasses a regular part of your diet.

HEALTHFUL HINT

Help for Wannabe Dads

Gentlemen, recent studies show that eating 1 to 2 ounces of dark chocolate per day can double both your semen volume and sperm count. Be sure to choose a brand that contains the lowest possible levels of sugar, preservatives, and other additives, and at least a 60 to 70 percent concentration of pure cocoa. This way, you'll get a potent dose of its magic sperm-boosting ingredient, L-arginine HCL. **Note:** Don't overdo it. If your chocolate consumption leads to weight gain, it could throw your body's testosterone and estrogen levels out of balance, thereby compromising your sperm count and putting you right back where you started!

★ A Spoonful of Sugar . . .

Stops hiccups in their tracks. When you swallow a teaspoon of sugar, it signals the nerves that control your diaphragm muscles to stop the spasms.

★ Chocolate Chases Wrinkles

We all know that modern science has debunked the myth that chocolate causes acne. Well, here's even better news: Not only does chocolate not harm your skin; it's one of the best friends your complexion ever had because it combats the cellular damage caused by free radicals. Believe it or not, just half an ounce of dark chocolate contains more wrinkle-fighting antioxidants than a glass of orange juice. **Note:** Make sure the brand you choose contains at least 60 to 70 percent cocoa.

★ Battle the Frizzies

Flyaway hair driving you nuts? Dissolve 1 teaspoon of lemon gelatin powder in 1 tablespoon of water. Dip a comb into the liquid, and run it through your hair, section by section, rolling each section onto a hair roller. Let your hair air-dry, comb it out, and presto—end of frizzies!

★ Jiggle Away Foot Odor

When your feet are, shall we say, less than sweet-smelling, march into the kitchen and grab a box of lemon or lime gelatin. Mix the contents with 2 cups of hot water, stirring until the gelatin dissolves. Add enough cold water to make a comfortably warm footbath, then soak your tootsies in the mixture until the gelatin begins to set. When

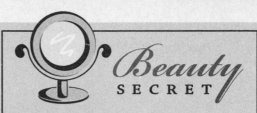

Beauty S E C R E T

SUPER-SIMPLE PEEL-OFF MASK

There's nothing like a peel-off facial mask to remove environmental toxins and embedded dirt from your pores. And the formulas don't come any easier than this one: Mix 1½ tablespoons of unflavored gelatin and ½ cup of 100 percent fruit juice in a microwave-safe bowl, and nuke it until the gelatin is dissolved. Put the container in the refrigerator until the contents are almost set, but still spreadable (25 minutes or so). Smooth the mask onto your face, avoiding the area around your eyes. Let it dry, peel it off, and follow up with your usual moisturizer. As for what kind of fruit juice to use, it depends on your skin type.

Oily skin. *Go with grapefruit, lemon, or tomato.*

Normal, dry, or mature skin. *Apple, pear, and raspberry are all good choices.*

you're done, wash your feet with warm, soapy water, rinse, and dry them thoroughly. Then run out and treat yourself to a new pair of sandals!

★ Face Up to Sugar

White granulated sugar might not be good for the inside of your body, but it can do a couple of big favors for your face. Reach for it the next time you want to perform one of these chores:

CLEAR UP PIMPLES. Just mix a spoonful of sugar with a few drops of water, and dab it onto the spots.

SUPERCHARGE YOUR CLEANSER. Simply add 1 teaspoon of sugar to the lather when you wash your face.

★ Reverse the Gray

Here's good news if you're spending time and money covering up the gray in your hair: Blackstrap molasses may actually reverse the graying process and restore your original hair color. The recommended dose is 1 tablespoon each day, first thing in the morning. You can take it straight from the spoon, spread it on toast, or mix it into herbal tea. You could start getting results in as little as two weeks, and within three to six months, there's a chance that your crowning glory will be back to its youthful shade. **Note:** Even if you don't see a color change, the minerals in molasses will make your hair shinier and healthier.

Fabulous Food Fix

HARD-AS-NAILS TONIC

Just like every other part of your body, your finger- and toenails reflect what you eat. If your nails are soft, chances are that you're not getting enough protein in your diet. This tasty supplement should solve your problem fast.

1 cup of milk
1 tsp. of blackstrap molasses
1 tsp. of unflavored gelatin
¼ tsp. of peanut oil

Heat (but don't boil) the milk, pour it into a mug, and stir in the other ingredients. Drink the potion three times a day, and you should start seeing results within a few weeks.

* If the gelatin doesn't dissolve, pop the mug into the microwave for 30 seconds.

★ A Sweet and Natural Hair Spray

Within a short time, residue from commercial hair sprays can build up in your hair, making it look dull and lifeless. Here's an all-natural, gunk-free alternative: Dissolve 1 tablespoon of sugar in 1 cup of hot distilled water, and mix in 1 tablespoon of vodka to act as a preservative. If you like a scented spray, wait until the water has cooled to room temperature, and add 3 to 5 drops of your favorite essential oil. Pour the potion into a plastic spray bottle, and use it as you would any other hair spray.

★ Super Sugar Hand Scrub

It always pays to have an extra-strength cleaner on hand for those times when work or play leaves you with grimy paws. To make one that's as gentle as it is hardworking, mix 2½ cups of white sugar, 1 cup of extra virgin olive oil, and 4 tablespoons of lemon juice to make a gritty paste. Pour it into a container with a tight-fitting lid, and stash it somewhere handy in your workshop, garden shed, or garage.

★ Remove a Fake Tan

Self-tanning products can give you a great faux glow—until it starts to fade, which leaves your skin dry, patchy, and flaky. You could resort to a commercial tan remover, or you could take a more natural approach. Mix 1 cup of raw sugar (available in health-food stores and some supermarkets) with ¾ cup of lemon juice. Rub the mixture over your skin, and leave it on for a few minutes. Rinse it off with warm water, and apply your usual moisturizer.

POTENT POTION

INTENSIVE MOLASSES HAIR CONDITIONER

This concentrated treatment works wonders for revitalizing dry, brittle, and heat-damaged hair.

3 tbsp. of cold-pressed sweet almond oil
1 tbsp. of blackstrap molasses
2 egg yolks
2 tsp. of aloe vera gel

Put the first three ingredients in a bowl, and whip vigorously with a wire whisk. Add the aloe and stir to form a smooth paste. Apply the mixture to your hair, and cover your head with a plastic shower cap, topped with a warm towel. Leave it on for 30 minutes or so, then rinse with warm water, and let your hair air-dry.

13 Lavender

If there's a lavender fan club in heaven, then its meetings must be real humdingers! Throughout the centuries, a motley crew of savvy folks ranging from Cleopatra and Pliny the Elder to Mary Magdalene and Queen Victoria have called upon, and treasured, lavender for its healing and beautifying powers. In recent years, lavender fell out of favor with the "in" crowd, who dismissed it as quaint and old-fashioned. But what goes around comes around. And today, thanks in large part to modern scientific research, this fragrant superstar is once again front and center on the health- and beauty-care stage.

Lusty Lavender

✔ Repel Mosquitoes

When skeeter season rolls around, keep the bloodthirsty bugs at bay with a coat of fragrant "armor." Mix 2 parts lavender oil (available in health-food stores and over the Internet) with 1 part rubbing alcohol in a plastic spray bottle, and spritz the potion onto your skin whenever you venture outdoors. You'll love the aroma, but mosquitoes won't go near it (or you)!

✔ When It's Too Late for That . . .

Lavender oil can reduce the itching, swelling, and redness of a mosquito bite. Just dab a drop or two on the affected area, and let it seep into your skin. Reapply as needed every six to eight hours until you feel relief.

✔ Say "Sayonara, Sunburn"

And "bye-bye" to other burns, too! Lavender oil is renowned for its ability to heal burns quickly and, often, with no scarring. Depending on the location and the extent of the burn, as well as your own personal preference, you have three excellent treatment options:

■ Fill a plastic spray bottle with cool water, add a few drops of lavender oil, and spritz the afflicted skin.

■ Dip a soft, clean cotton cloth into 1 quart of water with 5 or 6 drops of lavender oil mixed into it, and apply the compress to the burn site.

■ Mix 10 to 12 drops of lavender oil into a tub full of cool water, and soak in it for 20 minutes or so. **Note:** It goes without saying (I hope!) that this tip is intended for treating minor first-degree burns only. If your skin is broken or blistering, or the burn is on your face or covers a large part of your body, hightail it to the ER!

✔ Heal Burns from the Inside

Believe it or not, eating English lavender (*Lavandula angustifolia*) can help reduce the pain and speed the healing of burns, thanks to its potent load of analgesic, antibacterial, and anti-inflammatory compounds. The R_X from naturopathic physicians: Simply toss fresh or dried leaves, petals, and/or flower tips into salads, dressings, jams and jellies, soups and stews,

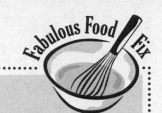
Fabulous Food Fix

BOUNTIFUL BREAKFAST SMOOTHIE

You couldn't ask for a tastier way to combine the healing power of lavender with the antioxidant punch of blueberries, bananas, and oranges.

1 cup of ice*
1 banana, peeled and sliced
1 can (14.5 oz.) of mandarin oranges, drained
1 cup of blueberries, fresh or frozen
½ cup of vanilla yogurt
2 tbsp. of honey
1 tbsp. of fresh lavender buds, chopped
½ cup of milk

Put the ice and fruits in a blender or food processor and process until finely chopped. Add the yogurt, honey, lavender, and milk and blend until smooth. Then drink up!

***Make-ahead tip:** Prepare the smoothie as directed, but omit the ice. Pour single-size servings into individual containers, and pop them into the freezer. Before bedtime, transfer one or more servings to the fridge, and they'll be thawed by morning.

YIELD: 5 (8-OUNCE) SERVINGS

POTENT POTION

LAVENDER BLISTER DUST

You never know where you'll be when blisters erupt on your hands or feet. So make up multiple batches of this remarkable remedy, and stash each container where you can grab it quickly when you need instant relief—whether you're mowing the lawn, hiking through the woods, or lining up a putt on the 15th hole.

Buds from 1 sprig of dried lavender, crushed*
4 tbsp. of cornstarch
4 drops of lavender oil

Mix all of the ingredients together, and store the mixture in an airtight container, where it will keep indefinitely. Then whenever the need arises, dip a cotton ball or swab into the mixture and dab it onto your blister(s).

* Either a coffee grinder or a mortar and pestle will do the job nicely.

YIELD: ABOUT ¼ CUP

vinegars, and wines—or drinks like the Bountiful Breakfast Smoothie (see page 169). **Note:** To retain the health-giving volatile oils of dried lavender, always store it in an airtight container in a cool, dark place (but not the fridge).

✔ Soothe Inflamed Skin

Whether the "culprit" that left your hands red, raw, and sore was a harsh cleanser or cold winter winds, this lovely lavender lotion will heal them in a jiffy. To make it, put ½ cup of dried lavender flowers and ½ cup of finely chopped fresh sage in a pan with 2 cups of water. Simmer, covered, on low heat for 20 minutes. Strain the liquid into a glass jar with a tight-fitting lid, let it cool, and add 8 drops of lavender oil. Put the lid on the jar, and shake it thoroughly to mix in the oil. Then gently smooth the lotion onto your skin with cotton pads or a soft cotton cloth. Repeat as needed until your hands are sore no more.

✔ Pack Up Poison-Plant Miseries

Sooner or later, just about everyone has a brush with poison ivy, oak, or sumac. So it pays to tuck this helpful hint into your memory bank (or write it down and keep the note in your medicine chest): Mix 3 drops of lavender oil with 1 tablespoon of apple cider vinegar, 1 tablespoon of water, and ½ teaspoon of salt. Then apply the mixture to the problem areas using a cotton ball. It'll ease the itch, dry out the rash, and prevent infection.

✔ Relieve Body Aches

When you go a little overboard at the gym or yank a few weeds too many out of your flower beds, don't pop pills to ease your pain. Instead, massage lavender oil into your sore joints and muscles. The oil's anti-inflammatory compounds will deliver deep-down relief. As a bonus, the lavender scent will relax you and might even take your mind off your aching body.

✔ Ease Aches from the Bottom Up

Believe it or not, soaking your feet in a lavender bath can pulverize muscle pain anywhere in your body. Just fill a basin with hot, but not scalding, water, and for every quart of H_2O, stir in 5 to 10 drops of lavender oil. Settle into a comfy chair, put your tootsies in the potion, and relax for at least 10 minutes. The fluid will get your blood flowing all through your system, just like an internal hot compress—and that's exactly what your muscles need for quick healing.

CAUTION ⚠️

For health and beauty purposes, *always* choose organically grown lavender or lavender oil that is labeled "food grade." Unless you're simply making potpourri or scented sachets, avoid the dried lavender that is sold in craft shops or on crafting websites. And never consume lavender flowers (or any other kind) that came from a florist or the supermarket's floral section. It's all but guaranteed that they've been sprayed with insecticides, fungicides, and/or chemical fertilizers.

✔ Conquer Coughing Fits

We've all been there: Your chest hurts like the dickens from nonstop coughing, and your airways are so congested that they seem to have solidified. That's when you need a lavender-eucalyptus chest rub. Mix 10 drops of lavender oil and 15 drops of eucalyptus oil with ¼ cup of olive oil, massage the potion onto your upper chest, and hop into bed. (Remember to put on an old T-shirt or pajamas to protect your sheets.) The lavender will relax your muscles and help battle the germs, while the eucalyptus will open your clogged breathing passages.

If you'd rather not go to bed with an oily chest, add 3 drops each of lavender and eucalyptus oils to a tub full of warm water, and soak for 10 minutes. You'll get the same benefits with none of the potential mess.

✔ Minimize Morning Sickness

As all you mothers and soon-to-be mothers know, your sense of smell becomes much more acute during pregnancy. Odors that you never even noticed before, like your dog's bed or a basket of dirty laundry, can send you rushing for a bucket. The solution: Arm yourself against trouble by carrying an aromatic antidote with you wherever you go. Either fill a small tin with dried lavender, or splash some lavender oil onto a handkerchief or bandanna, and keep it in your pocket. Then, whenever you catch a whiff of something that turns your stomach, pull out your fragrant defense mechanism, put it up to your nose, and breathe in deeply.

HEALTHFUL HINT
Breathe an Earache Away

There are plenty of things you can put in your ear to relieve an ache or infection, but lavender oil does the job through your nasal passages. Here's what you need to do: Pour 1 cup of boiling water into a heat-proof bowl, and add 3 to 5 drops of lavender oil. Hold a towel over your head and the bowl to make a tent, lean over the bowl (being careful not to burn yourself), and inhale for 5 to 10 minutes. Besides battling the infection and boosting your immune system, the lavender will help you relax—and that's a key factor in healing.

✔ Sanitize Your Hands

A little bottle of hand sanitizer is a mighty handy thing to tote around, especially during cold and flu season. But you don't need to buy a commercial product because it's a snap to make your own that's every bit as potent as the major brands, but free of chemicals and a lot better smelling to boot! Simply mix 2½ tablespoons of lemon-scented witch hazel, 1 tablespoon of tea tree oil, and 25 drops of lavender oil in a plastic spray bottle, and tuck it into your pocket, purse, or desk drawer. When the need arises, pull it out, spritz your hands a few times, and rub them together. **Note:** The ingredients have a tendency to separate, so you'll need to shake the bottle before each use.

✔ Inhale Asthma Away

Breathing in steam laced with lavender can also help stop an asthma attack. In this case, though, the delivery mechanism is a little different than it is for earache relief. At the first sign of symptoms, fill a pot with water, and for each quart, add 2 tablespoons of lavender flowers (fresh or dried). Boil the water, and inhale the rising steam. It will open your respiratory passages and relax your facial muscles in no time flat. Before you know it, you should be breathing freely again. **Note:** If you're having what you think is an asthma attack, and you are not already under medical care for the condition, call your doctor.

✔ Fight Finger Infections

Splinters, insect bites, and lesions of various kinds can all result in finger infections, but no matter what causes them, they're a lot like toothaches: Even when they're minor in nature, the pain they cause is way out of proportion to the size of the afflicted body part. The simple remedy: Boil 2 tablespoons of fresh or 1 tablespoon of dried lavender flowers in 1 quart of water for 10 minutes. Strain out the solids, let the potion cool to a comfortable temperature, and soak your sore digit for 5 to 10 minutes. Repeat the procedure several times a day until the problem is gone. **Note:** If you don't start to see progress after a few days, or if the infection reaches deep into your skin or the joints of your finger, get medical help.

Strike Oil

No medicine chest should be without lavender oil, so if yours is, go out and get a bottle now. You'll wonder how you ever got along without it. Don't believe me? Then just take a gander at some of the healing feats it can perform.

HEALTH PROBLEM	HOW TO SOLVE IT
Blisters	Apply 2 drops of lavender oil to a bandage and cover the blister with it.
Headaches	Put a drop of lavender oil on the tip of each index finger, and massage your temples with your fingertips for a minute or two.
Heat rash	Apply a drop or 2 of lavender oil directly onto the rash three or four times a day.
Stuffy nose	Put a drop of lavender oil under your tongue.
Weeping sores	Apply several drops of lavender oil to the sore throughout the day.*

* If your sore doesn't heal within a week, see your doctor.

✔ Lovely Lavender Tea

Lavender tea is a time-honored remedy for solving a boatload of health problems (see "Take Tea and See . . . ," below). The basic formula is the same as it is for any other herbal tea: 1 to 2 teaspoons of fresh or dried flowers (or more if you prefer a stronger brew) per cup of just-boiled water, with honey and/or lemon added to taste. But when you'll be taking multiple "cuppas" throughout the day for medicinal purposes, do yourself a labor-saving favor and make a batch of brew (by the quart) ahead of time. Then put it into the refrigerator, where it'll keep for three to four days, or freeze it in ice cube trays or plastic cups. When teatime rolls around, your potion will work the same magic, whether you warm it up, drink it cold, or eat it like an ice pop. Whatever you do, though, don't let this or any other herbal tea sit at room temperature for any length of time. Within a few hours, it'll start to go sour.

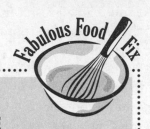

LAVENDER LEMONADE

You get all the health-giving power of lavender tea in this fresh twist on the classic summertime treat.

1 cup of fresh lavender flowers
2 cups of boiling water
2 cups of cold water
1 cup of fresh-squeezed lemon juice
1 cup of sugar
4 sprigs of fresh lavender

Put the lavender flowers in a heat-proof container, and pour in the boiling water. Cover the top with plastic wrap, and steep for 10 minutes. Strain the beverage into a pitcher, and add the cold water, lemon juice, and sugar, stirring until the sugar is dissolved. Refrigerate until chilled, pour into ice-filled glasses, and garnish each one with a lavender sprig.

YIELD: 4 (8-OUNCE) SERVINGS

✔ Take Tea and See . . .

How quickly and effectively lavender tea can perform heaping helpings of healing feats. Like these, for instance:

EASE ANXIETY. Drink 2 or 3 (or more) cups a day as needed to calm your nerves.

HEAL CUTS AND SCRAPES. Clean the wound, then dip a cotton ball or pad in lavender tea, and apply it to the "owie."

QUELL MIGRAINES AND HEADACHES. Sip the brew as needed throughout the day to tame the pain.

RELIEVE HEARTBURN AND INDIGESTION. Take 1 cup in the morning and another at bedtime.

STRENGTHEN YOUR GUMS. Swish room-temperature tea around in your mouth as you would any other mouth-wash. Used every day or two, it will make your gums stronger and health-ier—and sweeten your breath to boot!

VANQUISH VERTIGO. When a dizzy spell strikes, drink 3 or 4 cups a day until you're feeling steady on your feet again. **Note:** If you suffer from vertigo frequently for no apparent reason, it could indicate the presence of a seri-ous health problem, so see your doctor ASAP.

✔ Call It a Night

Studies have shown that consistently poor sleep can reduce your life span by (are you ready for this?) as much as 8 to 10 years. And we all know that even a few nights of tossing and turning can make you feel like a zom-bie—and act like one, too. Fortunately, no matter what's keeping you awake at night, the calming scent of lavender will beckon the sandman in a hurry. How you put that aromatic power to work is your call. Here are a few simple options:

■ Keep a vase of fresh or dried lavender on your bedside table.

■ Fill a small fabric pouch with dried lavender, and tuck it under your pil-low. Replace it when the scent fades.

■ On laundry day, put some dried lavender into a small zippered pillow-case or tightly closed cheesecloth bag, and toss it into the dryer with your bed linens. They'll emerge with a sleepy-time scent.

■ Pour cooled, strong lavender tea into a plastic spray bottle, and spritz your pillowcase and sheets. (Be sure you give them time to dry before you hit the sack.)

Looking for Stress Relief?

HEALTHFUL HINT

It's in your sock drawer. At least it can be if you try this terrific trick: Mix up equal parts of dried lavender, dried rosemary, and broken cinnamon sticks, all of which have aromas that are highly effective in lowering anxiety levels. Stuff a handful or so of the mixture into a clean sock until you have a ball that's about the size of a base-ball, and tie the top closed with yarn or ribbon. Then anytime you feel on edge, repeatedly squeeze the ball to release a blast of calm-ing scent. And if you keep this stress buster in your sock drawer, it'll remind you to start off every morning on an easygoing foot!

Lavender Loveliness

✤ Make White Flakes Flee

Dandruff got you down? Lavender oil can fix that in a jiffy. First, stir 15 drops of lavender oil into 2 tablespoons of olive oil, and microwave the mixture until it's lukewarm (about 10 seconds). Wet your hair with warm water, towel it dry, and massage the oil into your scalp. Pop on a shower cap, wait an hour or so, and then wash the oil out with your usual shampoo. Repeat two or three times a week until the flakes stop falling.

✤ Perfect Hair Perk-Me-Up

Refresh your hairdo and leave it smelling fresh at the same time with a gentle lavender spritzer. To make it, pour 4 cups of distilled water into a pot and bring to a boil. Add 3 drops of lavender oil, cover the pot, and remove it from the heat. Let the water cool, pour it into a plastic spray bottle, and use it whenever your hair needs a little pick-me-up.

POTENT POTION

COOLING SUMMER SKIN MIST
This antioxidant-packed potion will not only cool you down, but also protect your skin against the ravages of summer heat and junk-filled air.

1 cup of fresh lavender flowers
2 tbsp. of fresh peppermint leaves, chopped
4 tsp. of green-tea leaves
2 cups of distilled water, boiled
2 tsp. of aloe vera gel

Steep the first three ingredients in the freshly boiled water for 15 minutes. Strain out the solids and stir in the aloe vera gel. Pour the solution into a plastic spray bottle, and store it in the refrigerator. Spritz the potion onto your face and neck after cleansing, or anytime you feel the need to cool off.

YIELD: ABOUT 16 OUNCES

✤ Four Steps to Thicker, Softer Hair

The secret to this remarkable rinse lies in its all-star ingredient team: Lavender regenerates hair follicles, rosemary strengthens your hair shafts and helps them grow, vinegar strips out residue from styling products, and borax packs amazing softening power. Here's the DIY routine:

STEP 1. Gather the goods. You'll need ½ cup of dried lavender flowers, ½ cup of dried rosemary, 3 tablespoons of unfiltered apple cider vinegar, 1 teaspoon of borax, 4 cups of water, a large pot, and a 1-quart glass jar with a tight-fitting lid.

STEP 2. Bring the water to a boil, remove the pot from the stove, and stir in the vinegar and borax.

STEP 3. Add the lavender and rosemary, and mix until they're thoroughly wet. Cover the pot, and let it sit for at least two to four hours (longer if possible; the longer the potion steeps, the stronger it will be).

STEP 4. When the mixture has reached a caramel-brown color, strain out the herbs, pour the liquid into the jar, and tuck it into the fridge, where it will keep for up to two weeks.

To use your hair-improvement potion, shampoo as usual, then pour the rinse over your hair so that it's completely saturated. Rinse with clear water, and follow up with your normal drying and styling procedure. **Note:** You can omit the clear-water rinse if you like, but be aware that the brownish color may stain a light-colored towel.

✤ Rejuvenate Dry Skin

Whether your skin is naturally dry, or winter winds have left it chafed and irritated, there's an ultra-simple way to restore the moisture and relieve the irritation. What is it? Just stir 5 or 6 drops of lavender oil into a jar of your regular moisturizer, and smooth it on as usual.

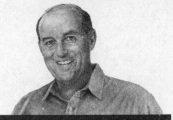

YOU DON'T SAY!

For many, if not most folks, the scent of lavender evokes thoughts of simpler, more innocent times. But lavender actually has quite a romantic (not to say racy) history. For instance, although Eve first enticed Adam with an apple, legend has it that the First Couple took lavender with them when they were banished from the Garden of Eden. Cleopatra wore lavender-scented perfume to seduce both Julius Caesar and Mark Antony. And now, we're seeing scientific evidence to back up the relationship between lavender and love. In a recent study by the Smell & Taste Treatment and Research Foundation, male subjects overwhelmingly found lavender to be one of the two most sexually arousing aromas of all. (The other was pumpkin pie—go figure!)

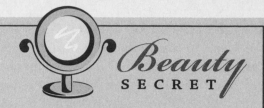

RELAX AND SOFTEN BATH BLEND

Combine the skin-softening power of milk and honey with the anti-inflammatory and relaxing properties of lavender, and what do you get? One delightful bathing experience—that's what! And it couldn't be simpler: Put 3 table- spoons of dried lavender flowers in a food processor or blender, and process them into a powder. Whisk it in a bowl with 1½ cups of whole milk and ⅓ cup of honey, and pour the mixture into a jar with a tight-fitting lid. At bath time, shake the jar to remix the ingredi- ents, pour half of the potion into the tub, and swish it around with your hand. Then hop in and soak your cares away. Store the leftover portion in the refrigerator, tightly covered, for up to a week.

✤ Scare Away Scarring

If you act quickly, lavender oil can reduce or even prevent the formation of scars. Immediately after an injury, proceed in whichever way you prefer:

■ Put a few drops of undiluted oil onto the wound.

■ Mix a few drops of lavender oil with a teaspoon or so of aloe vera gel, apply it to the injured skin, and cover it with a bandage.

✤ A Better Aftershave

Hey, guys—this tip is all yours! If you're tired of burning your freshly shaved skin with alcohol-based lotions, whip up this kinder, gentler alter- native: Mix 2 tablespoons of dried lavender flowers and 2 tablespoons of dried sage per 2 cups of witch hazel in a jar with a tight-fitting lid. Set the container in a very warm area for seven days, shaking it every day if you can. Strain out the solids, and pour the liquid into a bottle with a tight- fitting cap. Slap it on as you would any other aftershave. **Note:** Besides feeling and smelling great, the lavender will quickly heal any irritating razor nicks.

✤ It'll Suit You to a T

Lavender tea is just as good for the outside of your body as it is for the inside. Make it according to the instructions in "Lovely Lavender Tea" (see page 174). Then use it either as a stand-alone treatment or to prep your skin for one of the facial masks you'll find throughout this book. Whichever way you use the tea, dab it onto your face with a cotton pad, and let it air-dry. Or, to give your whole body a teatime treat, pour the potion into your bathwater. It'll soothe and cleanse your skin, reduce inflammation, and relax you all over.

✤ Instant Gratification

For those days when you need a nice soothing bath, but even brewing a cup of tea seems like too much of a hassle, opt for one of these more direct approaches:

■ Add 5 to 10 drops of lavender oil to a tub of water. (The temperature is your call.)

■ Stuff a cheesecloth pouch or old panty hose foot with fresh or dried lavender flowers, and toss it into the tub. **Note:** Never add lavender plant parts—or any other non-soluble substance—directly to your bathwater, or you'll wind up with a clogged drain.

Best of the Rest

★ Comforting Calendula Oil

If you grow calendulas (*Calendula officinalis*), a.k.a. pot marigolds, in your yard, you have the makings of a powerful, but oh-so-gentle—and oh-so-versatile—healer. It's terrific for treating minor cuts, scrapes, burns, and insect bites, and even massaging tired, achy muscles. To make a supply to keep in your medicine chest, follow this three-step procedure:

STEP 1. Put 5 cups of calendula blossoms in a pan, and pour in just enough extra virgin olive oil to reach 2 inches above the flowers.

STEP 2. Heat the mixture on low until it *almost* simmers. Let it continue to heat on low, uncovered, for six to eight hours, or until the oil has turned a deep golden-orange color and has a strong herbal aroma. (Just test for "doneness" every hour or so, and make sure the oil doesn't start to simmer.)

STEP 3. Remove the pan from the heat, and let the brew cool to room temperature. Strain it through cheesecloth or a sieve, and store it in a tightly capped bottle in the refrigerator. It'll keep for six months to a year.

★ Echinacea Evicts Cold Sores

Echinacea is renowned as a cold fighter, but it can also battle cold sores by boosting the antiviral immune fighters in your mucus membranes. The simple routine: Mix ¼ teaspoon of echinacea extract (available in health-food stores) in water or fruit juice, and drink it three times a day for as long as your symptoms last. **Note:** Do not use echinacea if you're pregnant or nursing, or if you have an autoimmune disease such as lupus, rheumatoid arthritis, or multiple sclerosis.

More Feverfew Equals Fewer Bee Stings

Correction: Make that *no* bee stings. Whether you're allergic to bee venom, or you simply want to keep the buzzers from spoiling your summertime fun, here's a tip that could make your backyard a safer and more pleasant place to hang out: Grow plenty of feverfew (*Tanacetum parthenium*) in your outdoor-living areas. Bees won't go anywhere near it. And don't worry that you'll be enhancing your safety at the price of downgrading the beauty of your landscape. On the contrary, this old-time perennial is one beautiful plant. It reaches about 2 feet tall; has lacy, light green leaves; and sports delicate, white, daisy-like flowers from early summer to early fall. It's hardy in Zones 5 to 9, and like most herbs, it's highly undemanding.

★ Feverfew Flattens Migraines

In numerous studies, it's proven effective in lessening the duration, severity, and frequency of migraine headaches as well as related symptoms such as dizziness, nausea, and vomiting. If you're prone to migraines, you can take your preventive medicine in one of two ways:

■ Eat one to four leaves of fresh feverfew each day.

■ Steep two to eight fresh leaves per cup of freshly boiled water for five minutes or so, and sip 1 or 2 cups of the tea each day.

Note: You may need to take feverfew for four to six weeks before you begin to see results.

★ Roses Ride to the Rescue

If you think roses are just beautiful flowers, think again. Those pretty petals are packed with plenty of healing power that can tackle a trio of common health problems. And here's more good news: The petals' medicinal power increases as the flowers fade, so you can make your "medicine" from blooms that you'd otherwise toss in the compost bin. Here's the scoop:

EASE JOINT PAIN (INCLUDING ARTHRITIS). Pull the petals from three or four over-the-hill roses, toss them into your bathwater, and settle in for a good soak. Just be sure to put a piece of cheesecloth or old panty hose over the drain, so you don't wind up with clogged plumbing!

SOOTHE A SORE THROAT. Make a concentrated tea using ¼ cup of petals per quart of water (see "Lovely Lavender Tea" on page 174), and drink 2 or 3 cups a day until you're feeling better.

STRENGTHEN WEAK, TIRED EYES. Throw a handful of faded petals into a pot, cover them with water, and bring to a boil over medium heat. Remove the pot from the stove, let the water cool, and strain out the petals. Soak a washcloth in the solution, and put it on your closed eyes for 15 to 30 minutes.

★ Calendula Conquers Foot Odor

Sweeten up your tootsies with an odor-fighting powder made from ¼ cup of finely chopped calendula flowers mixed with ¼ cup of arrowroot powder. Simply rub the combo into your skin, and sprinkle it between your toes.

POTENT POTION

MULTIPURPOSE MARIGOLD SALVE

This old-time country remedy is just the ticket for soothing all sorts of aches and pains, including bruises, varicose veins, and tired, burning feet.

1 cup of fresh marigold petals
½ cup of petroleum jelly

Put the petals and petroleum jelly in a pan, and cook on low heat for about 30 minutes. Strain the mixture through cheesecloth until it runs clear, and store in a glass jar with a tight-fitting lid. Just before you go to bed at night, massage the salve into your affected skin. Then, to keep the grease from staining your sheets, put on an old pair of soft cotton pajamas, or cover your bed with an old flannel sheet or blanket.

YIELD: ABOUT ½ CUP

★ Echinacea Ends Wrinkles

Well, not entirely, but these pretty purple coneflowers can protect the collagen that keeps your skin soft and vibrant, thereby lessening the onset of those crinkly lines. To make coneflower power work for you, put 1 teaspoon of dried echinacea flowers in a heat-proof bowl, pour 2 cups of freshly boiled water over them, and cover the bowl. When the tea has cooled to room temperature, soak a soft, clean washcloth in the brew, lay it over your face, and let the anti-aging fluid soak in for 5 to 10 minutes.

★ Super-Softening Body Oil

Roses and almond oil are both renowned for their ability to soften skin and reduce irritation. So get the dynamic duo on your beauty team with this simple formula: Put 1 cup of rose petals in a jar with a tight-fitting lid, crush them with a wooden spoon, and pour in 1 cup of almond oil. Cover and let the mixture sit for a week, then strain it into a clean container. Spread it all over your body when you step out of the shower. You'll feel— and smell—fabulous!

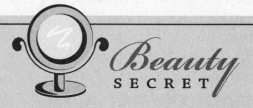

GRANDMA KNEW BEST

*Back in our grandmothers' day, rose water was a staple in every woman's beauty-care kit, and for good reason: It can purify and tone any type of skin, heal blemishes, hydrate dry skin, reduce redness and swelling, and do much more. You can buy rose water in health-food stores and over the Internet, but it's a snap to make your own. Just put 1 cup of rose petals into a heat-proof bowl, and pour in just enough boiling distilled water to cover them (about 2 cups). Cover the bowl, let the petals steep for 30 to 60 minutes, and strain the liquid into a bottle or jar. Store your rose water in the refrigerator, where it will keep for 7 to 10 days. **Note:** Rinse the petals well before you use them, and avoid any roses that have been sprayed with pesticides or foliar fertilizers.*

★ Shine Up Fair Hair

A calendula rinse makes blonde or light brown hair sparkle. Put 3 tablespoons of calendula flowers in a heat-proof container, and pour in 8 cups of just-boiled water. Let it steep, covered, until it cools to room temperature, then strain it through muslin or a superfine strainer. Shampoo your hair as usual, and massage the tea into your scalp as you rinse with it.

★ Put Rose Water to Work

Once you've made your rose water (see "Grandma Knew Best," at left), you can use it in the following ways:

■ Splash it on your face after cleansing.

■ Spray it on all over to cool and refresh your whole body.

■ Dab it onto your legs and underarms to soothe freshly shaved skin.

■ Pour ½ cup or so into your bathwater for a smoothing, softening soak.

★ Ravishing Rose Perfume

Why spend a fortune on perfume, when you can make your own for pennies? Just pack fragrant rose petals into a glass jar that has a tight-fitting lid, and pour in as much glycerin as the container will hold. (You can buy glycerin in health-food stores and most pharmacies.) Let it sit with the lid on for three weeks or so, then strain the liquid into a clean bottle with a tight-fitting cap.

POTENT POTION

ROSY VINEGAR SPLASH

The key to maintaining healthy, young-looking skin is water and plenty of it. In addition to drinking a steady supply of H_2O, using mildly astringent splashes like this one will help hydrate your skin, keeping it supple.

1 cup of rose petals
4 cups of white-wine vinegar,
    heated to near boiling
1 cup of rose water

Put the flowers in a sterilized glass jar,* pour in the vinegar, cover the jar with a lid or plastic wrap, and set it in a dark place at room temperature for 10 days, shaking it occasionally. Then strain the liquid into a fresh jar, and add the rose water. To use the potion, pour 1 tablespoon of it into a bowl, add 1 cup of warm water, splash it onto your face, and pat your skin dry.

* Fill the jar with boiling water, and let it sit for 10 minutes.

YIELD: ABOUT 5 CUPS

CHAPTER

14

Lemons

Lemons are nothing new on the healing scene. For thousands of years, they've been used for everything from soothing sore throats to lightening hair. What *is* new is that medical science has discovered just how crucial lemons are to our health and well-being. For one thing, they're packed with compounds called *phytochemicals* that are associated with the prevention and/or treatment of at least four of the leading causes of death in Western countries: cancer, cardiovascular disease, diabetes, and hypertension. What's more, although lemons are acidic, they increase the alkalinity of our bodily fluids—and an alkaline system is key to maintaining good health and good looks.

Lemon Aid

✔ Give a Headache the Heave-Ho . . .
And fast! How? Simply drink a cup of coffee with a few drops of fresh-squeezed lemon juice mixed into it. Sip it slowly, and before you know it, your headache will be history. **Note:** Do *not* use this remedy if you have a sensitive stomach!

✔ Conquer Cuts
When you cut yourself in the kitchen, help is close at hand. Slice a lemon in two, squeeze some juice onto the wound to disinfect it, then run cool

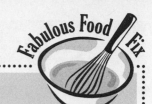

water over the area to stop the sting. Finally, sprinkle powdered cloves over the spot to reduce the pain and help the cut close up more quickly. **Note:** This treatment also works like a charm on paper cuts.

✔ A Glass a Day Keeps the Doctor Away

For generations of Americans, nothing has said—make that shouted—"Summertime!" like a tall, cold glass of lemonade. Well, it turns out that this sweet and tangy treat is a lot more than just a cooling beverage. Medical experts now tell us that drinking a glass of lemonade a day can help resolve or prevent a whole lot of health problems. Just take a gander at this (partial) list of fabulous feats:

■ Boost your immune system

■ Cleanse your system of toxins and impurities

■ Conquer cravings for cigarettes, alcohol, and junk food

■ Improve your mood

■ Increase your energy level

■ Prevent kidney stones

■ Protect against adult asthma and other respiratory ailments

■ Reduce acid reflux

■ Speed weight loss

For best results, make your own lemonade from scratch using fresh-squeezed lemon juice and sugar (see the Classic Lemonade recipe, at right).

CLASSIC LEMONADE

Whether you're making lemonade to address a specific medicinal purpose or simply to sip on your front porch as you watch the world go by, this is the ultimate, old-time recipe.

1 cup of water (for the simple syrup)
1 cup of sugar (or less to taste)
1 cup of fresh-squeezed lemon juice (4–6 lemons)
3–4 cups of cold water (to dilute)

Make a simple syrup by heating 1 cup of water in a pan, and then stirring in the sugar until it's dissolved. Mix the syrup and lemon juice in a pitcher, and add enough cold water to reach the desired strength. Refrigerate, covered, for 30 to 40 minutes. Then take a sip. If the lemonade is too sweet for your liking, add more lemon juice, and use less sugar next time. Serve it up in ice-filled glasses, garnished with lemon slices. **Note:** Feel free to multiply the ingredients if you're serving a crowd, but stick to the same proportions.

YIELD: 6 SERVINGS

POTENT POTION

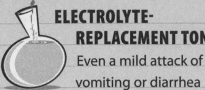

ELECTROLYTE-REPLACEMENT TONIC

Even a mild attack of vomiting or diarrhea whisks crucial fluids and electrolytes right out of a child's body. But this potion will put them back where they belong. Plus, it's healthier and a whole lot cheaper than commercial versions. By the way, adults will benefit from this tonic, too.

1 cup of warm water
2 tsp. of sugar
1 tsp. of sea salt
4 cups of lemon juice*

Pour the water into a jar or pitcher, add the sugar and salt, and stir until they're dissolved. Then mix in the lemon juice. Store the tonic, covered, in the refrigerator. After each occurrence of vomiting or diarrhea, pour 2 to 3 ounces of the tonic into a glass, and have the child sip it down.

* Preferably freshly squeezed, but in a pinch, frozen lemon juice will do.

YIELD: ABOUT 5 CUPS

✔ Stop Indigestion in Its Tracks

Spicy foods aren't the only kinds that cause acid indigestion. An overdose of sweet goodies can bring on that burning pain, too. Fortunately, there's a simple way to ease the discomfort. Just mix the juice of half a lemon in 1 cup of warm water, add ½ teaspoon of salt, and drink the potion slowly.

To treat chronic indigestion, drink the juice of one freshly squeezed lemon in a glass of lukewarm water after each meal. The lemon will stimulate the production of gastric juices and the activity of your stomach muscles.

✔ A Rummy Good Cold Stopper

If you enjoy a spot of rum now and then, you'll love this cold cure: At the first sign of symptoms, mix the juice of 1 lemon with 4 teaspoons of rum (either dark or light) and 3 teaspoons of honey. Pour the mixture into a glass of hot water, drink it down, and hop into bed. When you wake up, you should feel as fit as a fiddle.

✔ Give a Cold the Cold Shoulder

When you feel yourself coming down with a cold or flu, try this time-tested remedy: Fill your bathtub with water that's as hot as you can stand it. While the tub is filling, pour a jigger of scotch, rum, bourbon, or Irish whiskey into a glass of hot lemonade (preferably homemade using the recipe on page 185). Then ease into the tub and drink your hot toddy. When you're finished, dry off and dive into bed. Come morning, you'll be on top of the world again! **Note:** To avoid the risk of trading your cold symptoms for a bad cut, drink your tub-side tonic from a plastic glass.

✔ Calm a Sore Throat

Simply mix the juice of half a lemon and 1 teaspoon of pure maple syrup in 1 cup of warm water, and drink it down. It'll relieve the pain pronto. This same remedy loosens any mucus in your throat and nasal passages and cleanses your blood to boot!

✔ Bash Bronchitis

When a cold turns into bronchitis, and the tubes in your windpipe become so inflamed and swollen that breathing is a chore, reach for a lemon. Scrub it well, grate 1 teaspoon of the rind, and add it to 1 cup of just-boiled water. Let it steep for five minutes, and sip it down. It will help clear the mucus and bacteria out of your respiratory system. Repeat as needed throughout the day until you're breathing freely again. **Note:** Anytime you use citrus peels in an oral or topical remedy, opt for organic produce if at all possible. And, organic or not, always scrub the skins thoroughly (see "Scrub Pesticide Worries Away" on page 38).

✔ Nix the Nausea

The next time you feel as though you're going to vomit, mix a few drops of lemon juice, ½ teaspoon of sugar, and a pinch of baking soda in an 8-ounce glass of water. Drink it down, and heave a sigh of relief because the contents of your tummy will now stay right where they are.

Whoa, Charley!

HEALTHFUL HINT

There are few more annoying out-of-the-blue ailments than the shooting pain and stiffness of a charley horse. The next time you suffer an equine muscle attack, try this highly recommended healer: Chop three small lemons, two small oranges, and a small grapefruit, and toss them (peels and all) into a blender. Pulverize the fruits into a pulp, and mix in 1 teaspoon of cream of tartar. Pour the mixture into a jar with a tight-fitting lid, and store it in the refrigerator. Then take 2 tablespoons of the concoction mixed with 2 tablespoons of water twice a day, first thing in the morning and just before bedtime.

✔ Battle a Bladder Infection

If you've ever suffered from a bladder infection—or have one now—you know how important it is to drink plenty of water so that you can flush the impurities from your system. Well, here's a hot tip: You'll speed up that outflow and get back into the pink of health faster if you add a couple teaspoons of lemon juice to each glass of water.

✔ Purge Your Gallbladder

Your gallbladder's mission in life is to store the bile produced by your liver, largely to aid in the digestion of fats. But it doesn't always function smoothly, especially if you eat a lot of fatty foods. So if you wake up feeling tired and nauseated, there's a good chance that your gallbladder has gotten clogged with stale bile and other pollutants. The simple remedy: Take 3 tablespoons of lemon juice 15 to 30 minutes before breakfast each day for a week.

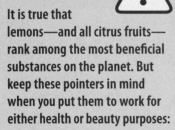

CAUTION

It is true that lemons—and all citrus fruits—rank among the most beneficial substances on the planet. But keep these pointers in mind when you put them to work for either health or beauty purposes:

■ The high citric acid content in lemons produces an intense reaction to light called photosensitivity. So in order to avoid a nasty burn, stay out of the sun for at least an hour after you've applied lemon juice, or any commercial lemon-based product, to your skin.

■ More is not always better. In particular, if you have sensitive teeth, go easy on citrus fruits and juices because they can aggravate your condition.

✔ Heal Hemorrhoids

There are scads of folk remedies for hemorrhoids, but legions of folks swear by this old-time favorite: Mix the juice of half a lemon in 1 cup of warm water, and add ¼ teaspoon of ground nutmeg. Drink the potion twice daily. It works its magic by shrinking the swollen blood vessels that cause the pain and itching, so you should be sitting pretty again in no time flat.

✔ Quick and Easy Does It

When you're wielding a weapon as powerful as a lemon, it doesn't take much to make a big difference in your health. Just look at some of the pesky problems a lemon wedge or a few drops of fresh-squeezed lemon juice can help you solve—*fast*.

BEE STINGS. First, get the stinger out, and then squeeze a few drops of lemon juice onto the sting site. If you've responded quickly enough, you'll head off any pain and swelling.

COLD SORES. Dab a little lemon juice on them. Yes, it will burn at first, but your discomfort will only last a few seconds, and the sores will soon be gone.

HICCUPS. Tuck a thin slice of lemon under your tongue. Suck it once, hold the juice for 10 seconds, and then swallow it (the juice, not the lemon). Your hiccups will be history!

MOTION SICKNESS. Whenever you head off on a car or boat trip, take along a supply of lemon wedges. Then, at the first sign of queasiness, pull out a wedge and suck on it for a minute or two. That should chase the butterflies away.

Boost Iron Intake

HEALTHFUL HINT

We all know that it's important for women of childbearing age to have a steady supply of iron in their diets. But teenage girls are at ultra-high risk for iron-deficiency anemia—especially those who have gone vegetarian or decided that they absolutely must lose a few pounds to fit into their size 1 jeans. If you have a daughter or granddaughter who falls into this category, here's one way to help her meet her iron quota: Serve her plenty of iron-rich, leafy greens, and douse them generously with lemon juice. Besides perking up the flavor, the lemon will help liberate the minerals, thereby enabling her body to absorb the iron more efficiently.

NOSEBLEED. Saturate a cotton ball with lemon juice, and gently insert it into the bleeding nostril. The flow should stop instantly.

TIRED, STRAINED, OR BURNING EYES. Mix a drop of lemon juice and 4 tablespoons of distilled water (not tap water!) in an eyecup. Wash your eyes with the solution, and you'll be back in business again.

✔ Corns, Be Gone

These annoying, often painful bumps are no match for lemon power. You can put it to work in a couple of ways:

■ Before you go to bed, place a slice of fresh lemon peel (white side down) over the toughened skin, and secure it with a bandage. Leave it on overnight, and remove it in the morning.

■ Dab lemon juice directly onto the corn several times a day.

In each case, repeat the treatment until your C-lumps are gone. (It shouldn't be long.)

POTENT POTION

CITRUS-POWERED TOOTH POWDER

This old-time formula will keep your gums and teeth clean, healthy, and sparkling white.

¼ cup of baking soda

2 tbsp. of dried, grated lemon and/or orange rind*

2 tbsp. of sea salt or kosher salt

Put all of the ingredients in a food processor, and process until you have a fine powder. Store it at room temperature in an airtight tin or jar. To use, pour out a small amount in the palm of one hand, dip your wet toothbrush into it, and go to town.

* Grate off only the top, colored layer of the skin, avoiding the white pith below. Transfer the gratings to a plate, and let them dry overnight, or until they are thoroughly dry. While you're at it, make an extra supply, and store it in a jar with a tight-fitting lid in a cool, dark place. That way, it'll be close at hand for use in other health and beauty treatments.

YIELD: ½ CUP

✔ Cut Your Risk of Skin Cancer

A study at the Arizona Cancer Center found that regularly drinking black tea with lemon slices added to it may reduce your lifetime risk of developing squamous cell skin cancer by (are you ready for this?) as much as 70 percent. Scientists speculate that the secret lies in d-limonene, an antioxidant in lemon peels that has been proven to kill cancer cells. So do as our English cousins do, and always take time for tea. Just remember, this is *not* intended as a substitute for sunscreen!

✔ Sniff Asthma Away

Studies show that the limonene in citrus peels seems to neutralize inhaled ozone, which often triggers asthma attacks. So if you're troubled by this nasty condition, grab a C-fruit (any kind will do), peel off the colorful skin, and sniff it early and often!

✔ Keep Your Gums Healthy

Lemon peel contains compounds that fight gum disease and whiten your choppers at the same time. The simple routine: Cut a wedge of the fruit, remove the skin, and wipe the inside of the peel over your teeth and gums. **Note:** Limes and oranges also perform the same dandy dental work.

Your Lemon-Fresh Looks

✤ Ward Off Warts

There must be a gazillion folk remedies for getting rid of warts, but one of the most popular is plain old lemon juice. Just dab it onto the offending site until the acids in the juice dissolve the unsightly growths.

✤ Eliminate Blackheads

Straight lemon juice is just what the beauty doc ordered for combating blackheads and pimples. At bedtime, rub lemon juice onto your affected skin. In the morning, wash your face with cool water and apply a rich moisturizer. Repeat the procedure for three or four evenings in a row, and you should see a major improvement in your complexion.

✤ Eradicate Acne

You can heal acne by dabbing lemon juice onto the spots. But if the condition covers a large area of skin, or if you (or your teenagers) have recurring problems, opt for this gentler approach: Combine equal parts of fresh-squeezed lemon juice and rose water, and smooth the mixture onto your skin: Leave it on for at least 30 minutes, and then wash it off with luke-warm water. Perform this routine in the morning and evening. **Note:** You can buy rose water in health-food stores and herb shops, but it's easy to make your own supply (see "Grandma Knew Best" on page 182.)

✤ Make Freckles and Age Spots Disappear

To get rid of these flatter, but just as bothersome, blemishes, dissolve a pinch of sugar in 2 tablespoons of lemon juice, and rub the mixture onto each blotch with a cotton ball or swab. Repeat the procedure every day until the spots have lightened up.

❖ It Takes Two to Tango

Rather, it takes these two natural beauty aids to both tone and soften your skin. Beat one large egg white until it forms peaks, and then fold in the juice of half a lemon. Spread the concoction onto your face and neck. Wait 20 minutes, and rinse it off with cool water. Pat dry, then use a cotton pad to dab on a little witch hazel.

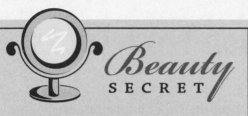

Beauty SECRET

AN EASY EVERYDAY ASTRINGENT

Lemon juice is one of Mother Nature's most powerful astringents, and it's fine to use it straight for jobs like spot-treating acne or blackheads. But it's too strong to use for a prolonged period of time. That's where this recipe comes in. It will invigorate and balance your skin, remove impurities, and unclog your pores. Plus, it's gentle enough to use every day! To make it, simply mix ½ cup of lemon juice, 1 cup of distilled water, and ⅔ cup of witch hazel in a clean bottle with a tight-fitting lid. Shake it well before each use, and apply the toner to your freshly washed face using a cotton ball or pad.

❖ Smooth Wrinkles

You don't need an expensive wrinkle-fighting cream to "iron out" your signs of experience. All you need is a trio of kitchen staples: 1 cup of milk, 2 tablespoons of lemon juice, and 1 tablespoon of brandy. Mix them in a saucepan, bring the combo to a boil, then remove the pan from the heat. When the mixture has cooled to room temperature, gently apply it to your crinkly lines. Let it dry thoroughly, then wipe it off with lukewarm water. Repeat the process every week or so to keep your skin youthful and vibrant.

❖ Ultra-Simple Facial Cleanser

Multi-ingredient DIY beauty treatments and leave-on masks are great, but who has time to fuss with them every day? Not many women I know—that's for sure! This recipe, on the other hand, takes just seconds to make, and you don't have to let it "cook" on your face. Just mix 1 tablespoon of dried, ground lemon and/or orange peels with enough plain yogurt to make a paste. (If you have dry skin, substitute olive or vegetable oil for the yogurt.) Then wash your face with the mixture, rinse with cool water, and pat dry. That's all there is to it! **Note:** For the scoop on grating and grinding citrus peels, see Citrus-Powered Tooth Powder on page 190.

❖ Terrific Treatment for Troubled Skin

If you're fighting rough, blemished skin, this is the mask for you. Grind ½ cup of uncooked oatmeal in a blender or coffee grinder, and mix it with 3 to 4 tablespoons of fresh-squeezed lemon juice. (Add a few drops at a time until you've got a smooth paste.) Apply it to your face, avoiding the area around your eyes. Let the mask dry, then rinse it off with warm water, and follow up with your usual moisturizer. The oatmeal will slough off dry, dead skin, and the lemon juice will reduce the appearance of dark spots as well as cleanse and purify your skin.

❖ Moisturize All Over

Here's a routine that'll moisten your skin from the tip of your nose to the tips of your toes. First, mix 1 tablespoon of fresh-squeezed lemon juice with ½ cup of baby oil, and set the mixture aside. Next, soak in a nice warm bath for 10 to 15 minutes (this will open your skin's pores in preparation for the treat that follows). Step out of the tub, and gently massage the lemony oil into your damp skin, beginning with your face and working all the way down to your feet. You'll feel soft and smooth all over.

POTENT POTION

VARIATIONS ON A THEME OF BEAUTIFUL

This fabulous facial mask works for any skin type—with one variation.

Juice of 1 lemon
1 egg*
¼ cup of nonfat dry milk
1 tbsp. of scotch, Irish, bourbon, or rye whiskey

Mix all of the ingredients together in a container with a tight-fitting lid. Smooth the mixture over your face, avoiding the eye area. Let it dry, and remove it with a warm, wet washcloth. Use it once a week or so to keep your skin soft, supple, and nourished.

* Here's the variation: For normal skin, use the whole egg; for dry skin, use only the yolk; and for oily skin, use only the white.

Fabulous Food Fix

LEMON-FRESH SMOOTHIE

In addition to skin-pleasing vitamin C, lemons contain phytochemicals (including some found in no other fruits) that help prevent cell damage. For that reason, many nutritionists recommend adding half a lemon to every smoothie, not only to bring out the full flavors of the other ingredients, but also to deliver a powerful passel of beauty (and health) benefits. Here's one of my favorite recipes.

2 cups of fresh baby spinach*
1 cup of honeydew melon, chopped
1 pear, sliced
½ lemon, peeled and sliced
1–2 tbsp. of chopped fresh mint to taste
½ cup of water

Place all of the ingredients in a blender, process until smooth, and drink to your good health and good looks.

* Or substitute other dark leafy greens of your choice.

✤ Soften Your Tootsies

Treat your cracked, dry feet to this enriched moisturizing formula: Combine 1 tablespoon of lemon juice with 1 ripe, mashed banana, 2 tablespoons of honey, and 2 tablespoons of soft margarine. Stir the ingredients until the texture is creamy, then massage the mixture onto your clean, dry feet. Pull on a pair of cotton socks, and head to bed. Come morning, rinse the stuff off. Repeat as needed until your feet are silky smooth and sandal-ready.

✤ A Penny-Pinching Pedicure

Why dump double-digit dollars on a beauty salon pedicure, when you can treat yourself to a refreshing, pre-exfoliating foot soak for a fraction of the price? Here's the routine: Fill a pan or foot basin with 10 cups of hot water, and mix in the juice of two freshly squeezed lemons, 1 cup of apple cider vinegar, and ½ cup of sea salt. Soak your dogs for about 15 minutes, pat dry, and use a pumice stone to slough off any dead or flaky skin. Then either hop into the shower to rinse off the salad-dressing aroma, or follow up with the "Sweet Treat Scrub," below.

✤ Sweet Treat Scrub

Your hands, feet, elbows, and knees work hard for you, day after day . . . after day. It's no wonder they get tired and rough. So deliver a big "Thank you!" with this refreshing, softening scrub. To make it, mix the juice of half a lemon, ½ cup of brown or raw sugar, and 2 tablespoons of almond oil in a bowl. If you like, add a few drops of essential oil.

Massage the mixture thoroughly onto your needy body parts, then rinse it off with warm water, and slather on body lotion to seal in the moisture.

❖ Show Dandruff the Door

Troubled by dandruff? Reach for the lemon juice. Apply 1 tablespoon of it to your hair, then shampoo as usual, and rinse with clear water. Rinse again, this time using a mixture of 2 tablespoons of lemon juice and 2 cups of water. Repeat every other day until the white flakes flee for good.

❖ Quick Fix for Oily Hair

Hair treatments don't come any faster or easier than this one: Mix 2 parts lemon juice with 1 part water, dip your comb into the solution, and run it through your hair. It'll remove excess oil without drying out your scalp.

POTENT POTION

SIMPLY CITRUS HAIR SPRAY

Tired of store-bought hair sprays that build up over time and leave gunky residue in your hair? Then try this pure and simple alternative.

1 lemon or orange, chopped but not peeled*
2 cups of distilled water
¼ cup of gin or vodka
6–8 drops of your favorite essential oil (optional)

Put the fruit into a small pan with the water. Bring it to a boil over medium-high heat, and continue boiling until the liquid is reduced by half. Strain the liquid into a measuring cup, and if necessary, add enough water to measure 1 cup. Let the potion cool to room temperature, and stir in the gin or vodka and, if desired, the oil. Pour the concoction into a spray bottle, store it at room temperature, and use it as you would any other hair spray.

* Lemon can lighten your hair when it's exposed to sunlight, so if your hair is dark and you want to keep it that way, opt for an orange in this formula.

YIELD: ABOUT 10 OUNCES

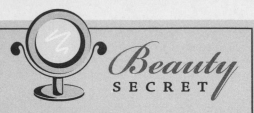

Beauty SECRET

FIGHT YELLOW WITH YELLOW

Prolonged exposure to sunlight, wearing nail polish for too long, and smoking can all turn your fingernails yellow. Fortunately, there's a lovely lemony solution. Just fill a shallow bowl with enough lemon juice to cover your fingernails, and soak them for five or six minutes. Then wash and rinse your hands, and apply your favorite moisturizer. Repeat the treatment once a day (or as close to it as your schedule allows). You should start seeing results in five to seven days. **Note:** *In this case, it's fine to use bottled or frozen lemon juice if you don't have fresh lemons on hand. Before you proceed, though, make sure your fingers are free of cuts or scrapes, or you'll get a stinging surprise!*

❖ Summerize Your Shampoo

Harsh sun, high temperatures, and muggy air—not to mention salt water and swimming-pool chlorine—can all leave your hair in need of a little extra TLC in the summertime. But that doesn't mean dropping big bucks at the beauty parlor. Instead, simply add 1 tablespoon of lemon juice and 1 teaspoon of aloe vera gel to your regular shampoo, and use it in the usual way. Your locks will stay clean, shiny, and bouncy all season long.

❖ Good Riddance to Body Odor

There's nothing more embarrassing than body odor. Fortunately, there's an ultra-easy way to flush out the toxins that cause the stink: Just drink at least eight glasses of water a day. And to make your deodorizing routine even more effective, every evening, add 1 teaspoon or so of fresh lemon juice and 1 teaspoon of chlorophyll (available in health-food stores) to your glass. This will help adjust the pH imbalance of your blood, which intensifies body odor, and also help get rid of odor-causing "bad" bacteria in your gut.

❖ Good Riddance to Breath Odor, Too!

Insufficient salivation or steady consumption of substances like alcohol, cigarettes, and certain spices can result in chronically sour breath. If your lifestyle has landed you with this problem, rinse your mouth several times a day with the freshly squeezed juice of one lemon mixed in a glass of lukewarm water. And do everything you can to kick your bad habits!

✣ Toughen Your Fingernails

All kinds of things, ranging from household cleaners to cold air, can draw moisture out of your fingernails, leaving them weak and brittle. Put the moisture and the strength back into them this way: Combine 1 tablespoon of fresh-squeezed lemon juice and 3 tablespoons of olive oil in a bowl, and heat the mixture until it's lukewarm. At bedtime, use a cotton swab to brush it onto each nail, including the underside and the surrounding cuticles. Put on a pair of soft, clean cotton gloves, and hit the sack. Repeat the procedure each night, until your "claws" are in fighting form again. **Note:** To avoid contamination from bacteria in your hands and fingers, make a fresh batch of strengthener each night. Also, if you don't start to see improvement within a couple of weeks, call your doctor. Fingernail problems can sometimes indicate an underlying health condition.

✣ Clean Your Hands

Whether your "paws" are stained from picking berries or aromatic from chopping onions or garlic, lemon can solve that problem lickety-split. Just wipe undiluted lemon juice onto your skin. Leave it on for a few minutes, then wash your hands with warm, soapy water. Repeat the process as necessary until the unwanted color or scent is gone.

Best of the Rest

★ Stop a Throbbing Headache . . .

And I mean *instantly*! How? Slice a lime in two, and rub one of the cut surfaces across your aching forehead. Zap—end of pain! **Note:** If this doesn't work and the ache continues for two days or more, call your doctor.

★ Lime Juice Dries Up Diarrhea

When you're rammed with a case of the runs, squeeze two or three limes, and pour the juice into an 8-ounce glass. Add enough water to fill it, and

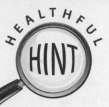

HEALTHFUL HINT

Super Citrus Cold Fighter

Talk about tasty medicine! This germ basher is so delicious that you might be tempted to fake a cold just to have an excuse to drink it! To make it, warm the juices of a grapefruit, a lemon, and an orange in a pan over medium heat. Stir in 1 tablespoon of raw honey, bring the mixture to a boil, and remove the pan from the heat. Let it cool a little, then pour it into a glass, and add a jigger of your favorite liquor. Toss the potion back, then crawl into bed and go to sleep. When you wake up, your cold will have flown the coop! **Note:** If you're taking drugs of any kind, speak with your doctor before you use this remedy. Grapefruit juice interacts with many prescription and OTC medications.

stir in 3 teaspoons or so of cornstarch (more if your "plumbing" is especially energetic). Add sugar to taste if you like, and drink up. Repeat once or twice if you need to (but you probably won't).

★ Sip a Sore Throat Away

There are scads of sore throat remedies, but this is one of the best tasting that I've ever found: Mix the juice of 1 freshly squeezed lime with 1 tablespoon of pineapple juice and 1 teaspoon of honey in a glass of water, and drink it down.

★ A Morning-After Cocktail

Don't get me wrong—I'm not suggesting that you try the old "hair of the dog" cure for a hangover! Instead, prop yourself up at the kitchen counter, and squeeze a glass of fresh orange juice. Then mix in 1 teaspoon of fresh-squeezed lime juice and a pinch of cumin, and drink up. You should be back in the land of the living in no time at all.

★ Orange Aid for Troubled Tummies

When a bout of nausea or stomach flu strikes, mix ½ cup of fresh-squeezed orange juice, 2 tablespoons of clear corn syrup, and a pinch of salt in ½ cup of water. Store the potion in a covered jar in the refrigerator, and take 1 tablespoon every half hour or so until your queasiness is gone.

★ Take Tangerine Tea . . .

And watch body aches flee. For many, if not most folks, the worst thing about the flu isn't coughing and congestion—it's the nonstop aching of every cell in your body. This remarkable remedy can help. Chop or coarsely shred the peel from three tangerines, toss the pieces into 1 quart of water, and bring it to a boil. Remove the pan from the heat, let the brew steep for an hour or so, then strain out the peel. Pour the tea into a container with a tight-fitting lid, and store it in the fridge. Drink a warmed-up "cuppa," sweetened with honey to taste, every five hours until you're ache-free.

★ Tangerines Cut Gas Emissions

If your system expels excess gas in burps and belches, rather than sending it out from the other end of your body, let tangerine tea fix the problem. Make it as described at left (see "Take Tangerine Tea . . . "), and sip it as needed. (By the way, if you're a collector of old folk remedies, this one definitely belongs in your archives: It dates back to the Taoists in the 6th century BC.)

★ Cellulite: It's a Wrap

Troubled by cellulite? Then try this copycat version of the herbal wraps that many fancy spas use: Mix ½ cup of grapefruit juice and 2 teaspoons of dried thyme with 1 cup of corn oil. Massage the mixture into your thighs, hips, and buttocks. Cover the area with plastic wrap, and hold a heating pad over each body part for five minutes. Repeat once a week or so, and after several treatments, you should see a definite improvement in your "cottage cheese" skin.

★ Put on Your Lime and Go to Sleep

Lime and milk team up in an overnight whole-body moisturizer that can't be beat. Just before you go to bed at night, bring 1 cup of milk to a boil, and mix in 1 teaspoon of glycerin and the freshly squeezed juice of 1 lime. Let the mixture cool to room temperature, then massage it into your face,

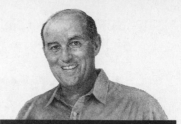

YOU DON'T SAY!

You probably know that the color orange was named after the fruit, and not the other way around. But how did the fruit get its name? According to a centuries-old legend recounted in *A History of Food* by Maguelonne Toussaint-Samat, it all started in ancient times when a hungry elephant came upon a tree filled with tempting golden fruit. He ate so much that he burst. Centuries later, a traveler found the fossilized remains of the poor pachyderm. Out of what had been the elephant's stomach had grown a cluster of trees covered with golden fruit. The astonished man exclaimed, "What an amazing *naga ranga!*" (which in Sanskrit means "fatal indigestion for elephants"). The trees acquired the name *naga ranga*, which became the Latin word *aurantium*, from which the English word *orange* is derived.

hands, and feet and hop under the covers. Store any extra moisturizer, tightly covered, in the refrigerator, and use it within a week or so.

★ Three for the Money

Whip up a triple-treat face cream that will remove makeup and clean and soften your skin. Mix the juice of 1 lime with ½ cup of mayonnaise (the full-strength kind, made with eggs and oil) and 1 tablespoon of melted butter (not margarine). Store the cream in a glass jar with a tight-fitting lid in the refrigerator. Use it as you would any facial cleanser, then rinse with cold water, and follow up with your usual moisturizer.

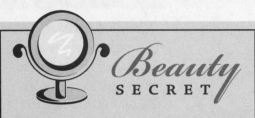

Beauty
S E C R E T

HEIRLOOM HAIR LIGHTENER

If you want to make your hair a few shades lighter, don't rush off to the beauty parlor and pay big bucks for a bleach job. Instead, whip up a concoction that beauty-conscious (and thrifty) women have been using for eons. Just mix the freshly squeezed juice of 2 limes and 1 lemon with 2 tablespoons of mild shampoo. Pour the solution onto your hair, massage it in, and go sit in the sun for 15 to 20 minutes. (Don't forget your sunscreen!) Then rinse thoroughly, and follow up with a good conditioner. Repeat the process as often as needed until you think you're blonde enough to have more fun!

★ Orange and Cornmeal Scrub

The orange in this delightful cleanser gives your skin a softening, wrinkle-fighting antioxidant kick, and the cornmeal leaves it smooth and free of dead skin. The simple formula: Mix the freshly squeezed juice of half an orange with enough cornmeal to make a paste (about ¼ cup should do the trick). Massage it onto your face and neck for three minutes or so, and rinse it off with warm water. Follow up with your usual moisturizer.

★ Cool Off and Wake Up

How would you like a facial mask that nourishes your skin, cools you off, and invigorates you all over? You've got it. Mix the juice of ¼ of an orange (about 2 tablespoons) with 1 teaspoon of plain yogurt. Smooth the mixture onto your face with your fingers, wait five minutes, and rinse. That's all there is to it!

★ Sock It to Stress

If stress and tension are your problems, here's the perfect solution: First, wrap a few chamomile tea bags in a panty hose leg or a piece of gauze, and cut an orange into thin slices. Suspend the tea pouch under your bathtub spigot, and let warm water flow over it. Float the orange slices in the water, climb into the tub, and soak your troubles away. **Note:** Be sure to cover the drain opening with gauze or a piece of panty hose, so the slices don't clog up your plumbing.

★ An A-Peeling Body Scrub

There's no doubt about it: Sugar- and salt-based body scrubs are effective, but when you don't have time to put one together—or you just don't feel inclined to slather on a grainy, potentially messy concoction—grab an orange. Peel it, and wrap the rind in a large piece of gauze or cheesecloth. Then hop into the shower, and rub the scrubber all over your body. The acid and vitamin C in the peel will firm and tone your skin.

POTENT POTION

CREAMY ORANGE FACIAL SPREAD

This sweet blend of goodness softens, "feeds," and helps detoxify your skin. Plus, it's so safe, you could eat it. Try it—you'll love it!

2 sections of a navel orange, peeled and chopped
2 oz. of full-fat cream cheese, softened
1 tsp. of honey
½ tsp. of fresh-squeezed lemon juice

Put all of the ingredients into a food processor, blend until the concoction has a soft, spreadable texture, and scrape it into a bowl. Apply a thin layer of the spread to your face and neck, and leave it on until it's hardened (15 minutes or so). Rinse it off with warm water, follow up with a few splashes of cold H_2O to close your pores, and gently pat dry. If there's anything left in the bowl, spread it on a toasted bagel, and enjoy!

15

Nuts

Back when fat phobia was sweeping the country, nuts became about as desirable as lumps of coal in a Christmas stocking. Now, though, nuts—from teeny-tiny pistachios to great big coconuts— rank high on every nutritionist's list of superfoods. That's because research has shown that nuts (including peanuts) contain vitamins, minerals, and plant compounds that help lower cholesterol, ward off cancer and heart disease, improve brain function, fight fatigue, and much more. Of course, any food that improves your health also improves your looks, so natural-beauty pros have added nuts (and nut oils) to their all-star rosters, too!

Say "Nuts" to Good Health

✔ Curb Your Appetite

Yes, while it's true that nuts are high in fat, much of it is monounsaturated (a.k.a. good) fat that fills you up without filling you out. In fact, studies show that folks who eat a handful of nuts each day are much less likely to be severely overweight than those who don't. The operative word here is *handful*—if you overindulge, you'll pack on the pounds.

✔ Don't Have a Heart(burn)

A natural chemical in almonds helps strengthen the sphincter that separates your esophagus from your stomach. And the stronger that muscle is, the better able it is to keep acid in your tummy where it belongs, instead of letting it seep upward. Your "workout" routine: Eat 10 raw almonds after each meal and snack.

✔ Beat the Blues

Feeling down in the dumps? Then reach for the nuts that are shaped like little smiles: cashews. Natural-health experts tell us that these tasty nuts work just as well as, if not better than, prescription antidepressants such as Prozac®. The secret lies in tryptophan, an amino acid that helps boost your mood, stabilize your thoughts, and produce a general mellow feeling. A large handful of cashews contains 1,000 to 2,000 milligrams of trypto-phan. Best of all, because nuts are food, and not drugs, they solve the problem at its root, rather than just temporarily removing your symptoms. Plus, the only side effect you'll have will be better health!

✔ More Mood Boosters

Cashews aren't the only nuts that can perform "funkectomies." Two other kinds are also highly effective at lifting low spirits:

Fabulous Food Fix

ANTI-ANXIETY PUNCH

No matter what's causing your stress level to soar toward the stratosphere, this relaxing (and tasty) beverage can help calm your turbulence.

10 raw almonds
Water
1 cup of warm milk
1 pinch of ginger
1 pinch of nutmeg

Put the almonds in a bowl with enough water to cover them, and let them soak for six to eight hours. Then liquefy them in a blender with the milk and spices, and drink the potion just before you go to bed. It should help you sleep soundly and wake up ready to face the day on a more even keel.

■ Brazil nuts are one of Mother Nature's best sources of selenium, a mineral that is likely to be lacking in your system if you're feeling depressed, anxious, irritated, and tired for no apparent reason. (Studies show that most people today are deficient in selenium.) Simply eating three Brazil nuts a day will provide your recommended daily dose of this essential nutrient.

■ Walnuts are high in serotonin, which has been shown to help lift your spirits when you're suffering from seasonal affective disorder (SAD), or simply battling a case of the blahs. The easy R_X: When you're going through a blue phase, eat a handful of walnuts every day or so.

Note: If you're suffering from severe depression, don't bother dosing yourself with nuts or any other homemade healer—get professional help ASAP!

✔ Coconut for Calm and Contentment

You don't have to be unhappy to feel the effects of stress. Whether your nerves are frayed from a long day at the office, a clogged rush-hour commute, or a mad dash to finish your Christmas shopping, coconut oil can help. Simply dip your finger into the jar, and massage a small amount onto your forehead and temples using circular motions. The soothing aroma of the oil combined with the gentle pressure of your fingertips will have you feeling better in no time at all.

✔ Cure a Headache

Almonds and walnuts are both packed with pain-relieving compounds that function much like aspirin—without any of the potential side effects. So the next time you feel that old familiar throbbing, grab a handful of nuts, and munch away!

✔ Relieve Migraines

As strange as this nut remedy may sound, it's powerfully effective for relieving the agony of a migraine attack. Put 2 tablespoons of pecans and 2 tablespoons of walnuts in a blender, and mix them with just enough water to make a thick puree. (Add the water a teaspoon at a time until you get the right

---

HEALTHFUL HINT

From Little Acorns . . .

Comes big relief for burns and poison-plant rashes. Long before commercial medications came along, the Iroquois Indians made a highly effective healer from the nuts of the oak tree. Centuries later, it still works. The updated formula: Put two dozen or so cracked acorns in a pot with 1½ gallons of water and boil, uncovered, until the H_2O is reduced by half. Then strain out the solids, and pour the liquid into sterilized, sealed quart jars (clamp-lidded canning jars are perfect). Store them in a cool place, and when the need arises, gently wash the affected skin with the healing water several times a day. **Note:** The Iroquois cracked their acorns using the blunt end of a tomahawk, but you'll probably want to use a nutcracker. No nutcracker? Then put the acorns in a plastic bag, and tap them with a hammer.

consistency.) Spread the mixture on two squares of gauze, and tape one to each of your temples. Then lie down in a comfortable spot for a few hours or until the throbbing stops—whichever comes first.

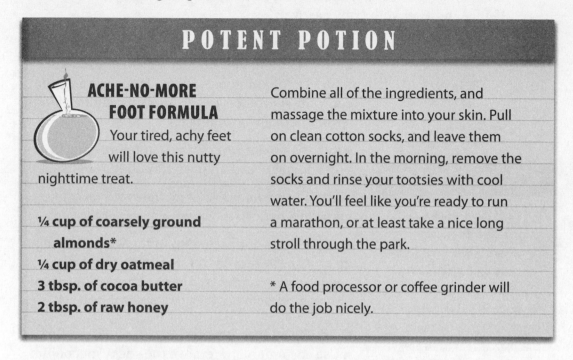

POTENT POTION

ACHE-NO-MORE FOOT FORMULA

Your tired, achy feet will love this nutty nighttime treat.

¼ **cup of coarsely ground almonds***

¼ **cup of dry oatmeal**

3 **tbsp. of cocoa butter**

2 **tbsp. of raw honey**

Combine all of the ingredients, and massage the mixture into your skin. Pull on clean cotton socks, and leave them on overnight. In the morning, remove the socks and rinse your tootsies with cool water. You'll feel like you're ready to run a marathon, or at least take a nice long stroll through the park.

* A food processor or coffee grinder will do the job nicely.

✔ Have a Heart-Healthy Handful

All nuts are packed with unsaturated fat that keeps your heart in good working order. In fact, studies have shown that people who ate a handful of nuts (especially walnuts, pecans, and almonds) five or more times a week cut their heart attack risk in half compared with folks who said "No thanks." How you eat your nut quota is up to you: You can snack on them; add them to salads, pasta, stir-fries, or smoothies; or use almond, walnut, and peanut oils for cooking and in salad dressings.

✔ A Sweet Solution for Sore Skin

Sweet almond oil is a super emollient for treating painful and itchy skin irritations, ranging from chapped hands to diaper rash, cold sores, shingles, and psoriasis. To put it to work, just mix 4 tablespoons of the oil with the juice of 1 lemon or lime, and apply the mixture generously to the afflicted skin. Repeat as needed until you feel relief. Then store any leftover salve in a tightly closed jar at room temperature.

✔ Attention, Expectant Mothers!

One of the handiest, healthiest helpers you could ever ask for is a big jar of organic coconut oil. Here are just some of the ways you can use it both before and after your baby's arrival:

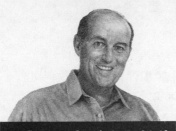

YOU DON'T SAY!

Unless you're a trained botanist, the whole business of classifying plants can be as confusing as all get-out. Take the coconut, for example. Botanically speaking, it's a *drupe*, or a kind of fruit that has a fleshy outer layer, which in this case is removed before the fruits go to market. The part we eat is the rich, flavorful nut-like endosperm inside. In fact, most of the "nuts" we eat regularly, including almonds, pecans, walnuts, pistachios, and macadamia nuts, are actually drupes. The Brazil nut is classified as a seed, and the peanut is (of course) a legume. Just about the only true nuts you'll see in the supermarket are hazelnuts and chestnuts.

While You're Waiting

■ Eat a teaspoon or two each day to boost your future child's immune system. The lauric acid in coconut oil protects the immune functions of both fetuses and newborn infants.

■ Rub the oil onto your stomach to prevent itchy skin and help head off unsightly stretch marks.

■ Mix a teaspoon or so of oil into your favorite herbal tea to keep morning sickness at bay.

■ Apply it to your perineum in the weeks leading up to labor to prevent tearing and possibly the need for an episiotomy. Then keep applying coconut oil after delivery to speed up healing.

Once Baby Has Arrived

■ Use coconut oil to remove the sticky meconium from your new baby's bottom, as well as any cradle cap that may develop on the infant's head. (In both cases, massage the oil onto the affected skin, leave it on for a few minutes, then gently wipe it off with a warm washcloth.)

■ Massage it onto your nipples to soothe pain and irritation. It's good for baby, too, and the tyke will love the taste!

■ Smooth the oil onto your infant's diaper rash. It's especially effective at healing rashes that are caused by yeast infections.

Note: If you have tested positive for allergies to any other tree nuts, especially hazelnuts or walnuts, check with your allergist first before you use coconut oil.

✔ Bang the Door on Mosquitoes

Brazil nuts are loaded with vitamin B_1 (a.k.a. thiamine), and skeeters tend to steer clear of people whose systems contain high amounts of it. So for several days before you head for a mosquito-infested area, chow down on Brazil nuts, and take a supply along with you. Not crazy about Brazil nuts? No worries—sunflower seeds are another potent source of vitamin B_1.

✔ Up Your Sperm Count

Hey, guys! If you and your wife are trying to conceive, but nothing's happening—and your doctors have found no medical reason—maybe it's time to go nuts. Specifically, start chowing down on almonds, Brazil nuts, and walnuts. All of them contain high levels of nutrients, antioxidants, and omega-3 fatty acids that increase both the quantity and quality of sperm. And if you're a fan of pumpkin seeds, you're in luck because they also offer the same reproductive benefits.

✔ Halt Hemorrhoid Havoc

As minor ailments go, hemorrhoids rank as one of the most widespread and bothersome. So it's no wonder that folks have come up with a gazillion home remedies for the nasty things. One classic cure is to eat three raw almonds each day, chewing each nut 50 times. To prevent hemorrhoids, the renowned psychic healer Edgar Cayce (widely regarded as the father of holistic medicine) also prescribed three almonds a day, but he didn't specify any chewing numbers.

Beauty in a Nutshell

❖ Beauty from the Inside Out

The same vitamins, minerals, and other compounds that make nuts so good for your health also make them a powerful addition to your beauty-care arsenal. If you need any enticement to add more nuts and nut oils to your daily diet, just take a gander at this list of beautifying nutrients:

ALPHA-LINOLENIC ACID. Walnuts are packed with this omega-3 fatty acid, which, among other feats, moisturizes your hair, nourishes and soft-

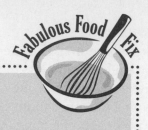

Fabulous Food Fix

WONDERFUL WALNUT DIP

You'll get all the beautifying, health-giving power of walnuts in this scrumptious dip.

1½ cups of toasted walnut pieces*
1 tbsp. of olive oil
1 tbsp. of sherry vinegar
Juice of 1 small lemon
1 tsp. of Dijon mustard
1 tsp. of kosher salt
½ tsp. of white pepper
4–5 tbsp. of water
2 tbsp. of fresh chives, chopped
Toasted walnut pieces for garnish
Chopped fresh chives for garnish

Put the first seven ingredients and 3 tablespoons of water in a food processor, and process until smooth. Add more water if necessary to get a smooth consistency. Stir in the chives, pour the dip into a bowl, and then garnish with the walnuts and chives. Serve with raw vegetables or your favorite chips.

* To toast: Spread the nuts in a single layer on a baking sheet, and bake at 350°F, stirring once or twice, for 10 to 12 minutes, or until lightly browned and fragrant.

YIELD: ABOUT 1¾ CUPS

ens your skin, relieves skin disorders such as acne and eczema, and helps fight aging.

SELENIUM. This mighty mineral helps hair grow thick and shiny. Among all foods, Brazil nuts rank as one of the most potent sources of selenium.

VITAMIN E. It aids in tissue repair, thereby slowing down your skin's aging process. Your prime dietary helpers: almonds, cashews, and peanuts.

ZINC. The big Z keeps your hair shiny, helps prevent hair loss, aids in healing acne and scabs on your skin, and guards against white spots on your fingernails and toenails. Almonds, cashews, pecans, and walnuts are all rich in zinc.

❖ Scrub Your Skin Soft

This A-rated facial scrub will clean and soften your skin at the same time: Grind 2 tablespoons of almonds in a blender or coffee grinder, and mix the powder with 2 teaspoons of milk, ½ teaspoon of flour, and just enough honey to make a thick paste. Rub it into your skin, then rinse with warm water and pat dry.

❖ Exfoliate Gently

All types of skin can benefit from regular exfoliating treatments to get rid of dead cells and make a more radiant complexion. But when your skin is beginning to reach a certain level of experience, it's important to treat it tenderly. This easygoing scrub does just that. (In fact, it's mild enough to use every day, but two or three times a week should keep your face looking smooth and vibrant.) Here's the routine: Blend a handful of shelled walnuts in a food processor with 3 tablespoons of plain yogurt until you've got a smooth consistency. Massage the mixture onto your freshly washed face, then rinse with lukewarm water, pat dry, and apply your usual moisturizer.

✤ Fresh-from-the-Kitchen Cleanser

Here's a facial cleanser that's perfect for all skin types. Plus, you can put it together in a flash and keep it on hand for daily use. Put 1 cup each of almonds, uncooked oatmeal, and dried orange peel in a blender or food processor, and chop the ingredients until they form a fine powder. Scoop some into the palm of your hand, add a few drops of water, and rub it onto your face. (Be careful not to get any in your eyes.) Rinse with warm water, pat dry, and follow up with your favorite toner and moisturizer. Store the mixture in an airtight container at room temperature.

✤ Pistachios Pack Eye-Improvement Power

For centuries, East Indian women have used these tiny nuts to remove unsightly dark circles under their eyes. Now you can, too! Just grind three or four shelled pistachios in a food processor or coffee grinder, and mix the powder with 1 teaspoon of whole milk. Dab it onto the delicate skin

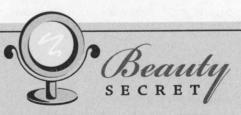

A MIGHTY MASK FOR AGING SKIN

Three age-defying all-stars team up in this simply sensational facial treatment: Grind 8 to 10 shelled almonds into a powder, using a food processor or coffee grinder. Mix the powder with 1 teaspoon of cold-pressed walnut oil and 1 drop of geranium essential oil to get a *smooth paste. Gently apply it to your freshly cleansed face and neck, avoiding your eye area. Leave it on for 20 minutes or so, then rinse it off with lukewarm water. Repeat once a week to keep your skin soft, supple, and younger looking.*

around your eyes, leave it on for 30 minutes or so, and wash it off with lukewarm water. Repeat once a day until your eye bags have bagged off. **Note:** Like many natural remedies, this one doesn't work overnight, so keep at it and don't give up too soon!

✤ A Pure and Simple Body Scrub

Department store cosmetic counters are filled with body scrubs that cost an arm and a leg—and contain chemicals that you can't even pronounce, much less recall from high school chemistry class. So give 'em a pass, and make your own scrub. Just melt ½ cup of coconut oil over very low heat,

POTENT POTION

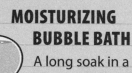

MOISTURIZING BUBBLE BATH

A long soak in a tub full of bubbles can make your troubles float away. Unfortunately, it can also dry out your skin. Enter this bubble bath blend, which actually softens your skin while you relax your cares away.

½ cup of soap flakes*
1 cup of boiling water
3 tbsp. of sweet almond oil
A few drops of your favorite essential oil (optional)
A glass of champagne (optional)

In a large heat-proof bowl, dissolve the soap flakes into the boiling water, stirring continuously. Add the almond oil and the essential oil, if desired. Keep stirring the mixture as you pour 4 to 5 tablespoons of it under the running spigot in your tub. Then pour yourself a glass of champagne, settle in, and enjoy your double bubbles. Store the remaining bath blend at room temperature in a container with a tight-fitting lid. It will keep for about a month, but you will need to shake or stir the mixture each time you use it.

* For bigger bubbles and maximum softening power, make your own soap flakes by grating a bar or two of glycerin soap using a blender, food processor, or hand grater.

YIELD: ABOUT 1 CUP

then pour it over 1 cup of brown sugar or coarse salt (whichever you have on hand), and mix thoroughly. If you like, stir in 5 drops of pure vanilla extract or your favorite essential oil. Massage the mixture into your skin from neck to toes, rinse it off with warm water, and pat dry. Follow up with your favorite body lotion.

❖ Beautiful Body Butter

Soften your skin all over with the magic-making combo of coconut oil and honey. It's a treat worthy of an ultra-fancy spa—for a fraction of the price. Here's the simple five-step routine:

STEP 1. Gather the goods. You'll need 2 tablespoons of extra virgin coconut oil; 1 tablespoon of raw honey; 2 drops of pure vanilla extract or peppermint oil (optional); a small bowl; and enough soft cotton bath towels to cover your body.

STEP 2. Mix all of the ingredients in the bowl. (If necessary, heat the coconut oil until it's soft enough to blend easily with the honey.)

STEP 3. Spread the towels out in your bathtub, and dampen them with water that's as hot as your comfort range will allow.

STEP 4. Rub the butter all over your body, settle into the tub, and wrap yourself in the hot towels. Then lie back and relax until the towels have cooled to room temperature.

CAUTION ⚠

If you're allergic to any particular kinds of nuts, I know (at least I hope!) that you wouldn't dream of using any oral remedies that contain them. Unfortunately, though, some websites that feature DIY beauty recipes would have you believe that it's okay for folks with nut allergies to use topical treatments. Well, friends, don't do it! Remember: What goes onto your skin goes into your body. If you know you're allergic to any ingredient in a potion, don't use it in any form. And allergy or not, before you use any kind of nut oil, do a sensitivity test by rubbing a dab into a small patch of skin. If no rash appears after a day or so, you're good to go.

STEP 5. Rinse yourself off, pat dry, and smooth plain coconut oil onto your skin to seal in the moisture. That's all there is to it!

❖ Shave Close, Shave Clean

Commercial shaving creams and gels (for ladies and gents) are expensive cocktails of chemicals that you don't need in order to get a nice clean shave on your legs, underarms, or face. The easy (and healthier) alternative: Simply smooth coconut oil onto your about-to-be-shaved skin. It will give you a close shave and leave your skin healthily hydrated.

✤ Let's Hair It for Peanut Butter

That jar of peanut butter in your kitchen cabinet is good for more than making sandwiches and cookies. In fact, it's one heck of a hair conditioner. But don't take my word for it—give it a try. Put ½ cup of creamy peanut butter into a bowl, and use a handheld eggbeater to mix in alternating teaspoons of extra virgin olive oil and raw honey until the mixture is smooth and light, but not runny (3 or 4 teaspoons of each should do the trick). Apply the blend to your hair, and cover it with a shower cap and a warm towel. Leave it on for an hour or so, then rinse it out and follow up with your usual shampoo. For maximum results, repeat the procedure once a week. The protein in the peanut butter will strengthen your hair shafts, while the olive oil and honey will provide deep-down moisture.

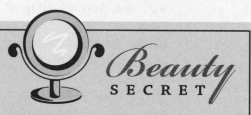

Beauty SECRET

MILK YOUR HAIR FOR ALL IT'S WORTH

Would you like to have thicker, fuller-looking hair in a jiffy? Then here's your single-ingredient formula: coconut milk. Simply pick up a can or carton of it at the supermarket (you'll find it in the milk aisle or in the international-foods section), and pour it into a plastic spray bottle. After shampooing, spray your still-wet hair with the C-milk, then blow-dry and style your mane as usual. Store the unused portion in the fridge, where it will keep for about a week.

✤ Make Room for Macadamia Oil

Chances are that unlike peanut butter, macadamia nut oil is not part of your standard pantry inventory. But it should be—if you want a no-muss, no-fuss conditioner that can soothe an irritated scalp and strengthen and shine your hair from the roots to the tips. Plus, it leaves no residual greasiness on your scalp, as some oils can do. The simple procedure: Heat a few tablespoons of the oil until it's slightly warm, and apply a thin layer to your scalp and the entire length of your hair. Leave the oil on for about two hours, then wash it out with a mild shampoo. Repeat as needed every week or so to keep your tresses smooth and shiny. You can buy macadamia nut oil in health-food stores and from numerous websites.

Best of the Rest

★ Flaxseed Fights Arthritis

Flaxseed contains compounds that help your body reduce the inflammation associated with both rheumatoid arthritis and osteoarthritis. All it takes is 1 tablespoon of seeds per day, and you can meet your quota in a couple of ways:

■ Grind the tasty seeds in a coffee grinder or food processor, and add the powder to a smoothie, mix it into yogurt or cottage cheese, or sprinkle it onto whatever you're having for breakfast, lunch, or dinner.

■ Take 1 teaspoon of flaxseed oil three times a day. Either sip it straight from the spoon, or mix it into food or beverages. (Keep the oil refrigerated to prolong its shelf life.)

Note: Like all natural remedies that go to the root of a problem rather than just masking symptoms, this one will take a little time to work. You can expect to wait at least a month for it to perform its pain-relieving magic.

★ Arthritis-Relief Rub

For a topical approach to easing arthritis pain, mix equal parts of sesame oil and ginger juice, and massage it into the painful areas. If the burning sensation produced by the ginger feels too strong, add more sesame oil to bring the heat down to a tolerable level. To produce ginger juice, grate a piece of fresh ginger, and squeeze the gratings through cheesecloth.

A Better Bladder Tonic

HEALTHFUL HINT

An old Russian folk remedy calls on pumpkin seed "tea" to relieve inflammation of the bladder and prostate. To make it, simmer ½ cup of whole (not shelled) pumpkin seeds in 1 quart of water for 20 minutes. Let it cool to room temperature, and pour it into a wide-mouthed jar with a tight-fitting lid. Do not strain out the seeds; just let them settle to the bottom of the jar. Stir thoroughly before using the potion. Drink 6 to 8 ounces three times a day, or as needed to relieve pain. **Note:** This is not a substitute for professional medical care. If you suspect that you have either bladder or prostate problems, see your doctor immediately.

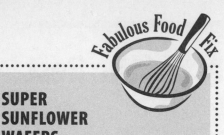

SUPER SUNFLOWER WAFERS

Eating a handful of sunflower seeds every day can help you quit smoking, lower your LDL (bad) cholesterol levels, relieve constipation, prevent tooth decay, improve your memory—and more. But you don't need to munch on seeds all the time. You can get all or part of your daily dose from these surprisingly tasty no-bake cookies.

2 cups of raw, shelled, unsalted sunflower seeds
Water
¼ cup of raisins (or to taste)

Grind the seeds in a food processor or coffee grinder to get a fine-textured meal. Moisten it with just enough water to make a thick dough, and mix in the raisins. Break off small pieces, and press them into half-dollar-sized wafers. Put them on a screen or cooling rack, and set it in a dry place (like the top of your refrigerator) for three to four days until the cookies are dry.

YIELD: ABOUT 16 WAFERS

★ Shrink Your Prostate

Medical statisticians estimate that one out of every three men over the age of 60 has some kind of prostate problem. And according to natural-health practitioners, one of the most effective ways to help relieve an enlarged prostate is to eat ½ cup of shelled, unsalted pumpkin seeds every day. One reason may be that the prostate gland contains 10 times more zinc than most other organs in your body, and pumpkin seeds are packed with that mineral. **Note:** If you're being treated for an enlarged prostate, or suspect that you have one, be sure to check with your doctor before you use this remedy.

★ An Asthma Antidote: Sunny and Sweet

Legions of chronic asthma sufferers swear by this classic prevention potion: Put 4 cups of shelled sunflower seeds in a pan with 2 quarts of water, and boil it until the water is reduced by half. Strain out the solids, add 8 cups of raw honey to the liquid, and boil it down to a syrupy consistency. Pour it into a sterilized glass jar with a tight-fitting lid (a clamp-top canning jar is perfect), and store it at room temperature. Then take 1 teaspoon of the syrup half an hour before each meal.

★ Seedy Cycle Regulators

Irregular menstrual cycles do not normally pose major health problems, but they sure are annoying (at least so I've been told by all the females in my life). Well, ladies, if you're eager to get your schedule back on track, two kinds of seeds can help. Each day, either eat 1 tablespoon of sesame seeds (chewing them thoroughly), or sprinkle 1 tablespoon of ground flaxseed onto your soup, salad, or cereal.

★ Turn Your Eyes to the Sun(flower)

For years, natural-health experts have sworn by sunflower seeds for strengthening your eyes and improving your vision. The action plan: Simply eat a handful of the seeds (shelled, raw, and unsalted) every day.

★ Put Your Sunny Face Forward

Sunflower oil is a key ingredient in many commercial beauty products for two reasons: It's rich in the moisturizing power of fatty acids and vitamins A, D, and E. Plus, it has a light texture that makes it easy for your skin to absorb. This mask is especially beneficial for dry or aging skin: Mix 2 tablespoons of sunflower oil with half a mashed banana, and apply the mixture to your freshly washed face. Leave it on for 20 minutes or so, rinse it off with warm water, splash on cool water, and pat your skin dry.

★ Soak in Sesame Oil

Relaxing, skin-pleasing bath routines don't come any simpler than this one: Add 2 tablespoons of sesame oil and 2 or 3 drops of your favorite essential oil to your bathwater, and settle into the tub. To maximize the softening effect, soak for five minutes first, then add the oils to seal in the moisture from the water.

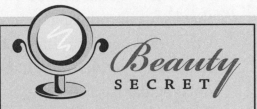

Beauty SECRET

SHINE SOME SUN ON DULL HAIR

When your locks have lost their luster, bring it back this way: Shortly before bedtime, mix 2 tablespoons of sunflower oil with 2 egg yolks, and massage the mixture into your hair. Cover with a shower cap, and leave it on overnight. (Put a towel over your pillowcase to catch any oil that might leak through your cap.) Come morning, wash the mixture out with your usual shampoo, then follow up by rinsing with a solution of 2 tablespoons of apple cider vinegar in 1 quart of warm water.

CHAPTER

16

Oatmeal

Historians reckon that we owe the ancient Greeks a great big thanks for introducing oatmeal to the world. For starters, the Mayo Clinic ranks oatmeal among the top five foods for lowering LDL (bad) cholesterol. And studies galore indicate that eating oatmeal on a regular basis can help reduce your risk for type 2 diabetes, lower your blood pressure, guard against heart disease and cancer, and boost your immune system. In addition, oatmeal has the amazing power to soften and nourish your skin, which alone would earn it superstar ranking in both the health *and* beauty categories.

Feeling Your Oats

✔ Jump-Start Your System

The next time constipation strikes, have a bowl of oatmeal for breakfast. It's loaded with a gummy fiber called mucilage, which soaks up water, softening stools and making them easier to pass. **Note:** Just don't top your cereal with bananas, which are noted for their internal binding power, or you'll never get off the mark!

✔ Say "Heck, No!" to Heartburn

This isn't the most appetizing heartburn remedy in the world, but it sure does work! When you get that fiery feeling, slowly chew a teaspoon or two of uncooked oatmeal, and then swallow it. The flames will flicker and die.

✔ Trouble Prevention on the Double

If you're prone to indigestion and/or flatulence, this "aperitif" can help: Add 1 cup of uncooked oatmeal and 1 cup of bran to a gallon of water. Let it sit for 24 hours, then strain out the solids, and store the liquid in the refrigerator. Drink a cupful of the potion (either cold or warmed up) 15 minutes before each meal.

✔ Quit Coughing

A number of ingredients in oatmeal can reduce bronchial inflammation and relieve coughing spasms. Make it according to the directions on the package, just as though you were making a bowl for breakfast, but reduce the water by ¼ cup. Add honey to taste, and eat 1 cup of warm cereal four times a day and at the start of each coughing spell. **Note:** For the sake of convenience, you may want to make your oatmeal in quantity ahead of time. If you do, then store it, covered, in the refrigerator, and warm up each "dose" before you eat it.

Slow Lane or Fast Track?

HEALTHFUL HINT

This may come as a surprise (I know it did to me), but the basic nutrient content of instant oatmeal is pretty much the same as it is for traditional, slower-cooking rolled oats. So when you're whipping up any of the health or beauty potions in this chapter, feel free to use whichever type you have on hand, provided your instant oatmeal is *plain*. Steer clear of any oatmeal that contains sweeteners, fruit, flavorings, or other ingredients.

Note: Unless otherwise specified in a tip or recipe, use uncooked oatmeal, straight from the container.

✔ Say "So Long" to Skin Troubles

There simply is no more effective remedy than oatmeal for relieving the pain, itch, and inflammation of skin problems ranging from windburn and sunburn to insect bites, poison-plant rashes, contact allergies, and eczema. How you need to use it depends on the location and extent of the affected area as well as your personal preference. You have a trio of pure and simple options:

■ Wrap about 1 cup of dry, uncooked oatmeal in cheesecloth and run cool water through it. Wring out the excess liquid, and apply the poultice to your burned skin for 20 minutes every two hours until you feel relief. (You can use the same oatmeal sachet over and over. Just put it in a plastic bag, stash it in the fridge, and give it a cold shower before each treatment.)

■ To soothe a burn or rash on your face, put a handful of uncooked oatmeal into a cheesecloth pouch or a clean, old panty hose foot, immerse it in a sink full of warm water, and squeeze the bag four or five times. When the water is cloudy, splash it onto your face a few times, and let it air-dry so that a thin film of the healing oat "tea" remains on your skin. If time's a wastin' and you need to use a towel, pat dry as gently as possible.

CAUTION ⚠

Although oatmeal is one of the healthiest substances you can put into or on your body, it can give you a major headache if it goes down a drain. So do your plumbing (and your pocketbook) a favor, and follow these trouble-avoidance guidelines:

■ Never pour either whole or ground oatmeal directly into a bathtub or sink, unless it's a kitchen sink with a garbage disposal attached to it.

■ Whenever you use oatmeal in a facial mask or other topical treatment, rinse it off over a pan or basin. Then dump the water down the garbage disposal or, better yet, onto the soil in your yard or garden. The nutrients in oats are just as good for your plants as they are for you!

■ When your affliction covers a larger expanse of your body—or you simply prefer a good soak—stuff a cotton drawstring bag or a panty hose leg with a cup or two of uncooked oatmeal. Toss it into your tub as you run cool to lukewarm water, then settle in and relax for 15 to 20 minutes. Again, if possible, let yourself air-dry when you're finished.

✔ Skin Relief Straight Up

You say you prefer showers to baths? No problem! Oatmeal can still help you conquer an all-over rash or sunburn. First, make an oatmeal pouch as described in "Say 'So Long' to Skin Troubles" (see page 217). Then put your showerhead on its gentlest setting, run cool to lukewarm water, and step into the tub. Gently rub the cereal soother over your affected skin, squeezing the bag periodically to release the milky essence of the flakes. When you're done, turn off the water and let your skin air-dry.

✔ Ditch the Discomfort of Yeast Infections

The same oatmeal bath that soothes skin rashes can also ease the internal pain and itching of a yeast infection. Simply fill a cotton sack or panty hose leg with uncooked oatmeal, and toss it into the tub as you run warm water into it. Squeeze the bag several times to extract the oaty goodness, and soak for

20 minutes or so. Repeat the procedure as needed until you're feeling better. **Note:** Although this treatment will relieve your irritating symptoms, it will not cure a yeast infection. If you've contracted one for the first time, call your doctor.

✔ Bottoms Up, Baby!

When your baby has been diagnosed with a yeast-infected diaper rash, oatmeal is just what the doctor ordered to alleviate the itch during the healing process. Bathe the child frequently in an infant tub filled with lukewarm water and a handful of uncooked oatmeal. Then let the tyke's bottom air-dry before you cover it with a clean diaper. And be sure to wash your and your baby's hands thoroughly after each diaper change because yeast fungi can spread to other areas.

POTENT POTION

FOOT-TO-HEAD WARM-UP TREATMENT

When Old Man Winter leaves you so cold that you just can't kill the chill, even in a nice toasty room, treat yourself to this sweet and spicy foot mask. It'll send its aromatic warmth up through your entire body.

½ cup of ground uncooked oatmeal*
1 tbsp. of fresh ginger, grated
1 tbsp. of honey
1 tsp. of olive oil
½ tsp. of cayenne pepper
½ tsp. of cinnamon
4 drops of sweet orange essential oil
4 tbsp. of warm water

Combine all of the ingredients in a bowl, and mix until you have a thick paste. Put your feet in a basin, and spread a thick layer of the mixture over each foot. Have two warm, damp hand towels ready. Wrap each tootsie in one of the towels, sit back, and relax for 15 minutes or so. Rinse the mask off with warm water, and pat your skin dry. Then park yourself in a cozy chair and think of spring.

* You can use either a coffee grinder or a food processor.

✔ Intensive Therapy for Sore Hands

Whether your hands are chapped from working or playing in the great outdoors or, worse, they're raw and sore as the dickens, here's your R_x: Mix 3 tablespoons of finely ground uncooked oatmeal (use a coffee grinder or food processor), 2 tablespoons of rose water, and 2 teaspoons of almond oil in a microwave-safe bowl, and nuke the mixture until it's just warm (not hot). Spread the paste on your hands and wrap them in plastic wrap. Leave it on until the salve has cooled, then rinse it off with warm water. Perform this routine as needed until your appendages are sore no more, which shouldn't take more than one or two treatments. By the way, this is a real neat treat for sore feet, too!

Oatmeal Magic

♣ Acne, Be Gone!

Troubled by acne? Treat your face to breakfast—so to speak. Just grind ¼ cup of uncooked oatmeal in a food processor or coffee grinder, and mix it with ¼ cup of boiling water to form a paste. Remove the pan from the heat, let the mixture cool to room temperature, and spread it onto your face. Leave it on for 10 to 15 minutes, and rinse it off with warm water. The oatmeal will draw out the inflammation without drying out your skin. **Note:** This treatment can also help remove any scarring and discoloration that may remain after the blemishes have cleared up.

♣ Oatmeal Conquers Oily Skin

Finding good facial masks for oily skin can be tricky because you need one that removes the excess oil without drying out your complexion. This formula strikes just the right balance: Mix 2 tablespoons of ground uncooked oatmeal (use a coffee grinder or food processor) and 1 teaspoon of turmeric in a bowl, and stir in enough water to make a smooth paste (start with 2 tablespoons, and add more as needed, teaspoon by teaspoon). Apply the mixture to your freshly washed face, avoiding the eye area. Leave it on for 20 minutes or so, then rinse it off with warm water, gently pat your skin dry, and follow up with your usual (preferably oil-free) moisturizer.

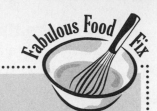

❖ On an Even Keel

An uneven skin tone can be just as annoying as dealing with skin that has a combination of dry and oily areas. That's where this facial comes in. It'll slough off dead skin cells, refine your pores, and even out the tone and texture of your complexion. To make the mask, mix 1 tablespoon of ground uncooked oatmeal (use a coffee grinder or food processor) with 2 teaspoons of fresh apple juice and 2 teaspoons of red wine to make a paste (add more liquid in equal proportions if necessary). Spread the mixture onto your face and throat, let it dry for 20 to 30 minutes, then rinse with warm water. Tone and moisturize your skin as usual, and you're good to go!

❖ A Bowl a Day Keeps Wrinkles Away

If you cook oatmeal for breakfast every day (whether for yourself or your children), this wrinkle-prevention plan has your name written all over it. Set aside a tablespoon or so of the cooked cereal until after breakfast. Then mix it with just enough olive oil or vegetable oil to make it spreadable, and massage it into your face and neck. Leave it on for about 30 minutes, and wash it off with lukewarm water. There's just one catch: This wrinkle-proofing trick works only if you perform the routine each and every day.

EASY OAT CRACKERS

Eating a bowl of cereal isn't the only way to get your daily dose of beautifying, health-giving oatmeal. These tasty crackers pack all the goodness of oats in a snackable, packable form.

¾ cup of uncooked oatmeal
½ tsp. of salt
1 tbsp. of butter, softened
5 oz. of boiling water
Additional uncooked oatmeal

Combine the oatmeal and salt in a bowl, add the butter and water, and mix to form a sticky dough. Let it sit for five minutes until the oatmeal expands. Then sprinkle a cutting board or other flat surface with a few tablespoons of additional oatmeal, turn the dough out onto it, and knead lightly. Roll the dough out as thinly as possible, sprinkling with more oatmeal as needed to prevent sticking. Cut it into squares or rectangles, and bake at 325°F for 15 to 20 minutes (until crisp and dry, but not browned). Enjoy them as you would any other crackers or chips.

YIELD: ABOUT 1 DOZEN SMALL CRACKERS

❖ Wake Up and Wash Your Face

Rather, I should say wash your face and wake up! This bracing but oh-so-gentle cleanser will get every morning off to a brisk start. Combine 2 tablespoons of ground uncooked oatmeal (use a coffee grinder or food processor), ¼ teaspoon of dried mint, and 2 pinches of dried rosemary, and mix the blend with just enough hot water to make a spreadable paste. Gently smooth it onto your face, avoiding the eye area. Let it dry, and remove it with a washcloth dipped in warm water. Rinse with cool water, and follow up with your usual toner and moisturizer.

❖ A Mask to Turn Back the Clock

In this fabulous facial treatment, oatmeal teams up with a trio of skin-rejuvenating ingredients to help hold back the hands of time. The simple process: Make a paste by mixing 1 teaspoon of uncooked oatmeal with 1 teaspoon each of honey and olive oil and 3 drops of dittany of Crete essential oil (available in health-food stores and online). Smooth the mixture onto your face, and leave it on for 20 minutes or so. Rinse it off with warm water, and apply a softening moisturizer.

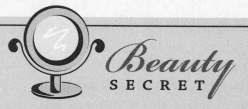

DEEP-CLEAN FOR COMBINATION SKIN

For women whose complexions are either dry or oily, skin care is a piece of cake: You just choose treatments that are tailor-made for your skin type. But when your face has both dry and oily zones, using a different product for each area can be a time-consuming nuisance, especially if you make your own beauty products. Enter this once-a-month cleansing mask that's good for all types of skin. The simple formula: *Grind up 1 cup of uncooked oatmeal in a blender. Add 1 egg white, ½ cup of skim milk, and 3 drops of almond oil, and blend to form a smooth paste. Spread the concoction over your face and neck (avoiding the eye area), and leave it there for 30 minutes or so. Rinse it off with lukewarm water, and apply your usual moisturizer.*

POTENT POTION

SOFTENING BODY SCRUB

Why pay a small fortune for a dry-skin body scrub, when this DIY version gives you all of the benefits at a fraction of the price—with no synthetic chemicals?

2 cups of finely ground
   uncooked oatmeal*
1 cup of baking soda
¾ cup of whole milk
½ cup of salt
¼ cup of honey
¼ cup of olive oil
1 tbsp. of vitamin E oil
20 drops of your favorite
   essential oil**

Mix the first five ingredients in a bowl, then stir in the oils. Pour the mixture into a wide-mouth jar with a tight-fitting lid. It will keep for about a week at room temperature and for up to three weeks in the refrigerator. To use it, scoop a handful of the scrub out of the jar, massage it into your skin, and rinse it off in the shower or tub. **Note:** Be sure to cover the drain with a piece of fabric to snag the oatmeal particles.

* You can use either a coffee grinder or a food processor; use more or less oatmeal to get the thickness you prefer.
** Tea tree, lavender, and geranium are especially good for dry skin.

YIELD: ABOUT 4 CUPS

✤ Oats, Milk, and Honey Bath Blend

Moisturizing, relaxing baths don't come any better (or easier) than this one: Put ½ cup of uncooked oatmeal, ¼ cup of dry whole milk, and 2 tablespoons of raw honey in an all-cotton muslin or cheesecloth bag. Tie it shut with a cord, and hang it under the spigot as you fill the tub. The running water will disperse the super-softening trio throughout your bath.

✤ Dry-Clean Your Hair

Here's the perfect helper to keep on hand for those times when your hair needs a little freshening, but you don't have the time or inclination for

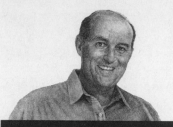

According to the folks who keep such statistics, an estimated 80 percent of American kitchens have oatmeal in their cupboards, and the most popular brand by far is Quaker Oats. It's been around for more than 130 years now, and it's racked up quite a few firsts in the cereal biz. For instance:

1877: First registered trademark (the name Quaker Oats and the image of a kind-looking gentleman in old-fashioned Quaker garb)

1882: First national advertising campaign

1890: First product "trial sizes" (½-ounce boxes of Quaker Oats were delivered to every mailbox in Portland, Oregon)

1891: The first premiums (pieces of chinaware) inserted in product packages and the first recipe to appear on a cereal box (for oatmeal bread)

a full-scale shampoo. Grind 3 tablespoons of uncooked oatmeal into a powder using a coffee grinder or food processor. Mix it with 3 tablespoons each of cornstarch and baking soda, and grind the mixture again to get the finest-possible texture. Store the blend in a large shaker (a powdered sugar shaker is perfect). Then whenever your "do" needs a quick pick-me-up, sprinkle a little of the powder onto your roots, and massage it into your scalp. Let it sit for a minute or two, and brush it out.

✤ Oatmeal-Lavender Soap

The oatmeal-lavender duo is a popular combination in commercial soaps, and for good reason: There are few healthier ways to clean, soften, and nourish all types of skin. The problem is that some of those bars, especially in the lower to middle price ranges, contain chemical additives that rank higher on the ingredient list than the star players do. The simple solution: Make your own soap using this six-step process:

STEP 1. Round up your supplies. You'll need dried lavender, water, grated pure castile soap, and uncooked oatmeal; plus, a heavy glass pot, a mold for each bar of soap you plan to make, and nonstick cooking spray or vegetable oil to lubricate your chosen mold(s).

STEP 2. Make a lavender tea by steeping 2 teaspoons of dried lavender in ½ cup of just-boiled water for 15 minutes, then strain out the solids, and let the brew cool to room temperature.

STEP 3. Place 4 tablespoons of the grated castile soap into the glass pot. Pour in the lavender tea, and melt the soap over low heat, stirring constantly. (If the soap clumps up, it means the tea was too hot.)

STEP 4. When the soap has dissolved, remove the pan from the heat, and let it cool slightly, stirring to keep it smooth. Then mix in ⅓ cup of uncooked oatmeal.

STEP 5. Lightly coat your mold(s) with cooking spray or vegetable oil, pour in the soap mixture, and refrigerate it overnight.

STEP 6. Invert the mold over a plate, and tap on the bottom. If the soap doesn't slide out readily, dip the mold in hot water for just a few seconds, and tap again.

Note: If you don't have a glass pot, substitute a heat-proof glass jar set in a pan of water. The recipe here makes enough to fill a small yogurt container, but you could also use soap or candy molds or silicone cupcake liners. Multiply the recipe as desired, but stick to the same proportions.

Best of the Rest

★ Bar(ley) the Door on Ulcers

Barley and barley water are renowned for their ability to soothe the pain of ulcers and help rebuild your stomach lining. To make barley water, boil 4 tablespoons of pearled barley in 6 cups of H_2O until the liquid is reduced by about half. Strain out the solids and drink the water, either warm or cool, throughout the day, adding honey and/or lemon if you like. Then eat the barley plain, or add it to soup or stew.

★ A Bran New Earache Remedy

There are few ailments more painful than an earache, and that's probably why so many folks have come up with ways to ease the agony. This is one of the best: Mix ½ cup of unprocessed bran (available in health-food stores and most supermarkets) with ½ cup of kosher or coarse sea salt. Wrap the mixture securely in a generous-sized piece of cheesecloth so that the stuff doesn't spill out all over the place. Then heat the pouch in the microwave or an oven turned on low until it's as warm as you can comfortably handle. Lay the poultice over the affected ear, and keep it on for 60 minutes or so. **Note:** If your ear is discharging fluid, get medical help immediately. It could be that your eardrum has ruptured.

★ Cure a Cough

A cough is generally caused by an irritation in your respiratory tract. It's Mother Nature's way of helping you loosen up the mucus and send it packing. Of course, knowing that doesn't help much when you're hacking up a storm—but this will: Cook 1 cup of barley according to the directions on the package. Stir in a tablespoon or so of water and the juice of one fresh lemon. Liquefy the mixture in a blender, and drink 1 cup every four hours.

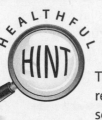

HEALTHFUL HINT

Give Corns the Boot

This old-time corn-removing formula sounds too good to be true, but a lot of folks I know swear by it. Just before your usual bedtime, put a slice of white bread, a slice of raw onion, and 1 cup of vinegar (any kind will do) in a bowl, and let it sit for 24 hours. The next night, put the bread on top of the corn, lay the onion on top of the bread, cover it with a bandage, and go to bed. There's a good chance the corn will fall off overnight. If it doesn't, repeat the procedure until the painful bump is history. It shouldn't take more than a couple of tries.

★ Slice Away an Ingrown Toenail

No, I don't mean you should cut the nail off. Rather, put a milk-soaked slice of bread in a plastic bag that's big enough to hold your foot. Put your foot into the bag and press the bread around the painful toe. Keep your foot in the bag for 30 minutes. Repeat as necessary until your nail has grown out.

★ Bread Beats Boils

Here's a remedy for boils that comes straight from the bread box: Soak a slice of bread in a bowl of milk until the bread is damp, but not sopping wet. Put the slice on top of the sore, fasten it in place with a strip of cloth, and leave it there for 20 minutes or so. Repeat several times a day until the boil has dried up.

★ Burning for Whiter Teeth

The next time you pop a piece of bread in the toaster and it comes out looking more like charcoal than toast, don't toss it in the trash. Instead, crush the charred bread into crumbs, mix it with about ½ teaspoon of honey, and brush your teeth with it. Then rinse thoroughly and admire your whiter, brighter choppers in the mirror.

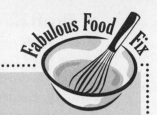

★ Back-to-Back Rice

Uncooked rice can also relieve a back-ache. For this use, fill a clean, thick sock with rice (a wool kneesock is perfect), and warm it up in the microwave on a medium-low setting for 30 to 60 seconds, until it's comfortably warm, but not hot. Then lie down, lay the DIY heating pad over the painful area, and relax until your ache has eased.

★ Rice Is Nice for Headache Relief

Headaches are an unfortunate fact of life—and that's why it pays to add this simple tool to your first-aid kit. Mix about 1½ cups of uncooked rice with 5 or 6 drops of lavender essential oil. Stuff the mixture into a soft, clean cotton sock and sew it closed. Then whenever that old familiar throbbing starts, lie down and lay the fragrant sock over your eyes. The lavender scent will soothe you, while the weight of the rice will provide massage-like pressure against your eyes and forehead to help stop the searing pain.

HANDY HYDRATOR

When you're suffering through a bout of diarrhea or stomach flu that's caused vomiting, it's important to replace the fluids and electrolytes you've lost. But you don't need to buy commercial sports drinks; whip up a batch of your own with this recipe instead.

4 cups of boiling water
½ tsp. of salt
1–2 cups of infant rice cereal

Pour the water into a large, heat-proof pitcher and add the salt. Then gradually stir in the cereal, mixing well. Drink 1 cup every hour to keep yourself in the pink of health. Cover and refrigerate the mixture between uses.

YIELD: ABOUT 4 CUPS

★ A Dynamic Duo for Oily Skin

Wheat germ and yogurt team up in this once-a-week facial that will balance and nourish oily or combination skin. And it couldn't be simpler to make—just mix together 1 tablespoon of each ingredient, and let the mixture stand for a few minutes to reach room temperature. Apply a generous coating to your face and neck, and leave it on for about 15 minutes. Remove the mask with a washcloth soaked in warm water. Douse your skin with warm water, then cool water. Pat dry, and follow up with your usual toner and moisturizer.

★ Bran Banishes Blemishes

Acne and blackheads don't stand a chance against this remarkable remover: Just mix 2 tablespoons of bran with enough water to make a paste. (Add it, a teaspoon or so at a time, until you get a spreadable consistency.) Smooth it onto your freshly washed face, avoiding the eye area, and leave it on for 20 minutes or so. Rinse it off with warm water, splash your skin with cool water to close your pores, and gently pat your face dry. Finish by applying your usual toner and moisturizer. Repeat this procedure once a week to keep your skin clear and fresh.

★ Beautiful Bran Body Scrub

Your skin couldn't ask for a healthier or more soothing scrub than this one. The easy formula: Mix ½ cup of bran and ½ cup of finely ground almonds in a heat-proof bowl, and gradually stir in 1 cup of hot green tea until you have a thick, but spreadable paste. Let it cool to room temperature, then add 10 drops of lavender essential oil, and mix well. Massage the mixture onto your body, and rinse with lukewarm water.

POTENT POTION

THYME-FOR-RICE TONER

Here's a kitchen-counter toner that's good for all skin types and gentle enough to use every time you wash your face.

2 tsp. of rice, crushed*
2 sprigs of fresh thyme, chopped**
½ cup of boiling water
Freshly squeezed juice of half a lemon

Mix the rice and thyme in a heat-proof bowl. Pour the boiling water over them, then stir in the lemon juice. Let the mixture steep for 15 minutes or so, and strain out the solids. Pour the liquid into a bottle with a tight-fitting cap, and store it in the refrigerator. Use the potion as you would any other toner.

* Use a spoon or a mortar and pestle.
** Or substitute ½ tablespoon of dried thyme.

YIELD: ABOUT 4½ OUNCES

★ Wheat for Feet

Say good-bye to rough, cracked skin on your feet with this soothing solution: Combine 1 teaspoon of wheat germ with 1 tablespoon each of almond oil and olive oil, and store the mixture in a bottle with a tight-fitting cap. Shake it well before using, then rub the softener generously onto your clean, dry feet, paying particular attention to your heels and other rough areas. Use this treatment once a day, and within just a few days, you'll see and feel the difference!

★ Tough as Nails

Wheat germ can also strengthen and shine your fingernails and toenails like nobody's business. Just mix 1 teaspoon of it with 2 teaspoons of castor oil and 2 teaspoons of salt, and pour the mixture into a bottle with a tight-fitting cap. To use it, give the bottle a good shake, and rub it onto your nails with a cotton ball or swab.

★ Fast Food for Your Hair

Make that *healthy* fast food. Most natural hair conditioning treatments need to stay on your head for anywhere from 20 minutes to several hours. But this one works almost instantly to add strength, shine, and body to your tresses. Just mix 1 tablespoon of wheat germ with 1 cup of plain yogurt, 2 tablespoons each of honey and almond oil, and a pinch of sea salt. Thoroughly coat your hair with the mixture, and massage it into your scalp for a few minutes. Then step into the shower and rinse it off. Follow up with a mild shampoo.

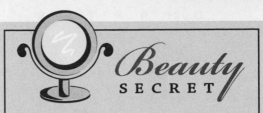

Beauty SECRET

POST-SUMMER HELP FOR LIGHT HAIR

A long, hot summer can turn blonde or light brown hair into a dull, drab, and dry mess. To pump nourishment into the shafts, replace the moisture, and bring back the oomph and shine, whip up this intensive treatment: Mix 2 tablespoons of wheat germ, 2 tablespoons of raw honey, and 2 tablespoons of pure lemon extract (not artificial) with ½ cup of olive oil. Work the mixture through your hair from the roots to the tips. Let it sit for 20 minutes or so, then comb it through your hair. Shampoo and condition as usual, then step up to the mirror and admire your sleek, shiny tresses.

17

Olive Oil

The Greek poet Homer called olive oil "liquid gold," and that moniker is just as apt today as it was all those centuries ago. Like many natural healers, olive oil was cast by the wayside when scads of commercial medications and cosmetics began to appear in the 1950s. Now, though, modern science has "discovered" that olive oil can help enhance the health and appearance of your skin, improve your long-term memory, lower your blood sugar and blood pressure, and cut your risk for just about every chronic disease under the sun. And that's just the tip of the olive branch!

A Mediterranean Marvel

✔ Relieve a Java Jolt
When a gulp of steaming coffee or any other hot beverage gives your throat a nasty burn, swallow 2 teaspoons of olive oil—it'll put out the flames fast! Then let the drink cool for a couple of minutes before you take your next sip.

✔ Hold Your Liquor
Olive oil can also protect your stomach from the effects of alcohol, thereby helping to head off morning-after miseries. The simple preventive measure: Before you head out to a party or to join the gang for an after-work happy hour, swallow 1 tablespoon of olive oil. **Note:** This trick is

only intended to help you avoid an upset stomach. It will do nothing to counteract alcohol's ability to impair your reflexes and mental processes.

✔ Take the Heat

You say you love hot, spicy food, but it always gives you indigestion? Well, you don't have to get out of the kitchen (or the restaurant). Instead, about 15 minutes before you sit down to eat a "high-risk" meal, sip 1 tablespoon of olive oil. It'll provide a protective coating so you can dig into your five-alarm chili without setting your tummy on fire.

✔ Toss a Toothache

For all-but-instant relief, mix 3 drops of olive oil with 1 drop of clove oil, and use a cotton swab to dab the mixture onto your aching tooth. Leave it in place until the pain is gone (which should be within a minute or so), and then rinse your mouth with clear water.

✔ Lubricate Your "Plumbing"

The same miraculous medicine that stops a cough can also get your stubborn bowels working smoothly again. Just take 1 tablespoon of extra virgin olive oil first thing in the morning and a second tablespoon an hour after eating dinner. Within a day or so, things will be moving right along.

✔ Heave the Hacking

How? Simply take 1 tablespoon of extra virgin olive oil in the morning and another tablespoon in the evening. If you like, chase each dose down with a glass of orange juice. Besides cutting the oily taste, it'll also give you a much-needed dose of vitamin C.

Only the Best Will Do

HEALTHFUL HINT

Most types of olive oil are tasty, and any kind will do when you're simply coating your stomach against the effects of hot beverages, spicy food, or liquor. But when you're buying olive oil for other health and beauty purposes, only one grade cuts the mustard: extra virgin. To qualify for that distinction, the oil must be extracted from the fruit by a method known as cold pressing, which ensures that the oil retains all of its health- and beauty-giving benefits. It contains no additives, and no solvents or other chemicals are used in processing the oil. That's why it's a key element in the Mediterranean Diet, an eating plan that's catching on with health-conscious folks from coast to coast.

POTENT POTION

HEALING OIL AND SALT SOAK

This all-purpose bath blend will draw toxins out of your body, calm your nerves, relieve aches and pains, and relax stiff, sore muscles. How could you top an act like that?

1 cup of Epsom salts*
2 tbsp. of extra virgin olive oil
½ tsp. of essential oil**

Mix all of the ingredients in a bowl, or shake them in a container with a tight-fitting lid. Pour the mixture into a tub of very warm (not hot!) water, settle in, and soak for 15 to 20 minutes. Then pat your skin dry, and follow up with your usual body lotion.

* For a larger, garden-size tub or hot tub, use 2 cups of Epsom salts, but stick to the same amounts of olive and essential oils.

** To choose an oil that has the healing benefits you want, see the table "Herbal Customizing Components" on page 234.

✔ Soothe Sunburned Skin

Olive oil can save the day by reducing sunburn pain, keeping your skin hydrated, and helping prevent peeling. For best results, apply the oil immediately after you've been exposed to the sun. Then wait at least a few hours before you wash, so the lubricant has plenty of time to penetrate your skin.

✔ Wallop Windburn

Cold, dry winter winds can be just as hard on your skin as the hot summer sun. When a session of snow shoveling or snowman building leaves your face as red as Santa's hat—and sore, besides—here's the fastest remedy I know of: Massage olive oil onto your face, wait about 10 minutes for it to sink in, then rinse with warm water and pat dry.

✔ Ease Eczema Flare-Ups

Olive oil is loaded with antioxidants that reduce inflammation. For that reason, it's a key ingredient in many commercial products that are designed to relieve eczema and other skin irritations. But guess what? Olive oil is just as effective all by its lonesome, plus it has none of the chemicals you often find in store-bought creams. The simple R_x: Gently rub on about 1 teaspoon of extra virgin olive oil per square inch of affected skin, and let the oil penetrate before you put on any clothing.

For an extra-intensive treatment,

cover your oiled skin with plastic wrap, and leave it on overnight. Just make sure you wear old pajamas and/or put a large towel over your sheets to protect your bedding.

✔ Good Riddance to Bad Rashes

All kinds of things, from environmental irritants and poison ivy to sweating, can make you break out in a rash. No matter what caused the condition, this simple remedy can speed up the healing process and restore the moisture that rashes tend to drain from your skin: Mix 2 tablespoons of extra virgin olive oil per 1½ tablespoons of beer, and gently apply the mixture to the affected area. Repeat several times a day until your skin is clear again.

✔ Extra-Strength Rash Relief

A severe case of poison ivy, oak, or sumac calls for a strong healer, and this triple-threat blend has been proven to be one of the best. Mix 3 parts extra virgin olive oil, 1 part sweet almond oil, and 1 part apricot kernel oil (available in health-food stores). Immediately after a bath or shower, gently pat your skin almost dry, and apply the oil mix to the affected area. Let it soak in for about 10 minutes or so before you put on any clothing. Repeat the procedure as often as needed until the rash has healed. **Note:** When any rash is crusting or blistering, get medical help immediately.

✔ Bathe Psoriasis Bye-Bye

Unfortunately, there is no permanent cure for this nasty skin condition. But there are plenty of ways to ease the pain and itching of the unsightly symptoms

Fabulous Food Fix

ITALIAN DIPPING OIL

The next time you invite the crowd over for a spaghetti or lasagna dinner, give the event a real Italian touch—and give your guests a healthy dose of olive oil—with this easy and delicious blend.

½ cup of extra virgin olive oil
1 tsp. of dried basil
1 tsp. of dried oregano
1 tsp. of dried rosemary, crumbled
1 tsp. of freshly ground black pepper
1 tsp. of garlic powder
1 tsp. of kosher or sea salt

Combine all of the ingredients in a jar with a tight-fitting lid, and shake well. Pour the oil into individual saucers, and serve it with slices of crusty Italian bread.

YIELD: ½ CUP

and help you recover more quickly from flare-ups. One of the best—and simplest—is to mix ¼ cup of olive oil in a large glass of milk, and pour the mixture into a tub of warm water. Then settle in and soak for 20 minutes or so. Repeat as often as needed to relieve your discomfort.

✔ Head for Psoriasis Relief

When psoriasis has flared up on your scalp, chances are you'd rather not soak your head in a bathtub for 20 minutes. Fortunately, there are several other effective remedies. Your best choice depends on how much time you have to spend on the project. Here are three excellent options:

A SHOWER-TIME TREATMENT. Pour 1 cup of olive oil into a bowl, and mix in 1 drop of oregano oil and 2 drops of calendula oil. Massage the mixture into your scalp, and shampoo as usual. Rinse with a half-and-half solution of apple cider vinegar and water.

A ONE-HOUR WONDER. Heat 1 cup of olive oil until it's just warm to the touch, pour it into a clean, empty shampoo or conditioner bottle, and mix

Herbal Customizing Components

Whether you're treating your aching body to an olive oil massage or the Healing Oil and Salt Soak on page 232, use this chart as a handy guide for formulating your own tailor-made healer.

TO GET THESE BENEFITS . . .	CHOOSE ONE OR MORE OF THESE ESSENTIAL OILS*
Antiseptic and healing	Calendula, eucalyptus, lavender, peppermint,** tea tree, wintergreen**
Energizing	Cyprus,** juniper berry,** lime, patchouli, peppermint,** rosemary,** rosewood, tangerine
Relaxing and sleep-inducing	Chamomile, geranium, lavender, rose
Especially beneficial during pregnancy	Catnip, chamomile, citrus oils (any), geranium, jasmine, lavender, rose

* All of these oils are available in health-food stores and online.
** Avoid these oils if you're pregnant or think you might be pregnant.

in 10 to 15 drops of tea tree oil. Apply the mixture to your scalp, and massage it in thoroughly. Cover your head with a plastic shower cap or, in a pinch, a plastic bag or plastic wrap. Leave it on for 60 minutes or so, then shampoo twice (because tea tree oil can dry out your hair) and follow up with a good conditioner. **Note:** Don't worry if your scalp tingles a little—that's a normal reaction to tea tree oil. But if you experience intense itching or burning, remove your head cover and wash your hair immediately.

AN OVERNIGHTER. Warm up ¼ cup of olive oil, and massage it into your scalp. Cover your hair with a plastic shower cap, and hit the sack. Come morning, shampoo as usual.

✔ Conquer Cradle Cap

Cradle cap, known in medical circles as *seborrheic dermatitis*, can be highly disturbing for new parents who are seeing it for the first time. The good news is that, as unsightly as this skin condition may be, it is both harmless and temporary. (It's essentially the infant form of dandruff.) But don't just sit there and wait for the child to outgrow it. Instead, massage a little extra virgin olive oil onto the tyke's scalp, and leave it on for 15 minutes. Then gently brush the flakes out with a soft brush. Follow up with a natural baby shampoo, and leave it on for a few minutes before rinsing to make sure you get all the oil off. Repeat the procedure as needed until the bough breaks and the cradle falls, so to speak.

Ease Teething Troubles

HEALTHFUL HINT

It's not easy being a baby. As if an itchy head and a sore bottom weren't enough, there's the agonizing process of "hatching" those first teeth. To relieve the pain, rub those sore little gums with extra virgin olive oil. Although the kiddo probably can't say "Thank you!" yet, you're sure to see a happy (mostly toothless) grin, or at least a pair of tear-free eyes.

✔ Stop Trouble at the Other End

It's probably safe to say that every infant on the planet suffers from diaper rash at one time or another. And according to legions of mothers and medical pros, the most effective natural remedy is extra virgin olive oil. To soothe the situation, whip 2 teaspoons of it (using either a wire whisk or a blender) with 1 teaspoon of water to form an emulsion. Then smooth the mixture onto baby's bottom, and wait a few minutes for it to penetrate before you cover the area with a fresh diaper.

✔ Rub Away Aches and Pains

No matter what's causing the discomfort in your muscles, joints, and tendons—a sports injury, arthritis, or simply a long day of working in the yard—extra virgin olive oil can help ease the pain. Just heat 1 cup of it in the microwave, or in a pan over very low heat, until the oil is comfortably warm to the touch. If you like, add 3 or 4 drops of the appropriate essential oil (see "Herbal Customizing Components," on page 234, for some good suggestions). Then massage the healer into your ailing body parts.

✔ Winter Wonder Bath

It's probably safe to say that even folks who love winter's crisp temperatures and snowy landscapes could do without the colds and flu—not to mention the chapped, dry skin—that come with the season. Well, take heart, my friend: Here's a bath blend that will help relieve your aches and pains, clear your clogged sinuses, and moisturize and soothe your raw, red skin. You can make it using this simple five-step process:

STEP 1. Gather the goods. You'll need 3 cups of extra virgin olive oil, 6 tablespoons of ground ginger, 4 tablespoons of dried rosemary, and a peppermint tea bag; a saucepan, wooden spoon, mixing bowl, strainer, and a jar with a tight-fitting lid.

STEP 2. Begin warming the olive oil over very low heat, and add the ginger and rosemary. Stir the mixture constantly, making sure it doesn't scorch.

STEP 3. Add the peppermint tea bag, stirring until it is completely submerged.

STEP 4. Cover the pan, and let the blend simmer for 15 minutes.

STEP 5. Strain the potion into a bowl, let it cool to room temperature, and pour it into the jar.

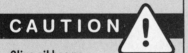

CAUTION ⚠

Olive oil has no known side effects or drug interactions. But oil *is* slippery, so use caution when getting into and out of the tub or shower if you're using an oil treatment.

At bath time, add ¾ to 1 cup of the mixture to very warm (not hot!) running bathwater. To maximize the sinus-clearing power, get into the tub while the water is still running, and take deep breaths of the rising steam. Soak for 15 to 20 minutes, then towel-dry, and toddle off to bed. Store any leftover blend in the refrigerator, where it will stay fresh for about a week. **Note:** This recipe makes about 3 cups of bath blend.

✔ Strike Oil for Sinus Relief

Is sinus congestion driving you up a wall? Well, climb down and grab a bottle of extra virgin olive oil. Pour 1 tablespoon of it into a bowl, and mix in 3 or 4 drops of peppermint oil. Massage the mixture onto your nose, cheekbones, temples, and forehead. Almost immediately, you should feel your sinuses beginning to clear up. Repeat two or three times a day, as needed, until you're breathing freely again. **Note:** If you don't have peppermint oil on hand, you can substitute eucalyptus, lavender, or rosemary oil. Whichever kind you choose, if you haven't used it before, test a drop or two on your wrist to make sure you're not sensitive to it.

One Alluring Oil

✤ Lush Lashes

Mascara will make your eyelashes look longer and fuller, all right. But this terrific treatment will strengthen and moisturize them at the hair follicles, so they really will be lusher and lovelier. The plan: Mix equal parts of extra virgin olive oil, coconut oil, and vitamin E oil in a clean, lidded container. Twice a day, dip a clean mascara wand or a cotton swab into the mixture, and swipe it across the base of your clean, mascara-free lashes. (Just make sure you don't get any in your eyes.) Store the conditioner, covered, at room temperature. It should keep indefinitely.

✤ Adios, Cellulite!

There are scads of anti-cellulite products out there, both commercial and DIY versions. But studies have shown the dynamic duo of extra virgin olive oil and juniper oil to be one of the most effective of all. Simply combine equal parts of the two oils, and massage the mixture into the affected area once a day. After three weeks or so, you should begin to see firmer, smoother skin and a definite reduction in your "cottage cheese" condition.

✤ Scrub and Soften

If you're like most women I know, you don't have a whole lot of free time on your hands. So why fuss with different products to clean, exfoliate, and moisturize your skin, when this triple-threat performer can do it all? To put it on your team, mix 2 tablespoons of olive oil with 1 cup of Epsom salts in an unbreakable container. Then step into the shower, scoop out handfuls of the mixture, and gently scrub your skin, paying special attention to any dry, rough, or itchy areas. When you're finished, rinse well and dry yourself off. **Note:** This combo is gentle enough to use on your face, but be careful not to get it in your eyes.

✤ TLC for Rough Hands and Feet . . .

And knees and elbows, too! This strong, but gentle treatment is just the ticket for exfoliating skin that's become overly rough and dry. First, pulverize ¼ cup of fresh ginger in a blender or food processor. Then mix it with ½ cup of lukewarm olive oil, ½ cup of coarse salt, and the juice of two limes to make a soft, gritty paste. Massage it into your skin using gentle circular motions. Rinse it off with warm water, and follow up with your favorite moisturizing lotion.

✤ Fill in the Cracks

Dry, cracked feet are no fun, and that's putting it mildly. Not only are they unsightly, but they can also be as sore as the dickens. The simple solution: this intensive overnight treatment. Just before bedtime, whisk ¼ cup of extra virgin olive oil and ¼ cup of mild, unscented body lotion in a bowl, and heat it in the microwave for 15 to 20 seconds. (You want it to be pleasantly warm, but not hot.) While the oil-lotion combo is heating, tear off two long sections of plastic wrap, and set them aside. Apply a generous layer of the mixture to one foot, and

POTENT POTION

AROMATIC OIL AND MILK BATH

This beauty of a bath blend will soften your skin, relax your muscles, lift your spirits, and delight your senses. Who could ask for anything more?

½ **cup of dry whole milk**
½ **cup of extra virgin olive oil**
1 egg
1 tbsp. of glycerin
6 drops of lavender essential oil
1 drop of jasmine essential oil
1 drop of rose essential oil
2 cups of distilled water

Beat the first four ingredients in a bowl, using a wire whisk or handheld eggbeater. Add the essential oils, and continue beating until a smooth paste forms. Gradually add the water as you keep beating. Then pour the mixture into a tub of toasty warm water, slip in, and enjoy!

cover it with plastic wrap to lock in the warmth and moisture. Repeat the procedure with your other foot. Then put on thick socks and head off to dreamland. Come morning, remove the socks and plastic wrap. If necessary, repeat the routine each night until your feet are silky smooth and sandal-ready.

❖ Preventive Maintenance

Once your feet are soft and crack-free, keep them that way using a lotion made from 2 drops of either lemon or lavender essential oil per tablespoon of extra virgin olive oil. Combine the oils in a sterilized bottle with a tight-fitting lid, and shake it until the solution is thick and milky. Store it at room temperature, and shake before each use. Massage the lotion into your feet a few times a week, or as often as needed to maintain picture-perfect tootsies.

❖ Soften Your Cuticles

When your hands spend a lot of time in water, whether it's in a kitchen sink or a swimming pool, your cuticles can dry out in a hurry. To replace the moisture, combine 1 teaspoon of olive oil with 1 teaspoon of vitamin E oil, and massage the mixture into your cuticles. Repeat as needed to keep them strong and supple.

❖ Moisturize Rough Lips

When winter wind or summer sun leaves your lips parched, dry, and sore, intensive care is right in your kitchen. Just mash a few slices of ripe banana

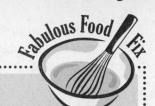

Fabulous Food Fix

FRENCH DRESSING

If you've ever wondered how French women manage to keep their skin beautiful and young looking well into their senior years, part of the secret lies in two words: olive oil. They use plenty of it to nourish and soften their skin from the outside *and* the inside. This classic salad dressing is one of the simplest ways to up your intake of beautifying olive oil. (You'll see that it bears no resemblance to the gooey orange stuff you find in the supermarket.)

1 tbsp. of wine vinegar or lemon juice
Salt and pepper to taste*
⅔ cup of extra virgin olive oil

With a wire whisk, beat the vinegar with the salt and pepper until the salt dissolves. Then whisk in the olive oil a drizzle at a time. Use it as a salad dressing, a topping for lightly steamed vegetables, or a dipping sauce for raw veggies or crusty French bread.

* If you like, add mustard, crushed garlic, and/or fresh herbs to taste.

YIELD: ⅔ CUP

with a couple teaspoons of extra virgin olive oil to make a thick paste, and rub it onto your lips. Leave it on for 15 to 20 minutes, and rinse it off with warm water. Repeat as needed until your kisser is in fine fettle again.

✤ Oil Acne Away

After washing your face with mild soap and hot water, apply a thin layer of olive oil, and let your skin absorb it—don't wash it off. Repeat the procedure three times a day, and within a week your skin should be smooth and clear. After that, use the treatment once a day to prevent further outbreaks and keep your skin looking its best.

✤ Spruce Up Your Hair

Here's a trick that will add sparkle to any color hair and reduce static at the same time: Mix 1 tablespoon of raw honey with 1 cup or so of extra virgin olive oil, and work it through your hair. Leave it on for at least 30 minutes (the longer the better), then rinse it out. Presto—gleaming locks that are soft and sleek, with no flyaway strands!

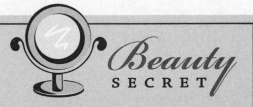

A MEGABUCKS MOISTURIZER...

Beauty SECRET

For only pennies on the dollar! You could go to a certain trendy spa out west and pay through the nose for a facial treatment that features a trio of moisturizing superstars. Or you could march into your kitchen and make that headliner yourself. Your action plan: Pour 2 cups of extra virgin olive oil into a large jar that has a screw-on lid, and tuck in two or three sprigs each of fresh basil and chamomile. Cover the jar opening with cheesecloth, screw on the lid, and let it sit for 30 days or so. Remove the cloth, leaving the herbs in the jar, and put the lid back on. To use the potion, dab a few tablespoons of it onto your face, as you would any other moisturizer, give it a few minutes to penetrate your skin, then remove it with a dry cotton cloth.

✤ Out with Chlorine!

Attention, frequent swimmers! I don't have to tell you what a mess chlorine can make of your hair. Fortunately, there's a simple way to undo the damage. Just blend 1 egg, 2 tablespoons of extra virgin olive oil, and ¼ of a peeled, chopped cucumber in a blender or food processor until it has a rich, creamy consistency. Spread the mixture evenly through your hair, and leave it on for 15 minutes or so. Then rinse thoroughly. Repeat once a month for ongoing damage control. **Note:** This treatment is also great for removing built-up residue from hair sprays and other styling products.

✤ Prevent Hair Loss . . .

Or at least slow it down. Even on the most well-endowed heads, hair falls out and regrows constantly. But if you seem to be shedding more and growing less, try this remedy: Combine equal parts of olive oil and rosemary essential oil in a bottle, and shake to mix thoroughly. At bedtime, massage the mixture into your scalp, and cover it with a shower cap. In the morning, wash your hair with a gentle shampoo, and rinse with 1 tablespoon of apple cider vinegar in 1 quart of warm water. Repeat the procedure each night for a few weeks. By that time, your hair income should exceed the outgo. **Note:** Some people claim this routine will even work to stop male-pattern baldness, but don't bet on it.

POTENT POTION

ALL-NATURAL SHAMPOO

Many commercial shampoos sport the word *natural* in big letters on the label, but when you read the fine print on the back, you usually see a bunch of ingredients that you can't even pronounce— much less buy at the grocery store. This shampoo, on the other hand, comes straight from Mother Nature herself. **Note:** This recipe must be made up just before you're ready to use it.

2 tbsp. of extra virgin olive oil
1 tbsp. of lemon juice
1 tsp. of unfiltered apple cider
   vinegar*
1 egg

Mix all of the ingredients thoroughly in a blender. Pour the mixture into a plastic bottle, bring it to the sink, tub, or shower, and use it as you would any other shampoo.

* Available in health-food stores and in the health-food sections of most supermarkets.

❖ Revitalizing Conditioner

Generations of women have sworn by this simple treatment to restore the shine and bounce to their hair: Heat ½ cup of olive oil until it's lukewarm. If you like, stir in a few drops of your favorite scented oil or extract. Using an eyedropper (or a spoon if you don't have a dropper), apply the warm oil to your hair, and massage it into your scalp so that your entire head is thoroughly oiled. Wait for three to five minutes, then shampoo as usual.

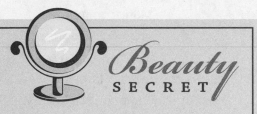

Beauty SECRET

CONDITION AND COLOR

If you have brown or auburn hair, this tip has your name (written in big red letters) all over it. Warm ½ cup of olive oil in a pan over low heat. Add 2 tablespoons of ground cloves, and heat until the mixture is hot, but not boiling. Remove the pan from the stove, put the cover on, and let it sit overnight. Strain it into a plastic bottle with a dispenser top (a clean shampoo or conditioner bottle is perfect). Squirt a bit of the mixture onto one of your palms, and rub it between your hands to warm it up. Work the potion into your scalp, and comb it through to the ends of your hair. Cover your head with a plastic shower cap, and go about your business for 20 minutes. Then rinse the oil out and shampoo as usual.

❖ Deep-Conditioning Treatment

Here's a five-step routine that will soothe a dry, irritated scalp, clear up dandruff—and soften and hydrate your hair at the same time:

STEP 1. Saturate your hair with extra virgin olive oil, and massage it into the roots.

STEP 2. Pile your hair on top of your head, and cover it with plastic wrap or a plastic shower cap.

STEP 3. Set your hair dryer on low, and "dry" your covered head for 60 seconds or so. Then wrap a warm towel around your head to lock in the heat.

STEP 4. Wait about 20 minutes, then remove the wrappings, and rinse out the oil.

STEP 5. Shampoo and style your hair as usual, and take a look in the mirror. You'll see a softer, shinier, and healthier mane.

✤ Solo Performances

For centuries, women in the Mediterranean region have relied on extra virgin olive oil as the key—and often only—product in their beauty-care routines. It'll work just as well for you. Here's a sampling of possibilities:

CONDITION YOUR HAIR. After shampooing, section your damp hair, and apply a light coat of oil from the roots to the ends. Then style your hair as usual. **Note:** This is an especially effective way to moisturize coarse gray hair and make it more manageable.

FADE SCARS. Rub a thin film of oil onto the marks every day. You won't see results overnight, but with time they should vanish, or at least greatly diminish in appearance.

MINIMIZE WRINKLES. Each night at bedtime, massage oil into the lined areas of your face and neck. In the morning, wash the oil off with luke-warm water, then splash your skin with cold water and gently pat dry.

MOISTURIZE DAILY. Use it as you would any other moisturizer. To avoid greasiness, smooth it on when your skin is damp, and blot the oil dry thoroughly before you apply any makeup.

REMOVE EYE MAKEUP. Simply moisten a cotton pad or ball with oil, and gently rub it across your eyelids and lashes.

SHAVE CLEAN, SHAVE CLOSE. Wipe oil onto your legs and underarms, and have at it. For guys, olive oil works just as well on your face, and it's a lot healthier than shaving creams that contain alcohol and who knows what chemicals.

SHINE YOUR LIPS. Put a dab of oil on your fingertip, and rub it across your lips to lock in the moisture and make them gleam. You can also apply the oil over your regular lipstick.

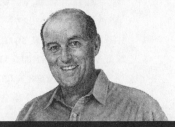

YOU DON'T SAY!

According to Homer, the olive tree has been offering its bounty to Greece for more than 10,000 years. The story of how it came to be there is one of my favorite legends. It seems that Zeus, the king of the Greek gods, held a contest between Athena, the goddess of wisdom, and Poseidon, the god of the seas, to determine who would control a newly built city in Attica. Zeus promised the land to whichever one provided the most useful gift to the people of the country. Poseidon pounded a rock with his trident, and salt water burst forth. Then Athena struck her spear on the ground, and it turned into an olive tree. The rest, as they say in Athens, is history.

Best of the Rest

★ Unpack the Wax

Wax is in our ears to trap dirt and dust particles and protect our ears from infections. But sometimes (especially as we get more, um, experienced), the wax can build up, become hardened, and block the ear canal. Fortunately, there's a simple way to keep the stuff soft, so it can move on out: A couple of times a week, put a few drops of vegetable oil into each ear.

★ Think "Oil" for Osteoarthritis

Gentle massage can help ease the pain in your joints. For even better results, put a little canola oil or vegetable oil on your fingertips, and work slowly around the affected area, forming small circles. Don't massage the joint itself; instead, stay above and below it. Perform this routine for three to five minutes every day if you can.

★ Relieve Skin Woes

As you know, if you have either eczema or psoriasis, these conditions are two of the most annoying skin afflictions on the planet. To moisturize those scaly patches, gently wipe solid vegetable shortening onto the affected skin. You'll feel almost-instant relief from the pain and roughness.

★ When You Need an Extra-Tough Hand Cleaner . . .

Like those times when you've got tar or pine sap all over your hands (or any other part of your body). What to do? Grab a can of vegetable shortening, and gently rub some of it into your skin. Then wipe the area with a soft cloth, and the sticky stuff will come right off. Follow up with soap and water.

★ It Works, by Gum!

You say your youngster just had a head-on collision with a wad of chewing gum? Or maybe you've been the victim of a little prankster. Vegetable oil can deliver first aid fast. Massage the oil into the gum, which will almost immediately begin to break down. Then comb the wad with outward strokes, starting at the hair ends. Be patient, and gradually work your way toward the scalp until you've removed all traces of the sticky blob.

★ A Short(ening) Course on Wart Removal

If the Guinness folks keep track of statistics for DIY healers, I have a hunch that wart-removal methods top the list. Here's another one: Mix 2 tablespoons of vegetable shortening, 1 chopped garlic clove, and ½ tablespoon of lemon juice in a bowl. Spread the mixture onto the wart, and cover it with a piece of duct tape. Leave it on for 12 hours, then remove the tape and wash the cream off. Repeat the process each day until the wart is gone.

★ Makeup Kit in a Can

During the Great Depression and World War II, very few women could find commercial cosmetics in stores, much less afford to buy them. So what did they use instead? Old-fashioned vegetable shortening like Crisco®, that's what! And it works just as well today. Here's a trio of handy, money-saving ways that you can put it to good use:

REMOVE YOUR MASCARA. Dab a little shortening onto your eyelids, then gently wipe it (and your eye makeup) away with a cotton pad.

SOFTEN YOUR FACE. Simply smooth a palmful onto your skin before bed, as you would any other night cream.

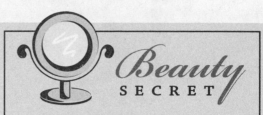

Beauty SECRET

**BRITTLE NAILS:
A PERMANENT FIX**

In order to fix dried-out nails for good, you have to address the root of the problem, which is too little moisture. So do what dermatologists recommend: At bedtime, massage either vegetable oil or vegetable shortening into your hands and nails, and put on a pair of rubber gloves, which will force the oil to penetrate into your skin. Leave the gloves on overnight and by morning, you should see signs of improvement. Repeat the treatment each night until your nails are in good shape. Then perform the procedure once every few weeks, or as needed, to maintain their strength and appearance.

SOFTEN YOUR HANDS. Pull the can out of the cupboard, scoop out a handful of shortening, and rub some into your rough "paws." It'll work every bit as well as the priciest brand-name product. Personal grooming couldn't get much easier (or cheaper) than that!

18

Onions

Folks have been cultivating onions for more than 6,000 years, and for eons before that, hunter-gatherers were plucking up the wild varieties. Throughout the centuries, the tangy bulbs have been used to do everything from fend off scurvy to clean bullet wounds. (You Civil War buffs may recall a telegram General Ulysses S. Grant sent to the War Department saying, "I will not move my troops without onions.") Today, the onion is touted far and wide as a "nutriceutical," meaning a nutritious food that also has powerful medicinal and health-promoting properties. And does it ever! The same compounds that make this papery-skinned veggie a health-care marvel also make it key to maintaining youthful good looks.

Medicine to Cry For

✔ Unclog Your Sinuses . . .

Fast! How? Slice an onion in two, hold it, cut side up, under your nose, and take a big whiff. Your nasal passages will be free and clear in no time flat! This same quick trick will also help when you're feeling faint.

✔ Exterminate an Earache

Heat half an onion in the oven until it's nice and warm (not hot). Wrap it in cheesecloth, and hold it against your sore ear. The chemicals in the onion will help increase your blood circulation and flush away the infection.

✔ Exterminate an Earache, Take 2

If you prefer a liquid approach to pain relief, steam or bake an onion until the skin is soft. Then crush the bulb to extract the warm juice. Use an eyedropper to put a few drops of the liquid into the affected ear, and plug it with a cotton ball. **Note:** Make sure the juice is just comfortably warm—not hot!

✔ Rout Out a Splinter

Don't even think about reaching for a sewing needle and a bottle of rubbing alcohol! Instead, grab a raw onion. Cut a slice that's about the size of a small postage stamp, place it over the splinter, and cover it with an adhesive bandage. Leave it on overnight, or for about eight hours. The onion will draw the sliver to the surface of your skin so you can easily grab it with a pair of tweezers and slide it out painlessly.

✔ Beat Bronchitis

One of the best bronchial medicines you could ever ask for is in the produce aisle of your local supermarket—or maybe growing in your own garden. That's right—it's onions! The pungent bulbs are a rich source of allicin and quercetin, two chemicals that help relieve chest colds, bronchitis, and even asthma attacks. Eat 'em raw in a salad, stir-fry them with other vegetables, or make yourself a big bowl of onion soup. No matter how you eat them, you should soon feel your airways clearing up.

POTENT POTION

ALL-PURPOSE COUGH SYRUP

This classic remedy has been stopping coughs for generations, and it remains one of the most effective treatments you could ever hope to find.

2 large sweet onions
2 cups of dark honey
2 oz. of brandy

Peel the onions, cut them into thin slices, and spread them out in a single layer in a large shallow bowl or baking dish. Pour the honey evenly over the slices, and cover the container with plastic wrap or anything else that fits (for instance, a pot lid or a wooden cutting board). Let it sit for eight hours or so, strain off the syrup, and mix it with the brandy. Pour the mixture into a glass jar with a tight-fitting lid, and store it in the refrigerator. Take 1 teaspoon every two to three hours, or as needed, to halt your hacking.

YIELD: ABOUT 2 CUPS

✔ Beat Bronchitis from the Outside

Even when you're feeling so lousy that you don't want to eat *anything*, onions can still break up your lung congestion. Here's the easy three-step routine:

STEP 1. Coat a cast-iron skillet with olive oil and add a handful of chopped onions, 1 teaspoon of unfiltered apple cider vinegar, and a pinch of cornstarch.

STEP 2. Cook the ingredients over low heat to make a paste. Let it cool to a comfortable temperature, and then spread it on a soft, clean cloth that's big enough to cover your chest.

STEP 3. Lay the cloth, paste side down, on your bare chest. Cover it with plastic wrap, add another cloth, and top everything with a heating pad set on low. Relax for an hour or so. The onion will be absorbed into your body and open up your bronchial tubes pronto.

You'll know the paste has penetrated into your system because you'll have the onion breath to prove it!

HEALTHFUL HINT

Onion Juicing 101

Onion juice is one of the most powerful, and versatile, healers you could ever hope to find. You can buy it in health-food stores and online, but it'll cost you a small fortune. Besides, the fresher it is, the better, and it's a snap to make your own supply, even if you don't have a juicing machine. Just grate a raw onion, or chop it finely in a food processor, squeeze the pieces through cheesecloth, and pour the liquid into a jar with a tight-fitting lid. You can store it in the refrigerator for up to 14 days. Just remember, the juice does lose its potency quickly, so for best results, make only as much as you'll use within a day or two.

✔ Quell the Common Cold

For centuries, onions have been known as one of the most potent healers on the planet. So it's only natural that folks have come up with scads of ways to use them to relieve cold symptoms. Here's a trio of options for you:

■ At bedtime, put a slice of raw onion on the sole of each foot, and hold the slices in place with thick wool socks. Overnight, the curative compounds in the onion will draw out the infection and lower your fever. (They'll also leave you with onion breath in the morning.)

■ Slice an onion in two, and set one half on each side of your bed so that you can breathe in the healing aroma as you sleep.

■ To break up congestion overnight, eat a whole raw onion just before you go to bed. It's fine to add the onion to a salad and/or sandwich—you don't have to munch on it like an apple.

✔ Fruit-of-the-Vine Fatigue Fighter

When a tough bout with the flu has left you so weak that you can barely function—or you're just plum tuckered out from a long period of work or play—try this old European folk remedy: Put ¼ cup of raw honey into a 1-liter jar, add a large chopped onion, and pour in enough white wine to fill the jar. Put the lid on and leave the mixture in a cool, dark place (not the fridge) for two weeks. Then strain out the onion, and take 1 tablespoon of the wine three times a day—before breakfast, lunch, and dinner. Before you know it, you'll be rarin' to go again. **Note:** If your fatigue persists, or you suddenly start feeling exhausted for no apparent reason, call your doctor.

✔ Protect Your Ticker

Medical science tells us that red wine and onions are both rich in compounds that help keep your heart in good working order. So why not combine those two powerful healers in one easy tonic? Simply add the juice of a medium-size onion to a bottle of red wine, and shake it for a few minutes. (For instructions on extracting juice from an onion, see "Onion Juicing 101," at left.) You may need to mix the two fluids in a slightly larger bottle or jar. Take 1½ to 3 tablespoons of the potion each day.

> **C A U T I O N** ⚠
>
> Onions lower blood sugar and slow blood clotting. So if you are taking either diabetes medications or anticoagulant drugs (including prescription doses of aspirin or ibuprofen), check with your doctor before you increase your intake of onions beyond the commonly eaten quantities. Also, the compounds in onions interact with lithium, so speak with your doc if you are on any drugs containing that chemical.

✔ Rev Up Your Circulation

Are your hands and feet always cold, no matter what season it is? Onion "tea" can send your blood flowing to those extremities. To make it, boil four to six chopped, medium-size onions in 1 quart of water for 10 to 15 minutes. Strain out the onions, and stir in 2 tablespoons of honey. Store the brew in the refrigerator, and drink 1 or 2 warmed-up cups each day. But if your circulation doesn't start improving within a couple of weeks, consult with your doctor. **Note:** This same bracing brew can also help soothe the burning sensation of a urinary tract infection.

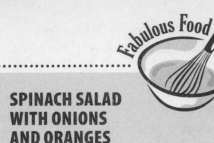

SPINACH SALAD WITH ONIONS AND ORANGES

We all need iron in our diets to maintain the oxygen supply in our blood, but it's especially important for women of childbearing age to replenish the iron they lose each month. Spinach and onions are both rich in that essential mineral, and this salad is a simple, delicious way to help meet your quota.

5–6 cups of baby spinach
1 cup of mandarin oranges,
   drained
½ cup of red onions, chopped*
2 tbsp. of red-wine vinegar
1 tbsp. of orange marmalade
⅓ cup of extra virgin olive oil
Salt and pepper to taste

Arrange the spinach leaves on four plates, and distribute the orange sections and onions among them. Whisk the vinegar and marmalade together. Gradually add the oil as you continue to whisk. Pour the dressing over the salad, serve it up, and pass the salt and pepper.

* Or substitute white sweet onions like Vidalia®, Texas Sweet, or Walla Walla.

YIELD: 4 SERVINGS

✔ Ease Asthma

A variation on All-Purpose Cough Syrup (see page 247) is just what the doctor ordered for relieving asthma symptoms. Slice or chop two large raw onions (any kind will do). Put them into a jar, and pour 2 cups of honey over the pieces. Cover the jar and let it stand at room temperature overnight. Beginning the next morning (and without removing the onion bits), take 1 teaspoon of the syrup 30 minutes after each meal and 1 teaspoon at bedtime.

✔ Fend Off Bruises

The next time you bang your leg on the coffee table, or maybe on your way down the stairs, grab an onion. The same chemicals that make your eyes water also flush excess blood from your system. So immediately after the unfortunate encounter, cut a slice of raw onion (the stronger, the better), put it over the bump site, and leave it on for 15 minutes or so. If you've acted fast enough, you should keep the black-and-blue blotches to a minimum.

✔ Season Your Singe

It seems to happen once or twice every summer (at least it does at my house): You accidentally brush up against your piping-hot barbecue grill and singe your finger. Well, don't run yelping to the kitchen for some first-aid ointment because help is probably right at hand. First, pour a little cold water on the burned area, or rub an ice cube over it. Then apply a slice of raw onion directly to the site. This simple makeshift poultice will cool the area, ease the pain, and act as an antiseptic to reduce the risk of infection. **Note:** Of course, this trick will work just as well if you're already in the kitchen when you burn yourself.

✔ Treat Bites and Stings

Onions can also relieve another frequent summertime occurrence: an encounter with the wrong end of a nasty insect. When a bug plants its stinger or blood-sucking mouth parts into your skin, grab a slice of onion (the juicier, the better) and lay it on the "crime scene." The powerful phytochemicals will reduce the pain and swelling. **Note:** If the culprit was a bee, there is no need to remove the stinger. Just tape the onion slice in place and leave it there for three hours or so. When you remove it, the "weapon" should come right along with it.

✔ Get Some Go Power

Having trouble urinating? Reach for some raw onions, and eat them in salads or sandwiches. They contain compounds that are gentle, but highly effective, diuretics. If you don't care for the taste of onions, slice one in half, and rub the cut surface on your loins (yes, you read that right). As odd as it may sound, it should start things flowing within a day or so.

✔ Whoops—Too Late!

When Chief Montezuma has already come a-callin' (see "Roam Happy Trails," at right), don't fret. Just mix 2 to 4 ounces of onion

---

Roam Happy Trails

HEALTHFUL HINT

Are you planning a trip to a foreign country? If so, then take a simple precaution to prevent that common traveler's affliction, bacterial dysentery (a.k.a. Montezuma's revenge or Delhi belly). Here's what to do: Beginning two weeks before your departure date, eat one good-size raw onion (weighing 8 ounces or so) every day. The simplest way to get your quota is to slice, dice, or chop an onion in the morning, and then add it to salads, sandwiches, guacamole, or whatever else you might eat throughout the day. **Note:** For an especially potent antibacterial wallop, mix a whole, finely diced raw onion in a cup of plain yogurt. Don't cringe! It tastes a lot better than you'd imagine. Somehow, the yogurt sweetens the flavor of the onion.

juice in 8 ounces of peppermint tea, and drink a cup every hour until your runs dry up. (For instructions on how to juice an onion, see "Onion Juicing 101" on page 248.) By the way, this remedy works just as well to alleviate any kind of diarrhea, no matter what caused it. **Note:** Although bacterial dysentery is usually more of a nuisance than a health threat, if your distress lasts more than 48 hours, see a doctor to rule out the possibility of either amoebic or viral dysentery, both of which are serious medical conditions.

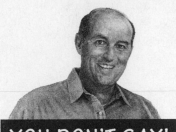

YOU DON'T SAY!

Over the centuries, every culture on earth has used and treasured onions, but nowhere have they been held in higher esteem than in ancient Egypt. For those folks, the tangy bulb was much more than a valuable source of food and medicine. Because of its many-layered, circle-within-a-circle structure, it symbolized eternity. Every Egyptian leader took his oath of office with his right hand on an onion. Paintings in pyramids and tombs show it on banquet tables at great religious feasts, and priests are often pictured holding onions in their hands or covering altars with the leaves. And mummies were sent off to the afterlife with a supply of onions, carefully swathed in bandages that resembled another little mummy.

✔ Ease a Kidney Infection
Simply eating plenty of fresh onions will help cleanse your urinary system and help prevent kidney problems. But when it's too late for preventive measures and you're battling an infection, wrap a cup or so of grated or finely chopped onions in a piece of cheesecloth, and place the poultice over your kidney area (on your back, just under your rib cage). Leave it on for an hour or so, and repeat as needed until your infection has cleared up. **Note:** If you're under medical care for a kidney infection, check with your doctor before using this or any other homemade healer. And if you suspect that you might have a kidney condition, but it has not been diagnosed, call the doc ASAP.

✔ Snag Some Shut-Eye
While we're on the subject of quirky remedies, a lot of former insomniacs swear by this sleep-inducing trick: Cut a yellow onion into chunks, put the pieces in a glass jar that has a tight-fitting lid, and keep it on your bedside table. Then, whenever the Sandman refuses to appear, or if you wake up in the middle of the night and can't get back to sleep, open the jar and take a nice big whiff. Then put the lid back on the jar, close your eyes, and hit the road to dreamland.

✔ Juicy Solutions

Some health issues are more convenient to treat using onion juice rather than the bulbs themselves. You can extract the fluid following the simple procedure outlined in "Onion Juicing 101" (see page 248). And here are juicy remedies for a handful of common problems:

ATHLETE'S FOOT. Massage the juice into your tootsies. Wait 10 minutes or so, rinse your feet in lukewarm water, and dry them thoroughly before you put on any footwear. Repeat the procedure three times a day until the fungus is no longer among us.

HEAT EXHAUSTION. First, get out of the sun. Then massage the juice onto your chest and behind your ears. You (or the victim) should start perking up almost immediately.

LARYNGITIS. Mix 2 parts onion juice with 1 part raw honey in a jar with a tight-fitting lid. Take 3 teaspoons of the mixture every three hours until you're warbling normally again.

RINGWORM. Apply a little juice to the affected areas, let it dry for at least an hour, and then wash it off. Repeat two or three times a day as needed.

TINNITUS. Put 2 drops of onion juice in each ear three times a week until the bells stop ringing.

Note: If you even suspect that heat exhaustion may be a case of full-blown heatstroke, call 911 *immediately*. As for the other conditions listed above, if you don't see signs of improvement within a week, give your doctor a call.

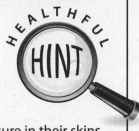

The Skinny on Skins

Like many other vegetables and fruits, onions hold health-giving treasure in their skins. Specifically, onion skins contain massive amounts of quercetin, a compound that has almost miraculous power to lower blood pressure and LDL (bad) cholesterol, reduce inflammation, fight allergies, relieve depression, treat some forms of cancer . . . the list goes on and on. Here are two simple ways you can tap into this medicinal gold mine anytime you make soup, stew, or rice:

1. Toss a whole, unpeeled onion or two into the pot, and fish the bulb out before you serve the dish.

2. Whenever you peel onions, save the skins in a paper bag. Then stuff a handful of the peels into a cheesecloth pouch, and put it into the cooking pot. At serving time, discard the skins. Wash and save the pouch for next time.

✔ Get a Breather from a Bellyache

This is not the most crowd-pleasing way to stop your belly achin', but it sure works wonders! Mix ½ teaspoon of honey and ½ teaspoon of black pepper in ¼ cup of fresh onion juice (see "Onion Juicing 101" on page 248), and toss it back. Just be sure that before you head out to mix and mingle with your pals (or welcome your spouse home with a big kiss), you spend some quality time with a glass of strong mouthwash!

✔ Marinate Your Calluses

Calluses do not pose a serious health hazard, but they can be as painful as the dickens. One simple—and quick—solution: Call Dr. Onion. Cut a slice that's big enough to cover the affected area, put it in a bowl, and pour in enough wine vinegar (either red or white) to cover it. Let the onion soak for four hours or so, then remove it from the bowl, lay it over the calluses, and secure it in place with plastic wrap. Put on a sock to contain the wrapper, and leave it on overnight. Come morning, you should be able to scrape away the thick, hard skin. Once you do, wash and rinse your feet thoroughly so you don't go around town smelling like a salad!

Fragrant Fascination

✤ Clear Up Your Face

Although acne is infamous for targeting teenagers, almost anyone can break out in annoying pimples. One simple cure: Slice a medium-size onion and simmer it in ½ cup of honey until the onion is soft. Then puree the mixture in a blender or food processor (or mash it by hand if you prefer) to make a paste. Let it cool to room temperature, and dab it on the blemishes. Leave it on for at least 60 minutes, and rinse it off with warm water. Repeat the routine every evening until a clear face stares back at you in the mirror.

✤ Another Way to Abolish Acne

To treat large areas of acned skin, give this full-face mask a try: Peel, chop, and heat seven plums until their flesh is soft. (You can do the job in either the microwave or a conventional oven.) Mash the fruit, and mix it with 1 tablespoon of onion juice (see "Onion Juicing 101" on page 248) and 2 teaspoons of olive oil. Wipe the mixture onto your just-washed face, and leave it on for 30 minutes or so. Rinse thoroughly, gently pat your skin dry, and follow up with your usual moisturizer.

Fabulous Food Fix

SWEET-AND-SOUR ONIONS

Here's a two-word secret to maintaining your youthful good looks longer: Eat onions. They pack a potent load of compounds that help to prevent the cellular damage that occurs in your skin over time. This simple side dish (a.k.a. *Cipolline in Agrodolce*) is a classic favorite in Rome, where women are renowned for their beautiful skin.

½ cup of raisins
Hot water
3 tbsp. of extra virgin olive oil
1½ lbs. of cipollini onions, peeled*
¼ cup of balsamic vinegar
1½ tbsp. of sugar
Kosher or sea salt to taste

Put the raisins in a bowl, cover them with hot water, and let them soften for 30 minutes. Heat the oil in a skillet over medium-high heat. Add the onions and cook for 8 to 10 minutes, or until they're golden brown. Then pour off the oil. Drain the raisins and add them, along with the vinegar, sugar, and salt, to the skillet. Stir until the sauce thickens (2 to 3 minutes).

* Available in many large supermarkets; or substitute either fresh or frozen pearl onions.

YIELD: 4 TO 6 SERVINGS

✤ Go Away, Warts!

Are you ready for another remarkable remedy for bothersome warts? Ready or not, here it comes! Just slice an onion in two, dip one of the cut sides in a dish of salt, and rub the surface of the tangy bulb over each wart. Perform this routine twice a day until the unsightly bumps disappear.

✤ Out, Out, Danged Spots!

Many middle-aged people, especially those with fair skin, develop large, flat brown marks (a.k.a. age or liver spots) on their face and hands. The marks may be caused by the sun or by a nutritional deficiency, and in most cases, they're perfectly harmless. But who needs the unsightly things? One simple way to get rid of them: Mix 1 tablespoon of fresh

POTENT POTION

A WELL-ROOTED TONER

Here's a farm-fresh facial treatment that will tone, nourish, and soften your skin at the same time.

1 tbsp. of carrot juice
1 tbsp. of olive oil
1 tbsp. of onion juice*
1 egg yolk

Combine all of the ingredients thoroughly, and spread the mixture onto your face and neck. Leave it on for about 20 minutes, and then rinse it off with lukewarm water. Repeat every week or so.

* See "Onion Juicing 101" on page 248.

onion juice (see "Onion Juicing 101" on page 248) with 2 teaspoons of unfiltered apple cider vinegar. Massage the mixture into the discolored areas twice a day until you no longer see spots before your eyes. **Note:** It may be a few months before you start to see results, but be patient; you can't expect them to vanish overnight.

❖ Lighten and Brighten

For an overall skin-lightening treatment, puree 2 tablespoons of onion juice (see "Onion Juicing 101" on page 248), 1 peeled, chopped pear, and ¼ cup of whole milk in a blender or food processor. Gently apply the mixture to your freshly cleaned face, and leave it on for 15 to 20 minutes. Rinse it off with warm water, and follow up with your usual moisturizer. Repeat two or three times a week.

❖ Take *That,* Wrinkles!

This intensive anti-wrinkle mask is especially tailored for dry skin. To make it, boil a peeled, medium-size potato in 1 cup of whole milk until the spud is soft. Mash it, and mix in 1 tablespoon each of onion juice (see "Onion Juicing 101" on page 248) and honey. After washing your face as usual, smooth the blend onto your skin. Wait about 20 minutes or so, then rinse thoroughly, gently pat your face dry, and apply your normal moisturizer.

❖ Save Your Hair

You would think that in a time when we have vaccines to prevent scads of deadly diseases, some genius would come up with a pill to prevent hair loss. Unfortunately, at least so far, there is no foolproof solution. There are, however, plenty of homemade formulas. According to folks who have used them, some of the most effective ones feature (you guessed it) onions in the starring role. Here's a trio of choices that just might keep the hair on your head from fading fast:

■ Slice a raw onion in two, and massage your scalp with the cut surface. Cover your head with a shower cap, and leave it on overnight. In the morning, shampoo and rinse your hair thoroughly. Repeat at least three times a week.

■ Mix ¼ cup of onion juice (see "Onion Juicing 101" on page 248) with 1 tablespoon of raw honey, and massage the mixture into your scalp thoroughly every day. Then shampoo and condition as usual.

■ Combine the juice of a medium-size onion with 1 tablespoon of raw honey and 1 jigger of vodka. At bedtime each night, rub the cocktail into your scalp, and put on a shower cap. When you wake up, follow your normal shampoo and conditioning routine.

Whichever method you use, expect to see results in anywhere from two weeks to two months.

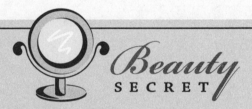

GIVE YOUR HAIR SOME SKIN(S)

*The same onion peels that deliver health benefits galore (see "The Skinny on Skins" on page 253) can also soften your hair and enhance its color. To make this super conditioner, put 2 ½ cups of lightly packed onion peels in a pan, and pour 1 quart of boiling water over them. Steep, covered, for 50 minutes. Strain the brew into a fresh container, and let it cool to room temperature. Then wash your hair as usual, and towel-dry it slightly. With your head over a basin to catch the runoff, rinse three or four times with the onion skin tea. Finish by rinsing with clear water. **Note:** When you use this treatment weekly, it will not only keep your hair amazingly silky, but it may also help minimize the appearance of any gray.*

✤ A Rummy Good Keeper

Once you've got your full head of hair back, help keep those locks in place with this simple routine: Chop a medium-size onion and soak it overnight, peels and all, in 8 ounces of dark rum (don't refrigerate it). Strain out the solids, and massage the liquid into your scalp. Then shampoo, condition, and style your hair as usual. Repeat the procedure every week or so, and your hair should stay well rooted for a long time.

✤ Keep Baldness at Bay

While it may not be possible to cure full-scale baldness, the compounds in onions have been proven to help remove toxins from your body and stimulate blood circulation. Both of those functions strengthen hair follicles, thereby minimizing hair loss and promoting beautiful, well-nourished locks. Best of all, tapping into that grow power is a snap. Just add a tablespoon or so of onion juice (see "Onion Juicing 101" on page 248) to a bottle of your regular shampoo, and use it as you always do. (Just be sure to shake the bottle well before you pour out your normal "dose.")

Best of the Rest

★ Send a Headache Packin'

When the congestion of a cold or flu gives you a headache from you know where, chive tea will end your misery fast. To make it, put 1½ tablespoons of finely chopped chives and ½ tablespoon of finely shredded fresh ginger into a mug or teapot, and pour 1 cup of boiling water over them. Cover the top, and let the mixture steep for 30 minutes. Strain out the solids, and drink the tea lukewarm. Your head should stop throbbing in 20 minutes or less. Repeat as often as needed during your illness.

★ Satisfy Your Salt Cravings

If you're on a sodium-restricted diet, and you really miss being able to let the salt flow freely, here's good news: Eating a scallion or two with each meal can be just the ticket to satisfy your appetite for salty foods. Trim and wash a bunch of scallions (a.k.a. green onions), wrap them in a damp paper towel, and stash them in the fridge, where they'll keep for up to a week. Change the moist wrapping every other day to maintain maximum freshness.

★ Take a Leek . . .

And use it to perform a couple of health-care feats, namely, these:

TREAT HEMORRHOIDS. An old folk remedy for these pains in your sitting area is to eat a large boiled leek every day, either as a snack or with dinner.

STIMULATE URINATION. Cooked leeks are a mild diuretic, and they're delicious in soups, stews, or simply sautéed in olive oil. But for stronger, faster action, eat them raw in salads, sandwiches, or dips. Before you know it, your system will be leaking normally again. (Sorry—I couldn't resist!)

★ Say "Phooey" to Flakes

Chives may look like one of the most mild-mannered plants on the planet, but their volatile compounds are murder on dandruff. To enlist them in your beauty-care posse, put 1 tablespoon of chopped, fresh chives in a mug, and add 1 cup of just-boiled water. Cover the mug, and let the mixture steep for 20 minutes or so. When it's cooled thoroughly, shampoo your hair as usual, and rinse with the chive tea. Repeat this routine daily, and after a few weeks, you'll find that your white flakes will have flown the coop.

POTENT POTION

LEEK LINIMENT

Whether you're a weekend warrior, or you simply spend a lot of time working in your yard, this lovely liniment is a must-have for treating muscle aches, pains, and sprains.

4 leeks, chopped
Water
4 tbsp. of coconut butter*

Put the leeks in a pan with enough water to cover them by 2 inches or so, and boil them until they're mushy. Pour off the water, reduce the heat to low, and add the coconut butter. Mix until you get a creamy consistency. Let the mixture cool to a comfortable temperature, and massage it into the painful area. Store any remaining rub in a tightly covered container at room temperature, and use within a week.

* Available in health-food stores and online (and not to be confused with coconut *oil*).

YIELD: ABOUT ¼ CUP

★ Good Riddance to Oniony Odors

It's no secret that all members of the onion (a.k.a. *Allium*) family, including leeks, shallots, and even chives, can leave an odor on your hands that ranges from merely unpleasant to downright rank. Fortunately, your kitchen is full of handy helpers that can remove the scent—like these, for instance:

BAKING SODA. Mix it with a little water to make a paste, and rub it thoroughly into your skin. Make sure you get in between your fingers and under your nails. When you're done, rinse your hands with clear warm water.

COFFEE. Grab a few beans, and roll them around between your hands. Or, if you don't have any beans, grab a handful of grinds left over from brewing this morning's joe and rub them into your skin. When the onion aroma is gone, wash your hands with soap and water unless, of course, you want to smell like a cup of coffee instead!

LEMON JUICE. Squeeze the juice of half a lemon into one palm, and rub your hands together vigorously. **Note:** If you don't have fresh lemons, the reconstituted stuff will work almost as well.

SALT. Simply massage plain old table salt into your damp skin, then rinse and dry thoroughly. In addition to being odor-free, your hands will feel softer and smoother.

Whichever scent remover you use, if you don't get total satisfaction on the first go-round, repeat the process until your paws pass the sniff test. Just one word of warning: If you have any cuts or scrapes on your hands, you may want to nix the lemon and salt treatments, or be prepared for the sting!

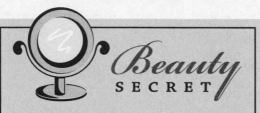

Beauty SECRET

RECHARGE YOUR HAIR COLOR

*If you have brown or reddish hair and you grow leeks in your garden, you have an almost-instant way to restore luster to your locks. Simply steep a pinch of leek seeds in a cup of just-boiled water for 10 minutes. Strain out the seeds, and let the tea cool to room temperature. After shampooing, pour the rinse through your hair. **Note:** Even if you don't have a garden, you might want to pick up some leek seeds at your local garden center just for this purpose.*

19

Parsley

Quick—think of parsley! Did your mind's eye see a frilly garnish on a restaurant plate? Well, think again. Today, health and beauty pros alike classify parsley as a true superfood, and for good reason. Eating as little as a tablespoon of the fresh herb a day (about the size of a typical garnish) can help fight fatigue, increase resistance to colds, relieve muscle and joint pain, prevent cancer, eliminate allergy symptoms, soften your skin, and much, much more. And here's a factoid for the vegetarians in our audience: Parsley has more protein than any other member of the vegetable kingdom.

The Power of Parsley

✔ Inhibit Indigestion

Nothing puts a damper on a good meal like a bout of indigestion. But you can nip your discomfort in the bud by nibbling on a few sprigs of fresh parsley. Got none on hand? Then stir ¼ teaspoon of dried parsley into a glass of warm water and drink up. Your tummy will feel better in no time.

✔ Can the Cramps

When your indigestion takes the form of painful stomach cramps, steep 1 teaspoon of dried or 1 tablespoon of chopped fresh parsley in 1 cup of just-boiled water for five minutes. Strain, and sip the tea slowly. **Note:** Parsley is a potent diuretic, so don't stray too far from a bathroom!

✔ Reduce Your Gas Emissions

You say your digestive problems tend to express themselves outwardly? Then this preventive medicine is just what the doctor ordered: Make a tea by steeping 1 teaspoon of parsley seed per cup of just-boiled water for 5 to 10 minutes. Drink 1 cup of the brew half an hour before each meal. (You can find parsley seed at herb shops, both online and in brick-and-mortar versions.) **Note:** Do not drink this tea, or use parsley seed in any form, if you are pregnant or think you might be pregnant.

Fabulous Food Fix

PARSLEY PESTO

This simple sauce is one of the most delicious ways I know of to pack more parsley power into your diet. It's a classic pasta sauce, but it also makes a terrific dip for crackers or raw veggies; a spread for crusty bread; or a topping for fish, chicken, or baked potatoes.

2 cups of fresh parsley, chopped
1 cup of shelled walnuts, chopped
½ cup of Romano or Parmesan cheese, grated*
3 garlic cloves, chopped
½ tsp. of salt
½ cup of extra virgin olive oil

Combine the first five ingredients in a blender or food processor. Process for about 30 seconds until the mixture is finely minced and just beginning to turn into a paste. Scrape the sides down. With the machine still running, slowly add the olive oil. Stop the machine, scrape the sides down again, and then process for another 30 seconds or so until the mixture is smooth. Serve it immediately or store it, covered, in the refrigerator for up to four days.

* For longer-term pesto storage (several weeks in the fridge or several months in the freezer), omit the cheese and mix it into the pesto just before serving.

YIELD: ABOUT 1¼ CUPS

✔ Build Stronger Bones

Attention, ladies of, um, a certain age! If you're taking calcium supplements to help fend off osteoporosis, here's something you should know: Those high doses of calcium can impair your body's ability to absorb manganese, which is a crucial bone-building compound. But that doesn't mean you should give up the calcium! Instead, simply include 1 tablespoon or so of parsley in your daily diet. It enhances manganese absorption, especially when you eat the herb with foods that are high in copper and zinc, such as shellfish, poultry, and whole grains. For a versatile and delicious way to tap into this manganese magnet, see the Parsley Pesto recipe (at left).

✔ Axe Arthritis Aches

The potent anti-inflammatory compounds in parsley can make quick work of reducing pain and stiffness in your joints. For fast-acting relief, steep 1 fully packed cup of fresh parsley in 1 quart of just-boiled water for 15 minutes. Strain out the solids, and refrigerate the liquid in a covered container. Drink ½ cup before breakfast, ½ cup before dinner, and ½ cup whenever your pain is especially severe.

✔ Keep Your Liver Lively

Your liver performs more than 200 crucial functions in your body, including eliminating toxic substances from your blood, converting food into chemicals that your body needs, and producing bile, which is essential for digestion. Simply making fresh parsley a regular part of your diet will help keep that vital organ running smoothly. But every once in a while, give it an extra boost with a cocktail made from ½ cup of finely chopped fresh parsley leaves and the juice of a medium-size carrot and half a raw beet. **Note:** If you don't have a juicer, you can substitute ½ cup each of organic carrot juice and beet juice.

POTENT POTION

ST. HILDEGARD'S PARSLEY WINE TONIC

The medieval German herbalist, St. Hildegard of Bingen, was a great fan of parsley. She prescribed this potent tonic to improve blood circulation, relieve heart conditions, and generally keep folks' tickers in tip-top shape.

1 qt. of red or white wine
10–12 large sprigs of fresh parsley
2 tbsp. of white vinegar
9 oz. of raw honey

Mix the first three ingredients in a saucepan, and boil for 10 minutes. Add the honey, reduce the temperature to medium, and stir until the honey is thoroughly blended in. Remove the pan from the heat. When the mixture is cool enough to handle safely, strain it and pour it into bottles with tight-fitting caps. Store them in a cool, dark place, and take 1 tablespoon of the tonic three times a day.

YIELD: ABOUT 4½ CUPS

263

✔ A Juicy Way to Relieve Asthma

For decades, naturopathic physicians have been prescribing various vegetable juices to help treat just about every health condition under the sun. A highly recommended blend for relieving asthma symptoms is 2 ounces each of parsley, carrot, and onion juices. Drink the concoction twice a day—but note that this is not a substitute for professional medical care.

To make parsley juice, simply puree the fresh herb in a blender or food processor, then strain it through cheesecloth or a very fine sieve to extract the juice. It should take 4 to 5 cups of fresh parsley to give you 2 to 3 ounces of juice. You can purchase organic carrot juice if you're not making your own, and to obtain onion juice, see "Onion Juicing 101" on page 248.

✔ Drink Green for Good Health

Like many other herbs, parsley makes a tea that's just the ticket for performing a passel of health-care feats. To make it, steep 1 teaspoon of dried or (preferably) 2 tablespoons of chopped fresh parsley per 8 ounces of freshly boiled water for 10 minutes. When the tea is ready to drink, it'll be a vibrant green color. Strain it, and (presuming you made it in quantity) store it, covered, in the refrigerator. Then drink 3 or 4 cups of the tea a day, either cold or warmed up, to work any of these wonders:

- Detoxify your kidneys, liver, and bladder
- Eliminate kidney stones
- Reduce prostate swelling
- Relieve urinary tract infections

Note: Consult with your doctor before you use parsley tea (or other homemade healers) to treat any of these conditions.

> **CAUTION** ⚠
>
> If you are pregnant or think you might be pregnant, do not drink parsley tea or juice, or use parsley seeds or essential oil. All of these contain high concentrations of the plant's volatile oils, which can cause serious problems. On the other hand, it's usually fine to eat either fresh or dried parsley in normal food portions. But just to be safe, ask your obstetrician how much of the herb you're allowed. Once your baby arrives, if you're nursing, go cold turkey on parsley because it can slow the flow of your milk. And steer clear of it entirely if you have kidney disease, high blood pressure, or edema.

✔ Banish Bruises

Minor bruises generally go away on their own, but it does take time. So why wait? Grab some parsley and speed up the process. It'll reduce the inflammation, relieve the pain, and make the colorful patches fade more quickly. You have two excellent treatment options:

■ Crush a handful of fresh parsley leaves, spread them over the bruise, and cover the area with a bandage to hold them in place. Change the dressing several times a day until you're black-and-blue no more.

■ Mix ½ teaspoon or so of chopped fresh parsley leaves per 1 teaspoon of butter, and gently rub the salve onto the discolored area. Then cover it with a loose bandage or a clean piece of cloth to keep the butter from staining your clothes or other fabric. Repeat as needed until the bruise is gone.

✔ Fast-Acting Sting Relief

You're puttering around in your yard on a fine summer morning when . . . OUCH! An insect plants its stinger (or its mouth parts) in your skin. What do you do? Well, if you grow parsley, just pluck a few of the leaves, and rub them on the bite site. The compounds will instantly relieve the pain and head off inflammation and swelling. **Note:** Of course, this remedy will work just as well if you use fresh parsley you bought at the supermarket.

✔ Bite Relief on the Dry Side

If all you have on hand is dried parsley, no problem! Just measure 4 teaspoons of the herb into a heat-proof container, and pour in 1 cup of boiling water. Cover, and let the mixture steep for 15 minutes, then strain out the leaves. Soak a soft cotton cloth in the tea, and apply it directly to the bite.

✔ Scram, Skeeters!

Don't let the disease-spreading vampires spoil your warm-weather fun. Make yourself some liquid "armor" by mixing 1 tablespoon of dried pars-

---

Help for the Frequently Bruised

HEALTHFUL HINT

Some folks seem to attract bruises the way dark clothes attract lint. If that sounds like you or the youngsters in your household, keep a supply of anti-bruise cubes on hand. To make them, just mix 1 cup of finely chopped fresh parsley with 2 tablespoons of water, and pour the slurry into an ice cube tray. Then, whenever someone bumps into a table or gets a black eye from a wayward tennis ball, pop a cube out of the tray, and gently glide it over the victim's "owie." The combination of cold temperature and parsley's healing power will send the bruise packin' pronto.

ley per ¼ cup of apple cider vinegar in a large jar that has a tight-fitting lid. Shake the jar to blend thoroughly, and keep it where you can get at it easily (don't strain out the parsley). Then before you venture outdoors, rub the lotion generously onto your exposed skin using a cotton pad. For extra protection, dip a bandanna or cotton scarf in the mixture, and tie it around your neck or hat.

✔ Easy on the Eyes

Styes do not generally pose a serious health threat, but these inflamed bumps on your eyelids are as painful as the dickens. Here's a fast way to relieve your discomfort: Steep a handful of chopped fresh parsley in 1 cup of just-boiled water for 10 minutes. While the parsley water is still hot—but not enough to burn you—soak a clean washcloth in it. Then lie down, put the compress over your closed eyelids, and relax for 15 minutes or so. Repeat the procedure just before you go to bed. **Note:** This same treatment is also excellent for soothing tired, irritated, or swollen eyes.

✔ Pampering Parsley Footbath

When your feet are dog tired and achy to boot, treat them to a feel-good footbath. To make it, steep ⅛ cup of dried parsley and 4 chamomile tea bags in 1 gallon of just-boiled water for 10 minutes. Strain the liquid into a basin or shallow pan that's big enough to hold your feet (warm up the tea on the stove first if it's cooled down too much to suit you). Add 4 drops of an essential oil of your choice. Peppermint, tangerine, and lime are energizing; chamomile, lavender, and rose will help you relax. For an ultra-soothing experience, put marbles or smooth river stones on the bottom of the basin, and slide your feet over them while they're soaking.

Gorgeously Garnished

✤ Exhale with Confidence

Parsley is a surefire cure for dragon breath, especially when it's caused by garlic or onions. If you frequently indulge in those odiferous foods, do yourself (and your friends and colleagues) a favor: Carry a small bag of fresh parsley sprigs or leaves with you and snack on them throughout the day.

❖ Swish Your Breath Clean

If you prefer your breath cleansers in liquid form, whip up a batch of this marvelous mouthwash: Bring 1 cup of hot water to a boil. Remove the pan from the heat, and add 1 teaspoon each of chopped fresh parsley and ground cinnamon and 1 whole clove. Let the ingredients steep for 15 minutes, then strain out the solids and stir in 1 teaspoon of your favorite extract. (Peppermint, vanilla, and orange are all good choices.) Pour the solution into a bottle that has a tight-fitting cap, and use it as you would any other mouthwash.

❖ Prevent Body Odor

The same compound in parsley that freshens your breath—namely chlorophyll—also makes the savory herb one of the most effective internal deodorants you can buy (or grow). Best of all, parsley power works whether you munch on fresh sprigs or chop the fresh leaves and toss them into quiches, omelets, salads, or soups.

❖ Shine Up Dark Hair

Is your dark brown or black hair looking a little dull? Here's a simple way to put back the razzle-dazzle: Place 3 tablespoons of dried parsley in a heat-proof bowl, and pour in 2 cups of just-boiled water. Let it steep until the water reaches room temperature, and then strain it into a clean, empty shampoo or conditioner bottle. After shampooing, rinse your hair with the potion, and massage it into your scalp. Use as often as needed to keep the luster in your locks. **Note:** If you don't happen to have dried parsley on hand, you can substitute either dried rosemary or dried sage.

❖ Grow, Grow, Grow Your Hair

Whether your hair is starting to get a little sparse, or it just doesn't have the healthy bounce it once

YOU DON'T SAY!

Parsley is far and away the most widely used culinary herb in the world, and it has been for centuries—that is, in most cultures. The ancient Greeks didn't eat it at all, except in medicinal potions. Hippocrates used it as an antidote for poisons and prescribed it to treat just about every ailment under the sun. No doubt folks expected nothing less than potent curative power from the herb, which they believed had sprung from the blood of Archemorus (a mythological prince who was supposedly killed by a dragon and later honored as a forerunner of death). For that reason, they considered it to be sacred, and they crowned the winners of major sporting events with wreaths made of parsley.

had, parsley can help. It stimulates the blood circulation in your scalp, which can lead to the growth of strong, healthy hair. To make a tonic with get-up-and-grow power, puree a big handful of fresh parsley sprigs with 2 tablespoons of water in a blender or food processor. Massage the mixture into your wet scalp, wrap a towel around your head, and go about your business for about an hour. Then shampoo as usual, and follow up with your normal conditioner. Repeat every week or so until your head is a growth industry again.

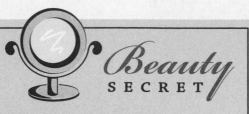

Beauty SECRET

MINTY PARSLEY HAIR RINSE

You say your hair is growing to beat the band, but your scalp is irritated? Or maybe your dry, fly-away strands make your hair look like it's always blowing in the wind. This remarkable rinse can solve either or both of those annoying problems. To make it, steep 2 tablespoons of chopped fresh parsley and 2 tablespoons of chopped fresh peppermint in 8 ounces of freshly boiled water for 10 minutes. Strain out the herbs, and pour the liquid into a plastic bottle. After shampooing, rinse your hair with the mixture, and then use your favorite conditioner. Follow this procedure twice a week, or as often as needed to keep your scalp healthy and your hair silky smooth. Note: If your hair is oily, add 1 tablespoon of lemon juice to the tea.

✤ Erase Dark Circles

Has your under-eye area gotten so dark that you refuse to leave the house without wearing concealer? Well, here's a remedy that may set you free from makeup prison: Blend a small handful of fresh parsley and 2 tablespoons of plain yogurt in a blender or food processor until you have a creamy paste. Apply it generously (and gently) to the skin under your eyes. Lie back and relax for 20 minutes or so, and then rinse the mixture off with lukewarm water. Treat yourself to this restful routine twice a week. After four or five treatments, you should start to see your skin getting lighter and brighter.

✤ Perfect Parsley Toner

If you're tired of spending your hard-earned money on expensive cosmetics, but you don't have time for elaborate DIY routines, give this ultra-simple toner a try. Just put ½ cup of chopped fresh parsley in a heat-proof bowl, and cover it with 1 cup of boiling water. When it's cooled to room temperature, strain the liquid into a glass jar that has a tight-fitting lid. Store it in the refrigerator, where it will keep for about three weeks. Then every morning and evening, sweep it over your freshly washed face with a cotton pad.

✤ Trouble-Prevention Toner

If you're in a place that has little, if any, fresh air circulating—like an airplane cabin or an office building with sealed windows—the germ-infested atmosphere can take a major toll on your skin. But here's a DIY liquid suit of armor that will fight off blemish-causing fungi and bacteria and stimulate the production of vital collagen. The easy formula: Pour 2 cups of boiling water over a handful of chopped fresh parsley, and let it steep, covered, for 10 minutes or so. Then strain out the solids, and mix the liquid

---

POTENT POTION

MOISTURIZING SKIN MASK

This facial treatment will soften and hydrate skin of any type and any age, but it's especially effective for skin that's reached a certain level of experience. As an added bonus, you can use the leftover oil as a stand-alone moisturizer.

⅛ cup of fresh parsley, chopped

3 tbsp. of extra virgin olive oil

1 tbsp. of full-fat sour cream

2 tsp. of unsweetened cocoa powder

Combine the parsley and olive oil in a small saucepan, and cook the mixture on *very low* heat for about 10 minutes.

Strain the oil into a small bowl, and set it aside. Put the parsley, sour cream, and cocoa powder in a blender or small food processor and blend thoroughly. Smooth the creamy mixture onto your freshly cleaned face and neck, and leave it on for 20 minutes or so. Then rinse with warm water and splash with cool water. Follow up with a light application of the parsley-infused olive oil. Store the remaining oil in a glass container with a tight-fitting lid, and use it as you would any other moisturizer.

YIELD: 1 MASK TREATMENT PLUS 4 TO 6 EXTRA APPLICATIONS OF PARSLEY-OIL MOISTURIZER

with ½ teaspoon of unfiltered apple cider vinegar and 20 drops of tea tree oil. Pour the mixture into a jar that has a tight-fitting lid or (if you're taking to the air) into small, TSA-approved bottles. When you're earthbound, the toner will stay fresh in the refrigerator for up to three weeks.

✤ Rejuvenating Facial Mask

Exfoliating skin treatments are designed to dissolve the bonds that hold dead skin cells together so that they slough off more easily—leaving you with a smoother, more radiant complexion. This one does the job like a champ. To make it, puree ⅔ cup of fresh pineapple chunks (at room temperature) in a blender or food processor. Pour in ¼ cup of extra virgin olive oil, and blend until the mixture is almost paste-like. Finally, add ¼ cup of chopped fresh parsley, and pulse a few seconds at a time, making sure the mask doesn't liquefy. Spread the mixture onto your face and neck, and leave it on for 15 minutes. Rinse it off with lukewarm water, and follow up with your usual moisturizer. Repeat every few weeks, as needed, to keep your skin dewy fresh and younger looking.

Best of the Rest

★ Calm a Nervous Stomach

When you feel like you're about to toss your cookies, add ¼ teaspoon of dried oregano and ½ teaspoon of dried marjoram to 1 cup of just-boiled water. Let it steep, covered, for 10 minutes. Then strain the tea into a mug, and sip it slowly. Two hours later, if your tummy still feels queasy, make another cup and drink it down to put your system back on an even keel.

★ Curb the Surge

To help control excessive menstrual bleeding, think thyme tea times two. Steep 2 tablespoons of fresh thyme in 2 cups of freshly boiled water. Strain out the herb, and drink 1 cup of the tea. Pour the other cup into a bowl, and add an ice cube or two. Soak a washcloth in the cold brew, then wring it out and lay it across your pelvic area. **Note:** If your periods are consistently heavy, get a medical checkup just to rule out any serious problems. And if you even suspect that you may be hemorrhaging, call 911 immediately!

★ Start the Flow

If your period is running late (and you know you're not pregnant), a strong basil tea can get the show on the road. Just steep 1 tablespoon of the chopped fresh herb in 1 cup of just-boiled water for five minutes. Then strain and sip. But first, make sure that you have a supply of tampons or sanitary pads on hand!

★ Sip Away Joint Pain

Basil, rosemary, and sage are potent pain relievers. So to get your joints jumpin' again, use one or all of them in the form of an herbal tea. Make it in the usual way—1 to 2 teaspoons of the dried or 1 to 2 tablespoons of the fresh herb per cup of just-boiled water, steeped for five minutes. Sip 2 cups a day, alternating herbs, until you find the one that works for you.

★ Thyme to Nix Nightmares

Are scary dreams waking you (or your youngsters) up in the middle of the night? Well, don't take that sleep-depriving nonsense lying down. Instead, drink a cup of thyme tea before you go to bed. It's an old-thyme, er, old-time trick for banishing bad dreams, and it works like a charm!

★ Scratch No More

No matter what has you scratching up a storm, thyme can be a timely cure. Just make a pint of thyme infusion (see Tea Times Two on page 99), and pour it into your bathwater. The herb contains a substance called thymol, which has antiseptic and antibacterial properties that can make your itch vanish in a flash.

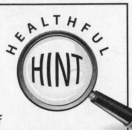

Shop with Care

HEALTHFUL HINT

If you want to get all the health and beauty benefits of dried herbs and spices, do yourself a favor: Avoid the little jars at the supermarket. Not only are the contents far from their peak of freshness (and highly overpriced), but in most cases, they've been irradiated to destroy any bacteria, viruses, and other microorganisms that might be present. Unfortunately, that process also destroys vitamins, minerals, proteins, and other nutrients. What's more, it can actually create damaging free radicals. In short, you'll be defeating the whole purpose of using herbs and spices in the first place! So always buy them in bulk from health-food stores, herb shops, or reputable websites that specialize in organic herbs and spices. Besides getting the active ingredients you want, you'll save a small fortune!

★ Dodge the Itch . . .

Of mosquito bites and—more importantly—the dastardly diseases they can deliver. How? Just put rosemary and sage to work. Skeeters hate the smell of both herbs. Any of these terrific tricks will keep the buggers at bay:

■ At your next barbecue, toss some fresh sage or rosemary sprigs on the coals.

■ Make insect-repelling candles. Melt grated white wax in a heat-proof container, and mix in a handful each of dried sage and rosemary. Pour the wax into molds (clean tin cans are perfect), and insert a wick in the center of each one. When they're dry, set them around your outdoor gathering areas.

■ Brew a strong cup (or more) of sage or rosemary tea, let it cool, and pour it into a spray bottle. Or, if you prefer, add 30 drops of sage or rosemary essential oil per 8 ounces of tap water. Then spritz it on your exposed skin whenever you venture into skeeter territory. **Note:** Test the oil on a small patch of skin before you make a batch of this repellent.

★ A Basil Beauty Trifecta

Basil is renowned for its ability to relieve skin irritations and breakouts, fade dark spots, and refine pores. Plus, it's chock-full of compounds that help fend off the effects of aging, such as fine lines and a dull complexion. Here's a trio of ways to use this heroic herb in your beauty routine:

CLEANSER. Crush 20 to 30 fresh basil leaves using either a mortar and pestle or a bowl and a wooden spoon. Mix in just enough distilled water to make a paste (½

Fabulous Food Fix

RASPBERRY-ROSEMARY SMOOTHIE

Talk about an herbal superstar! In addition to offering up a boatload of anti-aging antioxidants, rosemary can (among other feats) improve your memory and concentration, lift your spirits, aid your digestion, relieve muscle pain, and boost your immune system. This fruity treat is a delicious way to tap into that powerhouse.

1 cup of frozen raspberries
½ cup of frozen blackberries or blueberries
½ of a fresh or frozen banana
Leaves from 2 sprigs of fresh rosemary, chopped
1 cup of milk or water
Honey to taste (optional)

Put all of the ingredients in a blender, and blend on high speed for 30 to 45 seconds, or until the drink is smooth and creamy. Pour it into a tall glass, sip, and enjoy.

teaspoon or so should do the trick). Spread it on your face, leave it on for three to five minutes, and rinse with lukewarm water. Use this cleanser every other day.

MASK. Prepare the basil as described at left, but instead of adding water, mix the crushed leaves with 1 teaspoon of plain yogurt. Smooth it onto your face, wait about 20 minutes, and then rinse it off. Repeat the procedure every week or so or whenever your skin is irritated or breaking out.

EVERYDAY TONER. Again, crush 20 to 30 fresh basil leaves, but this time pour 1 cup of boiling water over them. Let the tea steep for 10 to 15 minutes, then strain out the solids. Pour the liquid into a glass bottle that has a tight-fitting cap, and store it in the refrigerator, where it will keep for about a week. Then each morning and evening, apply the toner to your freshly washed face using a cotton pad.

POTENT POTION

HERBAL SUPER SOAK

This bath blend does it all! It'll calm your frazzled nerves, increase your mental alertness, and stimulate your senses. Plus, it'll soften your skin and relieve any irritation caused by weather, insect bites, or allergies.

¼ **cup of dried rosemary, crumbled**
¼ **cup of dried sage, crumbled**
2 **tbsp. of coarse sea salt**
2 **tbsp. of dried parsley**
2 **tbsp. of uncooked oatmeal**

Grind all of the ingredients in a blender or food processor to make a coarse powder. Put ¼ cup of the blend in a muslin or cheesecloth bag or a clean panty hose foot, and tie the top securely.* Toss the pouch into the tub as you run hot—but not burning hot—water into it. Then step in, lean back, and relax. Squeeze the bag occasionally to release more of the potent essences into the water. When you've soaked to your heart's content, step out, dry off, and go conquer the world!

* Store leftover powder, either loose or in individual pouches, in a lidded container away from heat and light.

YIELD: 3 BATHS

★ A Thymely Cleanser

Here's a formula that's fabulous for cleaning and toning normal skin, and it's gentle enough to use every day. To make it, mix 2 sprigs of crumbled fresh thyme and 2 teaspoons of crushed fennel seeds in a bowl, and cover them with ½ cup of boiling water. Stir in the juice of half a lemon, and let the mixture steep for 15 minutes. Strain out the solids, pour the liquid into a jar that has a tight-fitting lid, and store it in the refrigerator. To use, simply dab it onto your face and neck with a cotton ball, then rinse with lukewarm water. Follow up with your usual moisturizer. **Note:** You can substitute ½ tablespoon of dried thyme.

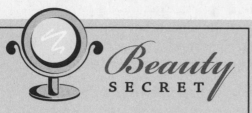

Beauty SECRET

THE GREAT GRAY COVER-UP

You say you'd like to conceal the silver strands in your hair, but you'd prefer not to fuss with time-consuming—and expensive—beauty shop visits? Then give this all-natural treatment a try: Bring 2 cups of water to a boil, and toss in a handful each of dried sage and dried rosemary. Reduce the heat, and let the mixture simmer for 30 minutes. Remove it from the stove, pour it into another container, and let it steep for several hours or (better yet) overnight. Strain out the herbs, massage the liquid into your hair, and let it air-dry. Then shampoo, condition, and style as usual. Repeat the procedure every three to five days, and before long, the gray should be gone, or it'll at least be a whole lot less noticeable.

★ Triple-Threat Rosemary Conditioner

This conditioner will de-tangle, nourish, and shine up your hair to beat the band. Just stand six to eight fresh rosemary sprigs upright in a heat-proof glass jar that's tall enough to hold them with an inch or so to spare on top. Pour in enough boiling water to cover the sprigs, and let them sit overnight. Come morning, pull out the herbs, and pour the liquid into a plastic squeeze bottle. Add about 2 teaspoons of unfiltered apple cider vinegar, and give the bottle a good shake. After shampooing, squirt the potion onto your head, and comb it through your hair. Then rinse with clear water, and dry and style your hair as usual.

20 Petroleum Jelly

For nearly a century and a half, petroleum jelly has been a staple in bathrooms from coast to coast. Over the years, scads of fancier health and beauty products have appeared on the scene, but when it comes to performing the jobs it does best, this skin-pleasing healer still can't be beat. Whether you choose the original Vaseline® or a generic version, you've got yourself a first-class first-aid helper.

A Gel of a Healer

✔ Send Psoriasis Plaques Packin'...

And fast! Twice a day, bathe the affected areas, pat them dry, and immediately rub on several layers of petroleum jelly—the more, the better! Within a week or so, at least 80 percent of your plaque problem should vanish.

✔ Bar the Door against Blisters

To fight the friction that causes blisters, smooth a light layer of petroleum jelly over each foot before you put your socks and shoes on. And be sure to lace up your shoes nice and tight, so your feet don't rub against your footgear. That way, you'll stay blister-free and rarin' to go!

✔ Give Hangnails the Heave-Ho

A hangnail is nothing more than a tiny piece of skin that's attached at the base or side of a fingernail. Unfortunately, it can pack a load of pain that's way out of proportion to its size. And it can cause even more pain after you've removed it—unless you do it the right way. The simple process: Soak your affected finger(s) for 5 to 10 minutes in a bowl of warm water with a few drops of olive oil added to it. Then cut the hangnail off at the base, using sharp, sterilized nail scissors (whatever you do, don't pull the hangnail out!). Dab the base with alcohol, apply petroleum jelly to the site, cover loosely with a bandage (to keep from staining the sheets), and go to bed. When you wake up in the morning, your trouble should be over. If any trace of the skin fragment remains, repeat the procedure.

To prevent future problems, rub the jelly onto your cuticles and the surrounding skin after each bath or shower, and anytime you've had your hands in water. Those painful projections should be gone for good.

✔ Dry Up the Drip

What's more annoying than postnasal drip? Not a whole lot that I can think of! So here's a simple formula that'll end the hassle fast. Melt ¼ cup of petroleum jelly in a small saucepan over medium-low heat, stirring frequently. Remove it from the stove and stir in 10 drops each of peppermint, eucalyptus, and thyme essential oils. When the mixture has reached room

POTENT POTION

ACHY MUSCLE MASSAGE GEL

Whether you got your muscle pain from hiking up a mountain trail, working in your yard, or standing on your feet for hours cooking Thanksgiving dinner, this ointment is your ticket to relief.

1 tbsp. of glycerin
1 tbsp. of petroleum jelly
1 tbsp. of water
½ tsp. of almond extract
⅛ tsp. of wintergreen essential oil

Mix the glycerin, petroleum jelly, and water in a microwave-safe container. Nuke the mixture on high for 30 seconds, then add the extract and oil, and stir until it's smooth. While it's still warm, massage the gel onto your sore body parts. If you have any leftover gel, store it in a jar with a tight-fitting lid, and warm it up before using it again. But it's best to make fresh batches two to three times a day and apply the gel until you're ache-free.

temperature, pour it into a clean glass jar with a tight-fitting lid for storage. Apply a small dab to the inside of each nostril one to three times a day. The secret to this trick: The petroleum jelly keeps the oils from being absorbed into your skin, thereby allowing you to inhale their drip-stopping essence over a prolonged period of time.

✔ Soothe Sore Hands and Feet

Dry, chapped, or calloused hands and feet are not only painful and unsightly, but also prime candidates for developing blisters and hot spots. Fortunately, this is one problem you can solve lying down. Just before bedtime, wash up the affected skin with warm soapy water, then spread a thin layer of petroleum jelly all over the area, and put on thick cotton gloves or socks. Then hit the sack. Come morning, pull off the coverings. Your skin will be noticeably smoother and softer. If necessary, repeat the procedure each night until the chapping and calluses are history.

HEALTHFUL HINT

Chuck Chub Rub

Runners, hikers, and workout enthusiasts are all at high risk for an amusing-sounding, but often agonizing condition called chub rub. It's caused when clothing constantly rubs against sensitive skin or when non-athletes', ahem, generous thighs brush against each other with every step. The chafing results in a painful, burning rash or even angry red welts. One excellent way to head it off: Cover the affected areas with a thick layer of petroleum jelly. It eliminates the friction, thereby allowing you to move freely with no fear of future misery. **Note:** Be aware that the jelly may stain your clothes, but folks who use this precaution tell me that's a small price to pay for pain-free movement.

✔ A Faster Route to Softer Skin

If you'd rather not wait all night for your skin to ditch its dryness, try this quicker fix: Mix equal parts of petroleum jelly and white sugar, and stir in a few drops of your favorite essential oil if you'd like. Wipe the mixture generously onto your freshly washed hands or feet, and put on cotton gloves or socks. Leave them on for 30 minutes or so, and then scrub the combo off with a pumice stone or brush. Gently pat your skin dry and apply a moisturizer. If your skin is still drier than you'd like, repeat the process every day until it's silky smooth and pain-free.

✔ Ditch Diaper Rash

You can pay a whole lot of money for diaper rash remedies, but you won't find any that are more effective than this doctor-approved DIY formula. Just mix equal parts of petroleum jelly and cornstarch to make a paste, and rub it on baby's sore bottom. Within 24 hours, all traces of the rash should be gone.

After that, keep trouble at bay by following the routine pediatricians recommend:

■ Change diapers frequently (at least every two hours for newborns) and the minute you know there's been some action.

■ Keep baby's skin cool and dry. The best way to do this: After you remove a soiled diaper, let the tyke spend some time in his birthday suit.

■ After the cooling-off period, coat the tot's bottom with a thick layer of petroleum jelly before you cover it with a fresh diaper.

> **CAUTION** ⚠
>
> While petroleum jelly can help burns heal faster, you should never use it on a fresh burn unless it is very minor, and only after cooling it completely as described in "Heal Wounds and Minor Burns," at right. That's because heat remains in your skin for some time after the initial impact and continues to damage the area. If you apply petroleum jelly (or any other kind of fat, including butter or oil) to a burn too soon, it will hold in the heat and cause more damage to the underlying tissue.

✔ Heal Wounds and Minor Burns

Petroleum jelly keeps the moisture level of the injured skin close to that of normal skin, which speeds healing. It also reduces inflammation, seals out infection-causing germs, and helps prevent scarring. Use it as follows:

WOUNDS. Clean the wound thoroughly, and apply an antibiotic ointment. Then cover it with a generous layer of petroleum jelly, and top that with a bandage. For a minor cut, change the dressing several times a day, or whenever it's gotten wet. If you're under medical care for a more serious injury, follow the schedule prescribed by your doctor.

MINOR BURNS. This treatment is only intended for minor first-degree burns—the kind you get from a brief encounter with a steam iron, hot pan, or barbecue grill. Run cold water on the burn site for at least five minutes. When it's cooled down completely, *very* gently rub petroleum jelly over the affected area. Then wrap the burn loosely in a single layer of light gauze, and tape it in place. **Note:** For anything more serious, get medical help ASAP (see the Caution! box above).

A Gem of a Jelly

❖ Make Up Some Makeup

Whether you've run out of a makeup essential on the eve of a special event, or you simply enjoy whipping up your own beauty products, here's a trio of DIY possibilities:

CREAM BLUSHER. Put 1 teaspoon or so of petroleum jelly in a bowl, and stir in a few scrapings of lipstick until it's well blended.

EYE SHADOW. Again, start with 1 teaspoon or so of petroleum jelly, but add a few drops of blue or green food coloring, and stir well.

LIPSTICK. Follow the same procedure described for eye shadow, but use red food coloring instead of blue or green. Better (and tastier) yet, go for a pinch or two of cherry or strawberry Kool-Aid® powder. Stir well to dissolve the powder.

Note: In each case, adjust the amount of colorant to create a darker or lighter cosmetic.

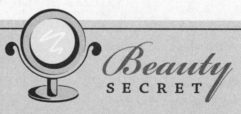

MIRACULOUS MATURE-SKIN CREAM

This ultra-simple formula is perfect for extra-dry skin, especially when it's reached a certain level of, um, experience. To make it, mix a 13-ounce jar of petroleum jelly, a 15-ounce bottle of baby lotion (not oil), and a 16-ounce jar of vitamin E cream (not lotion) in a large bowl. (If you like, nuke the jelly in the microwave for a few seconds to soften it up.) Mix well—the texture of the finished product should be somewhere between that of Cool Whip® and whipped butter. Store it in wide-mouth, lidded containers at room temperature, and use it as you would any other moisturizer. You should start seeing softer, more radiant skin almost immediately.

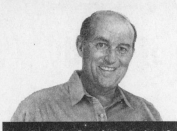

✣ Create a Luscious Lip Gloss

Would you like to have a moisturizing lip gloss that's your favorite shade *and* your favorite flavor? You can—and it's a snap. In a bowl, thoroughly mix 1 tablespoon of petroleum jelly, ¼ teaspoon of your favorite lipstick, and 2 to 4 drops of flavored extract. (Orange, rum, peppermint, and almond are all good choices, but the sky's the limit!) Scrape the mixture into a small, tight-lidded container. They're available at craft shops and health-food stores, but a clean, plastic throat-lozenge container will work well, too. Then tuck it into your pocket or purse, and use it as you would any other lip gloss.

✣ One Scrub Fits All

Here's an exfoliating scrub that works wonders for sloughing off dead cells and softening the skin on your whole body, including your face and lips. To make it, mix 1 part petroleum jelly with 2 parts brown sugar (add a little more petroleum jelly if the mixture is too thick to suit you). Scoop it out of the bowl with your fingers, and massage it thoroughly onto your skin. Then rinse it off, towel-dry, and follow up with your usual moisturizer.

✣ Tame Your Eyebrows

Before you pluck your eyebrows, lube up your skin with petroleum jelly. It'll make those stray hairs glide out smoothly and painlessly. And if your brows are unruly even after plucking, use petroleum jelly to instill a little discipline. Just put a dab of jelly on your fingertip or a soft toothbrush, and sweep it across each brow from the inside to the outside. The result: a neat, trim look with no muss and no fuss. **Note:** It goes without saying (I hope!) that you should not use the same brush that you use on your teeth.

POTENT POTION

SOLID PERFUME

This aromatic formula has three advantages over commercial perfumes: First, the petroleum jelly makes it glide onto your pulse points more easily and stay there longer; second, you can customize the scent to suit your taste; and third, it costs a whole lot less than commercial versions!

1 cup of petroleum jelly
1 oz. of beeswax*
1 tbsp. of essential oil**

Melt the petroleum jelly and beeswax in a glass pan or double boiler over low heat. Remove the pan from the stove, and stir in the essential oil for a minute or so. Pour the mixture into one or more dark-colored glass (not plastic) jars with tight-fitting lids, and let it cool until it's firm. It will keep just fine at room temperature for up to two years. Just one word of caution: Keep the perfume away from heat and sunlight, which can make the potency deteriorate quickly.

* Available in health-food stores and on numerous websites.

** Use whatever scent(s) you like best, but here are a few suggestions: A classic floral combo is 10 parts lavender, 4 parts rose, and 2 parts vanilla. If you prefer something outdoorsy, try equal parts pine and vanilla with a few drops of jasmine. A half-and-half blend of rosemary and lavender will give you an aroma that seems fresh from an herb garden.

YIELD: ABOUT 1 CUP

✤ Save That Scent!

Before you spray yourself with cologne or perfume, dab a little petroleum jelly onto your pulse points, like your wrists and the sides of your neck. That way, your scent will last through the entire day or evening.

✤ A Dandy DIY Deodorant

Forget commercial, chemical-laden deodorants! This simple concoction will keep you as fresh smelling as the priciest store-bought brand: Just mix

2 tablespoons each of petroleum jelly, baking soda, and baby powder in a pan. Heat the mixture on low until it's smooth and creamy. Then pour it into a jar that has a tight-fitting lid. Store at room temperature, and use it as you would any other antiperspirant.

✣ A Trick to Dye For

Rather, make that dye *with*. If you color your hair at home, keep the stuff from flowing into your eyes by rubbing a line of petroleum jelly above your eyebrows. For good measure, especially if you're using a dark-colored hair dye, wipe a layer of jelly all around your hairline to prevent hard-to-remove skin stains. **Note:** A line of jelly above the brows also works for keeping shampoo out of baby's (or Fido's) eyes at bath time.

✣ Seal Split Ends

When you've waited so long between haircuts that your ends have started to split—and you can't rush in for a trim—rub a little petroleum jelly between your palms, and wipe it onto the cracked strands. If necessary, use it all over your hair to hold frizzy flyaways in place. When the jelly's job is done for the day (or evening), wash it out with a clarifying shampoo, and follow up with your normal conditioner.

Best of the Rest

★ Keep Your Hands Warm

Baby, it's cold outside! But you've got a chore to do out there, and you can't do it with gloves on. So protect your bare skin by massaging your hands with baby oil before you head outdoors. It'll close up the pores and help prevent damage from the frigid air.

★ Foil Fungus

Whether foul fungi have infected the nails on your fingers or your toes, mentholated rub can charge to the rescue. Twice a day, coat the afflicted nail(s) and surrounding skin with mentholated rub. It should solve the problem in no time flat. **Note:** If the infection does not clear up after a week or two, call your doctor.

★ Give Bugs the Brush-Off

The same mentholated rub that's been easing chest colds since Hector was a pup is also a terrific insect repellent. Just smooth the stuff onto your skin (but not on your face) to fend off mosquitoes, ticks, and other bad blood-sucking bugs. Wash your hands if you're going to be handling any food though.

★ Oops—Too Late!

When a multilegged marauder has already zoomed in for the attack, put a dab of white (non-gel) toothpaste on the bite or sting site. It'll start working instantly to stop the itch and reduce any swelling.

Rub Out a Head Cold

HEALTHFUL HINT

When you're battling a ferocious head cold, but you need to be out and about, make yourself a portable "vaporizer." Just dip a cotton ball into a jar of mentholated rub so that it picks up a good dollop of the stuff. Put the coated ball into a clean pill bottle, cap it tightly, and tuck it in your pocket or purse. Then anytime you start to feel congested, remove the cap and take a few deep breaths. Bingo—your airways will be free and clear!

★ First Aid for Painted Hair

You say you were painting your ceiling, and some of the paint wound up in your hair? No problem! Pour some baby oil onto a cotton pad, wrap it around your paint-spattered locks, and wipe the offending stuff right out. Repeat as needed until you and your room are no longer color coordinated. Then shampoo your hair thoroughly to remove the oily residue.

★ Hold Your Hair in Place

Fresh out of hair gel? If there's a tube of gel toothpaste in the bathroom, you're in luck. These products contain the same water-soluble polymers that many hair gels are made of. Just squeeze as much paste as you need out of the tube, and style your hair as usual. **Note:** This is also a neat trick for making barrettes stay put in baby's ultra-fine hair.

★ Take a Powder

When you don't have time for a shampoo, or you simply don't feel up to the chore, reach for a shaker of baby powder. Sprinkle 1 tablespoon or so onto your head, rub it through your locks, and then brush it out. It'll leave your hair clean and fresh smelling all day long.

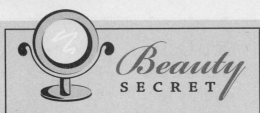

Beauty S E C R E T

PERFECTION FOR LESS

Every woman knows that translucent powder puts the perfect finishing touch on any makeup routine. But commercial powders can put a big dent in your pocketbook. Well, guess what? You can make your own version for about five cents' worth of ingredients that you probably have at home. All you need to do is mix 1 teaspoon of baby powder per ½ tablespoon of cornstarch. If you want a little color, add ⅛ teaspoon of powdered foundation. Store the mixture in a clean, lidded container, and apply it with a regular powder brush. The result: a professional-looking makeup job for pennies (or less) on the dollar!

★ Perform Dandruff Damage Control

Common dandruff is nothing more than cast-off skin cells from a dry scalp. And you don't need a special shampoo to get rid of the flakes. Instead, follow this three-step routine:

STEP 1. Rub baby oil into your hair and scalp until your hair is wet.

STEP 2. Massage the oil into patches of extra-dry skin to remove them—don't scrape them off!

STEP 3. Let the oil soak in for 30 minutes or so, then wash your hair with a regular, non-medicated shampoo. Let your hair air-dry, and style it as usual.

Note: Be aware that although this procedure will keep your "snowfall" to an absolute minimum, there is no permanent cure for dandruff. If you have a dry scalp, the condition is bound to reappear from time to time, especially if you live in (or visit) a dry climate. Whenever that happens, simply reach for the baby oil, and repeat this procedure.

★ A Toothy Solution for Brighter Nails

The same toothpaste that makes your teeth whiter and brighter can also shine up your fingernails and toenails like nobody's business. Just squeeze a little whitening toothpaste onto a soft toothbrush, and scrub-a-dub-dub. Repeat the procedure daily, or as often as needed to keep your nails clean and shiny. **Note:** Use a new, clean toothbrush for this job—but not the same one you use on your teeth!

★ Fast-Working Anti-Pimple Paste

It never fails: You've got a big event on the agenda tomorrow, and a pimple pops up from out of nowhere. Not to worry! At bedtime, simply cover the bump with a blob of white (non-gel) toothpaste. By morning, that zit should be history. **Note:** This trick is only intended to treat a spot or two. *Never* apply toothpaste to a large area of your face because it will make your skin red and irritated.

★ Stave Off Stretch Marks

When you're pregnant and your body is expanding to accommodate your fast-growing baby, the process can take a toll on your stretching skin. But you don't have to put up with those resulting, unsightly stretch marks. Just mix equal parts of baby oil and cocoa butter, and massage the mixture onto your extended tummy once or twice a day. Your skin will stay soft and mark-free.

★ Baby, Please Pass the Oil

It only stands to reason that a product that's gentle enough to use on an infant's tender skin is mild enough for even the most sensitive adult skin. In fact, baby oil could replace just about every fancy (and expensive) skin-care product you can name. Here's a trio of examples:

MAKEUP REMOVER. Use it to eliminate all traces of face and eye makeup.

MOISTURIZER. It will keep your skin soft and supple from head to toe.

SHAVING CREAM. It softens the hair on your legs and underarms, making easy work for your razor and leaving your skin silky smooth.

POTENT POTION

R & R BATH BLEND

Make a batch of this soothing bath oil, and reach for it whenever you need to relax and refresh after a long, hard day (or even a short, easy one).

½ cup of baby oil
¼ cup of whole milk
1 egg
2 tbsp. of honey

Mix all of the ingredients in a blender for about 45 seconds. Pour ¼ cup of the mixture into the tub as you fill it with warm water. Then step in, sit back, and say "Aaahh!" Refrigerate the leftover portion in an airtight container, and use it within a week or so.

YIELD: ABOUT ¾ CUP

21

Salt

Today when you walk into any supermarket or drugstore, you see aisle after aisle crammed with special remedies for every health and beauty problem under the sun (not to mention prescription drugs behind the pharmacist's counter). But not so long ago, most of those miracle lotions, potions, and pills didn't even exist. Instead, folks healed their wounds, cured their ills, and improved their looks with the same tried-and-true products their ancestors had used for centuries. One of those superstar performers was salt, and it's still worth having on hand for your health and beauty needs.

The Salt of the Earth

✔ Heal Bleeding Gums

When your gums start bleeding, you need to see a dentist ASAP. But while you're waiting for your appointment, salt can help stop the oozing. Just mix 1 part salt and 2 parts baking soda, and stir in a few drops of tea tree oil. Then three times a day, dip a damp, soft-bristled toothbrush into the moist powder and brush very gently.

✔ Tame a Toothache

You say your gums are just fine, but you've got a tooth that hurts like the dickens? No problem! Rinse your mouth with a mixture made from 1 tablespoon of salt, 2 tablespoons of apple cider vinegar, and 4 ounces of warm water. That should ease the pain until you can get to the dentist's office.

✔ Draw Out the Ouch

Long before commercial pain relievers came along, folks swore by hot, dry salt for treating a trio of common woes. It works wonders by drawing out pain quickly, safely, and inexpensively. Here's all you need to do: Heat a few tablespoons of salt in a dry frying pan until the salt is hot, but not too hot to touch. Either pour the salt into a clean cotton sock or wrap it up in a clean, dry dish towel. Then proceed as follows, depending on the location of the pain:

ARTHRITIS. Lay the poultice on your aching joint until you feel relief. To keep the salt comfortably warm, put a hot-water bottle or heating pad on top of it.

EARACHE. Simply hold the salty sock against your sore ear. By the time the salt cools off, your pain should be gone. If not, repeat the treatment.

HEADACHE. Hold the sock or pouch to the back of your head (yes, even though you feel the throbbing in the front), and rub it over your scalp.

✔ Clear Out Your Sinuses

Whether your stuffed-up airways are caused by a head cold or allergies, this trick will get the air flowing again: Mix ¼ teaspoon of salt and ¼ teaspoon of baking soda in 8 ounces of warm, distilled water, and fill a bulb (a.k.a. ear) syringe with the mixture. (You can find

---

POTENT POTION

TOXIN-TOSSIN' BATH BLEND

In addition to removing toxins from your body, this formula will soothe skin irritations, boost your magnesium levels, and relax you all over. For best results, use it in a warm bath just before bedtime.

¼ cup of baking soda
¼ cup of Epsom salts
¼ cup of sea salt
1 qt. of boiling water
⅓ cup of unfiltered apple cider vinegar
10 drops of lavender or peppermint essential oil (optional)

Dissolve the first three ingredients in the boiling water, and set the mixture aside. Fill your bathtub with warm water, and pour in the vinegar. Add the other ingredients, and swish the water around with your hand to disperse them. Then step into the tub, relax, and soak for 30 minutes or so. **Note:** You may feel a little light-headed, so be careful getting out of the tub.

bulb syringes in the baby products section of most drugstores.) Then lean over a sink, hold one nostril closed with your finger, and gently squirt the fluid into your open nostril. Blow your nose, and repeat the procedure on the other side. Bingo—you should be breathing freely again!

If you suffer from sleep apnea, a potentially dangerous condition in which your breathing is interrupted while you're sleeping, using this treatment at bedtime may help to keep your nasal passages open.

✔ Ring Out Ringworm

Contrary to its name, ringworm is not a worm; it's a fungus that causes circular, scaly patches on the skin. Unfortunately, it can spread like wildfire, even from one person to another. But there's a simple two-step way to douse the flames:

STEP 1. Soak a gauze pad in a solution made from 1 teaspoon of salt dissolved in 2 cups of distilled water, and put it on the affected area for about 30 minutes.

STEP 2. The next day, repeat the process using a gauze pad soaked in a solution made from 1 part apple cider vinegar mixed with 4 parts distilled water.

Alternate these compresses—salt one day, vinegar the next. In a week or so (depending on its severity), the foul fungus should be gone.

Fabulous Food Fix

EXCELLENT ELECTROLYTE ENHANCER

It seems that every time you turn around, there's another new "electrolyte-enhanced" drink on the scene. All that term means is that the beverage has been spiked with minerals like potassium and sodium, which help prevent dehydration when you're working or playing hard. This DIY formula works just as well at a fraction of the cost. And thanks to the agave nectar, it's quite tasty to boot!

2 tbsp. of agave
   nectar
½ tbsp. of sea salt
½ tsp. of baking soda
1 qt. of water

Mix all of the ingredients together thoroughly, and pour the potion into either a single quart-size water bottle or two or more smaller versions. Then take frequent sips as you hike, bike, or go mowing merrily along.

YIELD: ABOUT 32 OUNCES

✔ Say "Bye-Bye, Backache!"

As you know if you've ever suffered from back pain, there are few more debilitating conditions. One simple way to relieve the ache is to soak for 20 to 30 minutes in a bathtub of hot (but not burning hot!) water with a handful each of sea salt and dry mustard mixed in it. **Note:** If your back pain persists, especially if you don't know the cause, see your doctor to rule out a serious illness.

✔ Shoo a Shiner Away

Whether you got your black eye from a wayward tennis ball or a swinging door—or your youngster snagged a "souvenir" in a school-yard fistfight—this remedy will help it fade fast: Mix 2 tablespoons of salt with 2 tablespoons of vegetable shortening. Spread the mixture on a soft cotton cloth and lay it against the affected eye. It'll stimulate blood circulation, thereby helping to eliminate those bruised and blackened skin cells.

✔ Conquer Canker Sores

Canker sores do not pose a serious threat and, unlike cold sores, they are not contagious. But they sure can hurt! A simple way to solve the problem: Mix 1 teaspoon of salt, 1 teaspoon of baking soda, and 2 ounces of hydrogen peroxide, and rinse your mouth with the mixture four times a day until the sores disappear. If you find the tingle uncomfortable or the taste too strong, add 2 ounces of water to the formula.

✔ Fend Off Food-Borne Bacteria

Health-care pros tell us that wooden cutting boards are much more hygienic than plastic ones, which collect disease-causing bacteria by the zillions in the knicks and cuts that knives leave behind. Still, wooden versions can also pick up their fair share of bacteria. To avoid trouble, it's important to follow a routine maintenance plan: Every two to three weeks, cover the board's surface with a layer of coarse kosher or sea salt, then rub it thoroughly with the cut side of a lemon half. When you're finished, rinse the board with hot water, dry it, and wipe on a light coat of mineral oil. (Avoid vegetable oil, which may turn rancid.)

> **CAUTION** ⚠
>
> If you have high blood pressure or you're on a sodium-restricted diet, consult with your doctor before you use any oral remedies that contain salt. Likewise, if you are diabetic, speak with the doc before you use any foot treatments described in this chapter, or elsewhere in this book.

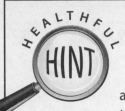

By Land or by Sea?

You hear a lot about sea salt these days, but is it really better than regular table salt? The answer is yes and no. Table salt is mined from land-based deposits and then processed to remove impurities and to make it flow freely from those familiar round boxes. On the other hand, sea salt is obtained by evaporating seawater collected in man-made pools near the shoreline. Unlike refined salt, the end product retains all of its original minerals, including magnesium, calcium, and potassium. Those elements are not present in sufficient amounts to make a difference in your diet, but they do impart a flavor that many folks prefer to that of refined salt. They also add extra oomph to many topical health and beauty remedies, as does the coarser texture of sea salt. Despite these differences, the bottom line is that both kinds are heroic healers.

✔ Deal With Diarrhea

When you're suffering from the runs, it's important to continuously replace the sodium, potassium, and chloride your body loses with each trip to the bathroom. One simple way to do that is to dissolve ½ teaspoon of salt (preferably sea salt) and 4 teaspoons of sugar in 1 quart of water. Stir in a tablespoon or two of orange, lemon, or lime juice for flavor and potassium. Then drink the whole quart over the course of the day.

✔ Treat Singed Skin

Whether it's a slight sunburn or very minor burn (nothing blistering), you can help heal the damaged skin with salt. First, run cold water over the area for about five minutes. Then mix 1 to 2 teaspoons of salt (preferably sea salt) in a glass of ice-cold milk, and sponge the solution onto your skin once or twice a day, or as needed, until the pain is gone. **Note:** If the burn is any more severe than a normal sunburn or very minor burn, or if your skin shows signs of becoming infected, get medical help pronto.

✔ Sayonara, Psoriasis!

Legions of psoriasis sufferers have found that frequent dips in the ocean can send the crusty, itchy patches packin' pronto. If you're not lucky enough to live by the sea, here's your best alternative: Dissolve ½ cup of sea salt per gallon of water in your bathtub, and soak your affected skin in the briny brew several times a day. **Note:** For best results, use Dead Sea salt, which you can find in some health-food stores and online.

✔ A Briny Bonanza

Psoriasis is far from the only health condition that salt water can cure. Just cast your eye on this list of remarkable remedies:

ATHLETE'S FOOT. Toss about ½ cup of salt into a basin filled with warm water, and mix it well. Then soak your feet for 5 to 10 minutes. This bath is also a great way to relax tired or achy feet and freshen up smelly ones.

HEAT EXHAUSTION. Mix 1 teaspoon of salt in a glass of water, and sip it slowly.

INGROWN NAILS. Soak your afflicted fingers or toes for 30 minutes in a solution of 1 tablespoon of salt per quart of warm water.

ITCHY SKIN. Whether it's caused by poison ivy, insect bites, food-allergy rashes, or post-sunburn peeling, mix ½ cup of salt in a tub of warm water, and soak for as long as you like.

JOCK ITCH. Pour a cup or two of salt into the tub, and soak for 15 to 30 minutes. Repeat two or three times a day until the itch is history.

LARYNGITIS. Gargle several times a day with a solution made of ½ teaspoon of salt in 1 cup of warm water. Don't use any more salt than that, or it may increase your throat irritation, rather than relieve it.

MOUTH OR TONGUE BITES. The next time you start to take a bite of food, but your teeth miss the mark and ding your

---

POTENT POTION

FOAMING ACHE RELIEVER

These colorful crystals are just what the doctor ordered for relaxing achy muscles or soothing frazzled nerves. So make a large batch and keep it on hand for those times when you need all-over relief.

6 cups of rock salt
½ cup of mild dishwashing liquid
1 tbsp. of vegetable oil
4 or 5 drops of food coloring (optional)

Put the rock salt in a bowl. In another bowl, mix the dishwashing liquid, vegetable oil, and food coloring together, and pour the solution over the salt. Stir to coat the crystals, and spread them out on wax paper. When they're completely dry (usually in about 24 hours), put them in a jar. Come bath time, pour ¼ cup of the crystals into the tub under running water.

YIELD: ABOUT 24 BATHS

tongue or cheek instead, mix 1 teaspoon of salt in 1 cup of warm water. Swish it around in your mouth until the wound feels better, which shouldn't take more than a minute or so.

SORE THROAT. Mix 1 teaspoon of salt in about 2 cups of warm water. Then tip your head back and gargle that pain away!

UNCOMFORTABLE NEW DENTURES OR BRACES. Rinse your mouth with a solution of 1 to 2 teaspoons of salt in a glass of warm water. If your oral tissue is still tender after a few days of this treatment, call your dentist or orthodontist.

Sleek and Salty

❖ De-Grime Your Hands

Sometimes, after a day of working hard in the yard, it almost seems like there's more dirt on your hands than there is in the ground. Don't worry. Simply add about 1 teaspoon of salt to the soap lather as you wash up, and your paws'll come out as clean as a whistle!

❖ Sea Spray Volumizer

Oily hair that's also limp and fine-textured can be a nuisance to maintain. If your tresses fall into that category, this is your magic bullet: Fill an 8-ounce spray bottle about a third of the way with sea salt (not table salt). Add ⅓ teaspoon of lemon juice and 3 drops of lavender essential oil. Fill the balance of the bottle with water, and shake until the salt is dissolved. Spray the mixture onto your wet hair, and then blow-dry and style it as usual. Or if you prefer, simply let your hair air-dry. The potion will add body and also soak up some of the oil, so you won't have to shampoo as often.

❖ Super Scalp Scrub

Whether you're plagued by dandruff, an itchy scalp, or hair loss, I have a two-word solution for you: sea salt. Just pour out a handful of it, and massage the granules into your scalp. It'll make dandruff and dead, irritating skin cells vanish and also stimulate your blood circulation, which is essential for healthy hair growth. When you're done, shampoo and condition your hair as usual. Perform this procedure two or three times a week until you see the results you want. (How long that will be depends upon the nature and severity of the problem, but you *will* see results—guaranteed!)

✤ Deflate Your Eyes

Eating overly salty foods can cause your eyes to become puffy and swollen. On the other hand, applying salt to the outside of your eyes can relieve puffiness, no matter what caused the problem. So mix ½ teaspoon of salt in 1 quart of warm water, and dip two cotton pads in the solution. Then lie down, put a pad over each closed eyelid, and relax for 10 to 20 minutes. Bingo—poof go the puffs!

✤ Face Up to Salt

You couldn't ask for a better facial cleanser than this one: In a bowl, mix ⅛ cup of finely ground sea salt and 1 to 2 teaspoons of finely chopped fresh mint. Drizzle in just enough unfiltered apple cider vinegar to make a thick paste. (An eyedropper is ideal for this job.) Gently massage the mixture onto your face and neck, and rinse well with warm water. Refrigerate any leftover formula, and use it within three days.

✤ Detoxifying Toner

Sea salt naturally absorbs impurities from your skin, which makes it an ideal toner for oily or problem-prone complexions. To put sea power to

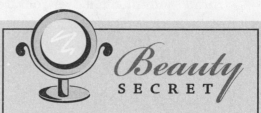

Beauty SECRET

BEACHY-KEEN WAVES

One popular hairstyle features waves that look like they've been made by salty sea breezes—but they're usually made by commercial sprays that contain harsh chemicals and sport hefty price tags to boot. If you're fond of that look (or have a daughter who is), a gentler DIY spritzer can supply it at a fraction of the cost. Here's how to make it: In a spray bottle, mix 2 teaspoons of coarse sea salt, ¼ teaspoon of warm coconut oil, and 1 teaspoon of hair gel in 8 ounces of warm water. Shake the bottle to blend the ingredients thoroughly. Spritz the mixture onto your freshly washed, towel-dried hair, scrunching handfuls of strands as you spray. Then go round up the gang for a game of beach blanket bingo (even if it is in your own backyard).

work for you, mix 1 teaspoon of sea salt per ¼ cup of warm water in a bottle that has a tight-fitting cap. Give it a shake and let it sit overnight so the salt can dissolve completely. Then dampen a cotton pad with the brine, and smooth it over your freshly washed face. Follow up with your usual moisturizer. **Note:** If you find this toner too drying to use every day, use it only as needed to keep your skin not too oily and blemish-free.

❧ Shrink Your Pores

Looking for a mask that will tighten up enlarged pores? This one couldn't be simpler: Mix equal parts of buttermilk and sea salt into a paste. Apply it to your face, and massage well. Leave it on for about five minutes, rinse with warm water, and pat dry.

❧ Soften Your Knees . . .

And elbows, too! Simply mix 1 heaping tablespoon of sea salt with 4 tablespoons of olive oil in an unbreakable container. Then step into the shower, massage the mixture into your dry joints, and when you're done, rinse it off. Pat dry with a soft towel, and apply your usual body lotion. **Note:** The olive oil can make the tub slippery, so be careful getting out of the shower.

❧ A Simple, Smoothing Softener

Looking for a basic, down-home way to make your skin softer and smoother? Here it is: After a shower or bath, but before you step out of the tub, grab a handful of sea salt (or plain table salt in a pinch), and rub it vigorously onto your

---

POTENT POTION

SWEET AND SALTY BODY SCRUB

Here's an all-over body cleanser that will open up and clean out clogged pores, help clear up any skin irritations, and leave you with soft, healthy, glowing skin from head to toe.

1 cup of brown sugar
½ cup of sea salt
2 tbsp. of coconut or olive oil
2 tbsp. of freshly squeezed
    lemon juice
1 tbsp. of essential oil*
1 tbsp. of raw honey

Mix all of the ingredients in a bowl to form a paste. Using your finger-tips, massage the mixture onto your skin in circular motions. Rinse thoroughly with warm water, and apply your usual moisturizer.

* Geranium, lavender, and rose are great skin-pleasing choices.

still-wet skin. When you rinse it off, it'll take all the dry, dead cells along with it and leave your skin soft and silky all over.

❖ Wintertime Foot Freshener

Your feet can develop unpleasant aromas at any time of the year, but they're at especially high risk when you wear boots all day, as many women do in the winter. That's when it pays to have this four-step trick up your sleeve:

STEP 1. Mix 1 cup of coarse sea salt, 5 tablespoons of olive or coconut oil, 1 tablespoon of cocoa powder, and 1 tablespoon of peppermint extract in a bowl, stirring just until blended.

STEP 2. Soak your feet in a basin of warm water for 10 to 15 minutes.

STEP 3. Starting at your toes, massage the salt mixture into your skin with your fingertips, making small circular motions. Pay special attention to your soles and any rough areas.

STEP 4. Rinse thoroughly, pat dry, and apply your favorite moisturizer.

Repeat the procedure as often as needed to keep your tootsies feeling—and smelling—as fresh as spring daisies.

❖ Get Ready, Get Set . . .

For sandal season! As summertime approaches, treat your feet to this super-softening scrub: Mix 1 cup of sea salt, ¼ cup of coconut oil, ¼ cup of vitamin E oil, and 3 or 4 drops of essential oil (rose, lavender, and orange blossom are all excellent choices). Massage a tablespoon or so of the mixture into each foot, then rinse with cool water. Store the blend at room temperature in a jar with a tight-fitting lid, and use it as needed to keep your tootsies sleek, smooth, and ready for warm-weather action.

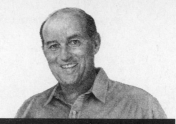

YOU DON'T SAY!

We all know the old adage that spilling salt brings bad luck. Well, as with most superstitions, this one has some basis in fact: In ancient times, when this belief arose, salt was such a rare and valuable commodity that losing even a little bit of it really was bad luck.

As for what you're supposed to do to stop the bad luck—toss a pinch of salt over your left shoulder—there's a reason for that, too. In most cultures, folks believed that good spirits followed you on your right side and evil spirits lurked behind you on the left. So, they reasoned, if you tossed some salt over your left shoulder, it would hit that bad guy square in the eye and distract him from his dirty tricks.

Best of the Rest

★ Mustard Cuts the Mustard . . .

When it comes to curing a trio of common health problems—namely these:

MINOR BURNS. When your hand brushes up against a hot pan or the edge of your barbecue grill, run your singed skin under cold running water for about five minutes. Then slather on a nice thick layer of yellow mustard. The pain will vanish instantly.

NASAL CONGESTION. Rub a generous amount of spicy brown mustard on your chest, and top it with a hot (but not burning hot!), damp cloth. The aroma of the hot mustard will clear your airways within minutes, and you'll be breathing freely again. **Note:** This decongestant works by encouraging your clogged nasal passages to drain, so be sure you've got plenty of tissues close at hand!

SORE THROAT. Combine 1 tablespoon each of prepared mustard (any kind will do), salt, and honey with the juice of half a lemon in a heat-proof container. Then pour in ½ cup of boiling water, and mix thoroughly. Let the mixture cool to lukewarm, and gargle with it two or three times. Fair warning: This remedy won't win any awards for good flavor, but it'll put your throat back in the swing of things fast!

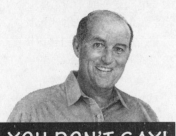

YOU DON'T SAY!

When heartburn has you in a pickle . . . eat one. Believe it or not, a dill pickle will put out the fire fast. Not in the mood to munch? Then swallow a tablespoon or so of pickle juice instead. It'll douse the flames just as fast. **Note:** This same tasty remedy is also just the ticket for relieving an upset stomach or muscle cramps.

★ Cool It!

On a hot summer day, biting into a spicy pickle probably isn't the first thought that leaps into your mind. But maybe it should be. That's because hot, spicy foods actually cool your body in two ways: They increase blood circulation, and they cause you to sweat, which releases excess heat from your system. Any kind of hot pickled veggies will do the trick—not just cucumbers. So when the temperatures start rising, pick up a few jars of your favorite pickled peppers, onions, or cauliflower. Then whenever you feel too darn hot, help yourself to a few of them, and feel your internal AC kick in!

★ A Must(ard) for Muscle Relief

Attention, weekend warriors! Here's how to stop those muscle cramps you get on the golf course, tennis court, or jogging track—and make good use of the extra mustard packets that come with your lunchtime sandwiches. Keep a supply of the little envelopes in your golf or gym bag, and whenever you feel a cramp coming on, open the package, swallow the contents, and chase it down with water. Repeat every two minutes until the twinges stop. **Note:** If you're at home when a cramp strikes, just take your medicinal mustard straight from the jar.

Fabulous Food Fix

CRISPY PICKLED CHARD STALKS

Before summertime sets in, make up a batch or two of these ultra-simple pickles and keep them in the fridge. They'll cool you down fast when the weather turns steamy and also give you a healthy dose of probiotics that'll help keep your digestive system running smoothly.

1 bunch of Swiss chard stalks
3 tbsp. of raw honey
1 cup of unfiltered apple cider vinegar
3 tbsp. of sriracha hot sauce*
16-oz. glass canning jar

Clean and cut the chard stalks about an inch shorter than the depth of the jar, and pack them in tightly. In a medium microwave-safe bowl, warm the honey on a low setting just until it is runny. Then mix in the vinegar and hot sauce, stirring until the honey completely dissolves. Pour the mixture over the stems so they're covered. Close the jar tightly, and store it in the refrigerator for at least a week so the flavor can develop fully. Your pickled chard will keep in the fridge for up to a year as long as the stems are completely covered with vinegar.

* Available in the Asian-food section of most supermarkets and online. Or substitute your favorite hot sauce.

YIELD: 1 PINT

★ More Mustard Muscle Magic

I know plenty of folks who wouldn't dream of eating straight mustard no matter how much their muscles hurt. And that's okay, because I've got a handful of topical healers that'll get the job done just as well. Depending on the nature and location of your aches and pains, try one of these mustardy muscle soothers:

ALL-OVER ACHES AND PAINS. Mix 2 tablespoons of mustard with 1 teaspoon of Epsom salts, and pour the mixture under the spigot as you run warm water into the tub. Step in, sit down, and relax for 20 minutes or so. Then take a quick shower so you don't walk around smelling like a ballpark hot dog!

TIRED, ACHY FEET. Dissolve 1 tablespoon of mustard in a basin of warm to hot (but not burning hot!) water. Soak your pooped puppies for 20 to 30 minutes, then dry them off and get ready to skip around the room.

PULLED MUSCLE. Make a paste by mixing 1 part mustard to 2 parts flour. Spread the mixture on a piece of cheesecloth, and fold the sides over to make an envelope. Lay the plaster on the affected area, securing it with a bandage. Leave it in place for 20 to 30 minutes (no longer!), and your pain should pack off. If necessary, repeat the process once or twice a day until you feel relief. But if the discomfort persists for more than a week, see your doctor.

> **HEALTHFUL HINT**
> ### Mash a Migraine
> The minute you feel an attack coming on, open a jar of strong mustard—the hotter and spicier, the better. Slowly inhale the aroma three or four times, and your pain should be gone in a flash.

★ Mayo for Your Mane

Plain old mayonnaise makes a great hair conditioner. Start by shampooing your hair as you normally do. Then towel it dry, and massage regular mayo (*not* the low-fat kind and *not* the miracle salad dressing!) into your hair. Let it sit for a good 15 minutes or so, shampoo again, and rinse thoroughly. Style your hair as usual, and get ready for compliments on your shiny locks.

★ Intensive Hair Help

Here's an extra-strength treatment that's tailor-made for dry or damaged hair: Puree a banana in a blender until it's smooth and free of lumps. Add about 1 tablespoon each of mayonnaise and olive oil to it, and blend until creamy. Massage the mixture into your hair, wait 15 to 30 minutes, rinse with warm water, and shampoo as usual.

★ Homemade Cold Cream

Here's an easy-as-pie formula that will remove makeup and clean and soften your skin: Just mix ½ cup of mayonnaise (the full-fat kind), 1 tablespoon of melted butter, and the juice of one lemon or lime, and store the cream in the refrigerator in a tightly closed glass jar. Use it as you would any facial cleanser, and rinse with cold water. It'll give you results that are as good as those of commercial products, but at a fraction of the price.

★ A Skin-Care Miracle

Before all those fancy skin exfoliators came on the scene, legions of women used Miracle Whip® salad dressing to remove dead, flaky skin. Well, it does the job just as well today, and it also helps balance excessively oily skin. Here's all you need to do: Apply a thin layer of the cream to your face and neck, avoiding the eye area. Leave it on for 10 minutes, and then massage gently, using small circular motions. Rinse with warm water, and follow up with your usual facial routine. Repeat the procedure two or three times a week, and within a month or so, you should see an amazing improvement in your skin's texture.

★ A Pickle a Day . . .

Keeps wrinkles away! Well, maybe not forever (nothing can do that).

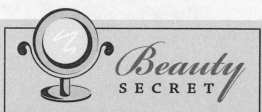

Beauty SECRET

REAL HELP FOR DRY SKIN

The very same mayonnaise that adds zing to sandwiches can also provide deep-down moisture to your skin. Simply mix 2 tablespoons of real mayo (not the low-fat variety) and 1 teaspoon of baby oil in a container. Smooth the mixture onto your face, neck, and any other part(s) of your body that could use some softening. Leave it on for 20 minutes or so, and then rinse thoroughly with lukewarm water. Presto, change-o—sleek, soft, supple skin!

But it will keep your skin fresher and younger looking longer. That's because pickles—and pickle juice—are packed with antioxidants that prevent cell damage. For that same reason, pickles and their juices help reduce your risk of cancer and heart disease. Plus, they have zero calories. Who could ask for anything more? **Note:** If you are watching your sodium intake, try this trick with only half a pickle a day because most pickles are loaded with salt.

22

Tea

An old Chinese adage says, "Drinking a daily cup of tea will surely starve the apothecary." And with each passing day, scientists are finding out just how true that saying is. Study after study has shown that tea, whether black, green, white, or oolong (all of which are made from the leaves of the *Camellia sinensis* shrub), can fight inflammation, boost your immune system, preserve your brain-power, and help prevent diabetes, osteoporosis, and many types of cancer—and that's just for starters! As for tapping into tea's beautifying power, we might amend that opening line to include "and the cosmetic manufacturer."

Tea-Totalin' Health

✔ Bash Boils . . .

And cold sores, fever blisters, and plantar warts, too! Several times a day, hold a warm tea bag on the painful bump for about 15 minutes. Before you know it, the nasty thing will vanish.

✔ Make Corns Disappear

Once each day, tape a moist tea bag on the spot and leave it on for 30 minutes or so. Within about two weeks, the annoying corn should be gone. You can use either a freshly soaked tea bag or a cooled one that's left over from your morning "cuppa."

✔ Give Blisters the Runaround

Sweaty feet can lead to blisters fast. So if your tootsies tend to be wet, shut off the waterworks this way: Steep five tea bags per quart of just-boiled water for four to five minutes. Let the tea cool, and soak your feet in it for about 30 minutes. Repeat the routine every other night for a week, and you'll say "Bye-bye" to blisters. Keep in mind that this remedy works just as well to dry up sweaty, blister-prone hands.

✔ Head Off Colds and Flu

As the cold and flu season approaches, start guzzling black tea. Studies at Harvard University show that people who drank 5 cups of black tea each day for just two weeks made the T cells in their immune systems pump out 10 times more virus-fighting interferon. Can't quite meet the 5-cup-per-day quota? Then just drink as much as you can manage. The tea's antioxidants should still rev up your immune system enough to help it fight back when trouble strikes.

✔ Put a Headache on Ice

Take a tip from the German Tea Association and freeze brewed green tea in ice cube trays. Then whenever a headache hits, wrap one of the cubes in a paper towel, and press it alternately against your neck, temples, and forehead. Hold it in place for at least 15 seconds in each spot, and your ache should ease off. **Note:** This same remedy can also relieve stress, whether it's accompanied by a headache or not.

Fabulous Food Fix

COLD-CLOBBERING TEA

Keep this recipe on hand and reach for it at the first sign of a cold or the flu. It'll mitigate your miseries fast!

3 tsp. of coriander seeds
6 black peppercorns
4 cups of water
2 black-tea bags*
2 tbsp. of raw honey
1 tbsp. of fresh-squeezed lemon or lime juice

Put the spices in a teakettle with the water, and bring it to a boil. Lower the heat, and let it simmer for 15 minutes. Add the tea bags, honey, and juice, stirring to dissolve the honey. Let the mixture steep for 10 minutes, then strain it into another container. Sip the brew, warmed up, throughout the day, and bid your symptoms adieu.

* Or 2 teaspoons of loose tea

YIELD: 4 (1-CUP) SERVINGS

✔ Thwart a Migraine

If you're troubled by migraines, do your head a favor and drink more tea. It's a routine treatment in China, where traditional medical hospitals boast recovery rates as high as 92 percent. The simple R$_X$: When the pain and throbbing start, brew a strong cup of black tea (two tea bags per cup of boiling water, steeped for 20 minutes). Drink it while it's still very warm, but not hot enough to burn your tongue or mouth. The caffeine in the tea will constrict the blood vessels in your head, almost instantly taming the turbulence.

✔ Tooth Extraction Made Easier

Even in these days of high-tech dentistry, having a tooth pulled is no picnic. And neither are the pain and swelling that often follow. Well, here's an old-time way to soothe those sore gums. Just put a cool, moist tea bag against the affected area, and hold it there for 15 minutes. Repeat the procedure four times a day for three or four days, and your gums should be back to normal. (If they're not, call your dentist.) By the way, this trick works just as well to comfort youngsters who are waiting for the tooth fairy to show up.

✔ Stop Bleeding Gums

To stop your gums from bleeding, rinse your mouth with black tea for one minute. Studies show that if you do this 10 times a day, you may decrease plaque buildup, which could be the cause of the bleeding. Compounds in the tea also suppress the growth of cavity-causing

---

HEALTHFUL HINT

Lessen Cataract Problems

No nutrient can cure cataracts, but studies show that quercetin, a powerful antioxidant, may help delay their formation or slow their development. And dried tea leaves (both green and black) contain more quercetin than any other food. There's just one catch: Brewed tea contains almost no quercetin. But you can still enjoy its benefits in two ways:

■ Brew your tea using loose leaves, and don't strain it before sipping. Just drink it down, leaves and all.

■ Add a teaspoon or two of tea leaves to a delicious smoothie recipe, or stir them into your favorite yogurt.

There is no specific recommended dosage for cataract avoidance—so make tea leaves part of your regular diet, along with the other quercetin-rich foods like apples, cranberries, onions, and peppers.

bacteria and inhibit acid production. **Note:** After a week or so, if your gums continue to bleed or feel tender, see your dentist ASAP.

✔ Bag Sore Eyes

Tea bags, whether left over from a brewed pot or pulled straight from the box and moistened, can work wonders for a trio of common eye problems. Each one demands a slightly different treatment, so here's the rundown:

PINKEYE, A.K.A. CONJUNCTIVITIS. Lay a warm (not hot), unsqueezed black-tea bag on the affected eye for 15 to 20 minutes (or as long as a young victim will tolerate). Squeeze the bag once in a while so the tea puddles on the closed eyelid. Don't worry if the tea gets into the eye—it will actually help the healing process. Repeat the procedure three or four times a day until the problem clears up. You can expect major improvement during the first day.

STYES. Moisten a tea bag, put it on your sty-afflicted eye (closed, of course!), and keep it in place with a bandage. Leave it on for as long as possible. Repeat the procedure once or twice a day as needed until the inflamed bump has cleared up.

STRAINED, SORE EYES. When you've had a sleepless night or spent too many hours at the computer, lay a cold, wet tea bag over each eye, then lie down and relax for half an hour. When you get up, you'll be rarin' to go!

✔ Ditch the Itch of Eczema

Studies show that polyphenols in tea relieve itching for many eczema sufferers. Drinking 3 cups of the brew each day, one after each meal, generally

POTENT POTION

ANTI-ITCH BATH
Whether you're suffering from eczema, hives, or a poison-plant rash, a soak in this comforting "cocktail" is just what the doctor ordered for quick relief.

3 or 4 green-tea bags
3 drops of chamomile essential oil
3 drops of geranium essential oil
3 drops of lavender essential oil

Add all of the ingredients to a tub of warm water, then settle in and relax for 20 minutes or so. Gently pat yourself dry and kiss the itch good-bye! **Note:** The oils may make your bathtub a little slippery, so be careful getting out.

does the trick. If that doesn't entirely solve the problem, it should, at the very least, greatly improve your comfort level. While some people find black tea most effective, others have better luck with green or oolong tea. So experiment and see which kind works best for you.

CAUTION ⚠️

Black tea is perfectly safe for most adults, but drinking too much can cause side effects ranging from nervousness and sleep problems to heartburn and diarrhea. How much is too much varies from one person to the next, but in most cases, up to 5 cups a day is fine. The caffeine in tea can also interact with many drugs, and too much caffeine can cause problems during pregnancy. So if you are pregnant, or think you might be pregnant, or if you're taking medications of any kind, ask your doctor how much tea (or any other caffeinated beverage) is safe for you to drink on a daily basis.

✔ Take Your Sunburn to Tea

Correction: Take tea to your sunburn. Depending on the size and location of the affected area, you have a couple of tea-time delivery options:

■ Steep six black-tea bags in 1 quart of just-boiled water for five to six minutes. Put the tea in the refrigerator or, for faster action, the freezer until it's nice and cold. Then soak soft cotton cloths in the brew, and lay them on the affected skin.

■ Soak the burned part of your body in the icy cold tea. (Increase the quantity as needed, but stick to the same proportions of six tea bags per quart of water.)

In either case, repeat the procedure until you feel relief, rechilling the tea and/or the cotton cloths as needed.

✔ Heal Neglected Lips

You say that most of your body is burn-free because you slathered it with sunscreen—but you forgot about your lips? No problem! Just dunk a tea bag in cold water until it's soaked through, and hold it between your lips for 15 minutes. Repeat the process four times a day, or as often as you can, until your lips are sore no more.

✔ Attention, Nursing Mothers!

You know how baby's eager mouth can make your nipples sore. Well, here's a simple way to ease the ache: Steep two tea bags in a cup of freshly boiled water for three to four minutes. Remove the bags without squeezing them, and let them cool to lukewarm. Then apply one to each nipple, and leave them on until the bags have cooled completely. Presto—problem solved! Repeat as needed between mealtimes to keep your feedings pain-free.

✔ Vanquish Vaccination Pain

There's no getting around it: Shots hurt, especially when the "victim" is a baby or small child. Fortunately, there's an easy way to stop the pain—and the tears. Just put a cool, wet tea bag over the injection site, and hold it there until the crying stops. (It won't be long.) You might want to try this trick yourself the next time you get your annual flu shot.

✔ Fend Off Osteoporosis

Here's good news, ladies! Studies show that drinking as little as 1 cup of black or green tea a day may preserve your bone density well into your senior years. The reason is that as your natural estrogen levels decline during menopause (thereby hindering your bones' ability to absorb calcium), the natural phytoestrogens in tea can take over to boost your absorption of this essential mineral. Of course, it's best to start your cup-a-day routine in the year or so leading up to menopause, when your body starts to produce less and less estrogen.

Loverly Leaves

✤ Tea for Aromatic Tootsies

The tannic acid in black tea helps close the sweat glands, thereby starving the bacteria that cause foot odor. Your game plan: Brew two tea bags in 1 pint of boiling water for 15 minutes, add the tea to 2 quarts of cool water, and soak your feet for 20 to 30 minutes. Do this for 10 days straight, and your feet will turn out sweet—guaranteed!

✤ Beat Bad Breath

There are more breath-freshening formulas than there is tea in China, but one of the most effective—and most pleasant—is, well, tea. Scientists tell us that the polyphenols in tea can stop the growth of microbes that cause halitosis, as well as the bacteria's production of odiferous gas. Don't believe me? Then try tea and see!

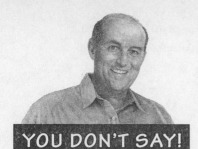

❖ Odor-Free Hands

To get rid of unpleasant aromas, just rinse your hands with brewed tea, or rub your skin with a couple of used tea bags. It works like a charm to remove odors left by fish, onions, garlic, or other strong-smelling foods.

❖ A Teatime Toner

Tone and firm any type of skin with this simple trick: Pour 1 cup of boiling water over 4 teaspoons of loose green-tea leaves or two green-tea bags. Let it steep for 10 to 15 minutes to get a nice strong brew. When the tea has cooled to room temperature, pour it into a bottle with a tight-fitting lid, and keep it in the refrigerator. Once or twice a day, dab some toner onto your face and neck with a cotton pad or ball, and follow up with your usual moisturizer.

❖ Invigorate Dry Skin

If your skin is very dry, this intensive-care facial routine will rejuvenate your skin, leaving your complexion soft and radiant: Mix ¼ cup of brewed green tea and two crushed vitamin C tablets. Apply the mixture to your face using a cotton ball or pad, and smooth on a thin layer of petroleum jelly to lock in the moisture. Leave the mask on for 20 minutes or so, and rinse it off with warm water. Then look in the mirror and admire the "new" you!

❖ Tone Down the Oil

You say your skin is as oily as a pipe on a West Texas drilling rig (or at least feels like it)? No problem! Your road to radiance couldn't be simpler. Just put 1 teaspoon of black tea in a mug, fill it with boiling water, and let it steep for 15 minutes. Strain out the tea leaves, immerse a soft washcloth in the brew, squeeze it out, and cover your face with the compress. Leave it on for 20 minutes, then rinse with lukewarm water, and apply your usual moisturizer. Repeat the procedure every three or four days, and your pores will be tighter and your face as fresh as a daisy. **Note:** This treatment also soothes irritated skin and prevents pimples.

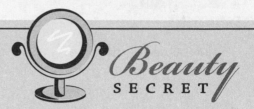

ANTI-AGING FACIAL CLEANSER

Green tea contains compounds called polyphenols that protect your skin from the sun's destructive rays and flush out cell-damaging free radicals. Sugar sloughs off dead skin cells and attracts moisture that keeps your skin hydrated. Putting this age-defying duo to work is a snap. Just bring ½ cup of distilled water to a rolling boil, pour it into a heat-proof bowl, and add two green-tea bags. Let them steep until the water is cool to the touch— about 15 minutes. Then stir in 3 tablespoons of granulated sugar. Saturate a clean washcloth in the solution, and gently massage your skin using small, circular motions. Rinse thoroughly with lukewarm water, and apply your favorite moisturizer. Repeat the process once a week to keep your skin clear, glowing, and younger looking.

✤ De-Puff Your Face

For many women, a puffy face is as much a part of summertime as baseball and corn on the cob—only a lot less welcome, of course! If that description fits you, here's good news: Ice cubes made from green tea and pureed blueberries can deflate your kisser faster than a speeding bullet. Well, almost as fast. Here's the four-step routine:

STEP 1. Pour 2½ cups of boiling water over three green-tea bags and steep them for about 10 minutes. Remove the bags and stir in 3 tablespoons of raw honey.

STEP 2. While the tea is cooling, puree ½ cup of fresh or frozen blueberries and 2 tablespoons of freshly squeezed lemon juice in a blender until the mixture is mushy, but not liquefied.

Fabulous Food Fix

A SMOOTH-SKIN SMOOTHIE

A beautiful complexion comes from the inside out. The antioxidants in green tea help prevent cell damage, thereby fending off wrinkles and keeping your skin soft and smooth. This delicious drink is one of the simplest ways to enjoy all the benefits of this internal-beauty powerhouse.

½ cup of brewed green tea, chilled*
1 large peach, sliced and pitted
½ banana
1 tbsp. of raw honey

Puree all of the ingredients in a blender or food processor, and drink to your good looks and good health!

* To speed up the process, make your tea by the quart, keep it in the fridge, and simply pour out as much as you need when it's time for a smoothie break.

STEP 3. Mix the puree with the tea, pour the blend into an ice cube tray, and put it in the freezer.

STEP 4. When the cubes are frozen, pop one out of the tray and rub it all over your face, concentrating on the puffiest areas, until the ice has melted (or you're tired of rubbing). Blot your face lightly with a paper towel, but leave the slightly sticky residue on your skin for 20 to 30 minutes. Then rinse it off with warm water. Not only will your face be de-puffed, but your pores will also be tighter and your skin softer, brighter, and younger looking. **Note:** Blueberries stain any fabric they touch, so perform this procedure over a sink while you're wearing expendable clothing!

✤ Meet Your Match(a)

Matcha (sometimes spelled maccha) is nothing more than green-tea leaves ground into a fine powder. It delivers all of the skin-nourishing benefits of regular green tea, but in a highly concentrated form. For that reason, it's become a key ingredient in many top-of-the-line beauty products. But it's easy, and a lot cheaper, to make your own. Here are some examples.

ANTI-INFLAMMATORY FACIAL RINSE. Dissolve 1 teaspoon of matcha power in 2 cups of distilled water, and splash your face with it as needed to reduce irritation or blemishes.

EXFOLIATING, MOISTURIZING MASK. Mix 3 teaspoons of matcha powder with 1½ teaspoons of distilled water and 1 teaspoon of raw honey to form a paste. (Add more matcha or water if necessary to get the right texture.) Smooth the paste onto your face, and leave it on for 15 to 30 minutes. Then gently massage it into your skin, and rinse with lukewarm water.

HYDRATING, CLEANSING MASK. Mix 3 teaspoons of matcha powder, 2 teaspoons of raw honey, and 5 teaspoons of plain yogurt in a bowl, and spread the mixture over your face and neck. Leave it on for 15 to 30 minutes, and rinse with lukewarm water.

SOFTENING, TONING BATH SALTS. Combine equal parts of matcha powder and either sea salt or Epsom salts, and store the mixture in a tightly covered container at room temperature. At bath time, pour ¼ cup of the blend under the spigot as you run warm water into the tub. Then settle in and soak for 20 minutes or so.

You can find matcha in the Asian food sections of many supermarkets, as well as in health-food stores and (of course) online. Or, if you prefer, simply put regular green-tea leaves in your coffee grinder, and hold the "on" button down until you get a fine green powder.

✤ Brighten Up Dark Hair

If your black or dark brown strands are looking a little lackluster, try this old-time trick to bring back the high-wattage shine and rich color. Steep two black-tea bags in 2 cups of boiling water for 10 minutes. Let the tea cool to room temperature, wash your hair, and immediately pour the tea over your wet head,

POTENT POTION

DARKENING COLOR RINSE

There are plenty of commercial dyes that will darken your hair either at home or in a beauty salon. But this simple rinse will do the job for a lot less money, and with none of the harsh chemicals.

2 cups of boiling water
2 black-tea bags
¼ cup of dried sage leaves
3 tbsp. of dried rosemary leaves

Pour the water over the tea bags, and steep, covered, in a pan for 15 minutes. Remove the tea bags, squeezing out the liquid. Reheat the tea to just the boiling point, take it off the stove, and add the herbs. Steep the brew, covered, for 60 minutes, and strain the liquid into another container. Holding your head over a basin to catch the runoff, pour the tea through your freshly washed and rinsed hair. Repeat several times, working it through your hair, then dry and style your tresses as usual.

rubbing it through your hair as you would shampoo. Leave the rinse on for 10 minutes, then shampoo again and apply your usual conditioner. The result: soft, shiny, and more manageable hair. Repeat the process once a week, or whenever you feel in need of a shine boost.

Best of the Rest

★ Wind Down with Wine

If you're going through a period where bedtime has become tossing-and-turning time, don't rush off to the drugstore for sleeping pills. Instead, put 2 cups of white wine in a pan, and heat it until it's *almost* boiling. (Don't let it boil!) Remove the pan from the heat, add 4 teaspoons of dill seeds, and let it steep, covered, for half an hour. Drink it, lukewarm, 30 to 45 minutes before you hit the sack and you should have no trouble sleeping.

★ Sleepy Time Cough Medicine

When you've got a cough that's keeping you awake at night, reach for this simple sleeping aid: Heat 1 cup of red wine (don't let it boil!), and stir in lemon juice, cinnamon, and sugar to taste. Sip it while it's hot, and you'll sleep like a baby—guaranteed!

★ Chase a Charley Horse Away

Ouch! You're sound asleep when, out of nowhere, a painful leg cramp jolts you wide awake. Well, don't just lie there squirming. Instead, hobble into the kitchen, pour an 8-ounce glass of tonic water, and drink it down. The quinine in the fizzy mixer should be enough to uncramp your muscles. If you don't care for the taste of plain tonic, jazz it up with a squirt of orange juice, a wedge of lime—or a shot of gin!

★ A Tropical Arthritis Cure

As quirky as it sounds, this Puerto Rican folk remedy has proven amazingly successful for many folks: First thing each morning, mix the freshly squeezed juice of a large lime into a cup of black coffee, and drink it while it's hot. That may just get rid of your aches and pains for good. **Note:** Don't use this treatment if you have a sensitive stomach!

★ Can Your Bunions

About to open an ice-cold can of beer or soda pop? Before you pull the tab, give your sore tootsies a treat: Lay the can sideways on the floor, slip off your shoes and socks, and put your aching foot on the can. Then roll it back and forth for several minutes. The cold will help reduce inflammation, and the motion will give your foot a good massage. Just be sure to let the can rest upright for a few minutes before you open it, or you'll get a fizzy shower!

★ Hangover Help from the Big Easy

On "the morning after the night before," some folks will settle for nothing less than the "hair of the dog." If you're part of that crowd, give this old-time New Orleans remedy a try: Combine 1 ounce of Pernod, 1 ounce of white crème de cacao, and 3 ounces of milk in a blender. Add three ice cubes, and blend on high speed. Then pour the potion into a glass, toss it back—and cross your fingers!

★ An Old-Time Flu Stopper

Here's a formula that dates back to the worldwide flu pandemic of 1918. For many folks, it was literally a lifesaver. To make it, put ½ pound of peeled, chopped garlic and 1 quart of 90-proof cognac in a dark brown bottle. Put on the cap, and seal it with heavy tape to make sure it's airtight. During the day, keep the bottle in a light, warm spot (preferably in the sun). Then move it to a cool, dark place for the night. After 14 days and nights of this routine, open the bottle and strain out the

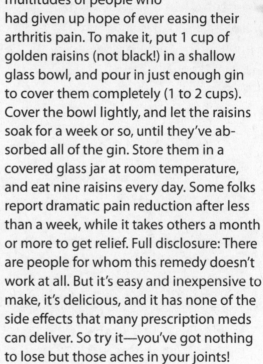

The Gin-Soaked Raisin Remedy

Over the years, this folk remedy has given relief to multitudes of people who had given up hope of ever easing their arthritis pain. To make it, put 1 cup of golden raisins (not black!) in a shallow glass bowl, and pour in just enough gin to cover them completely (1 to 2 cups). Cover the bowl lightly, and let the raisins soak for a week or so, until they've absorbed all of the gin. Store them in a covered glass jar at room temperature, and eat nine raisins every day. Some folks report dramatic pain reduction after less than a week, while it takes others a month or more to get relief. Full disclosure: There are people for whom this remedy doesn't work at all. But it's easy and inexpensive to make, it's delicious, and it has none of the side effects that many prescription meds can deliver. So try it—you've got nothing to lose but those aches in your joints!

garlic. Pour the infused cognac back into the bottle, and label it with the date (it should retain full potency for a year). Then use it as follows:

POTENT POTION

HANDY HAND SANITIZER

Heaven knows, there are plenty of commercial hand sanitizers out there. But when you read the labels, you wonder whether some of the ingredients could do you more harm than the bacteria you're trying to kill. At least I do. That's why I use this simple—and safe—DIY spray.

¼ cup of vodka
¼ cup of water
20 drops of lavender essential oil
20 drops of tea tree oil

Mix all of the ingredients together, and pour the potion into a 4-ounce spray bottle or two 2-ounce bottles. Tuck one into your pocket or purse, and spritz the liquid onto your hands as you would any other sanitizer.

YIELD: 4 OUNCES

■ To prevent the flu, take 10 to 15 drops, mixed in a glass of water, three times a day (one hour before each meal) for the duration of the flu season.

■ If you already have the flu, take 20 drops an hour before each meal for five days. That should send the virus packing. Then switch to the prevention plan described above.

★ Hair's to Beer!

One of the most versatile hair-care products you could ever ask for is probably right in your fridge. What is it? Beer! Here's a trio of ways to give your head a beautifying brewski:

■ Add volume and shine to your hair with this trick: In the shower, after shampooing, pour a bottle of beer over your head. (For best results, use a dark, rich brew that has a high yeast content, which means no "lite" brands!) The yeast and hops will swell your hair shafts and pump up the cuticles, while the beer's acidity will help remove any built-up product residue. Then rinse briefly with cool water.

■ Beer also works wonders as a setting lotion. Pour it into a spray bottle and spritz your hair before styling it into the "do" of your choice.

■ Hops (one of the main ingredients in beer) is an old-time cure for dandruff. So to get rid of the flakes, just add a good squirt of beer to your regular shampoo, then lather up and rinse well.

★ Join the Club

Has swimming in a chlorinated pool turned your blonde hair green? Not to worry! Just grab a bottle of club soda, and use it to wash those nasty chemicals right out of your hair.

★ Rev Up the Red

Want to put red highlights in your brown hair, or ramp up the brightness of your auburn tresses? After shampooing, rinse with strong black coffee that's been cooled to room temperature. Leave it on your hair for 15 minutes, and then rinse thoroughly with cool water.

★ Ginger Nails It

To make your fingernails lighter and brighter, soak them for 10 minutes twice a week in a small bowl of ginger ale. The soluble salts, like sodium benzoate and potassium sorbate (found in most commercial ginger ales), act as natural bleaching agents. They'll quickly clean up dingy nails and keep them whiter.

★ Soak Your Cares Away

Just pour 4 cups of red wine and 1 cup of raw honey into your bathtub as you fill it with very warm water. Settle in and relax for 30 minutes. The warm, steamy air will open your pores so they can absorb the wine's beautifying antioxidants and complex amino acids. The honey will help your skin retain moisture. When you're done soaking, rinse off with clear water, and pat dry.

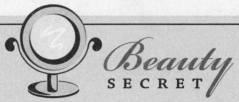

Beauty SECRET

HAIR-CONDITIONING DUO

In the natural-beauty biz, beer and honey are renowned as all-around champs. Here they team up in a conditioner that softens, shines, moisturizes, and strengthens your hair. To make it, pour a can or bottle of beer (preferably a dark, full-bodied brew) into a non-breakable bowl, and let it go flat. In a separate container, mix 1 teaspoon of raw honey in 4 cups of warm water. After shampooing, pour the flat beer onto your hair, work it through the strands, and let it soak in for about two minutes. Rinse with cold water, and apply your usual conditioner. Then rinse again with the honey solution, and let your hair air-dry. Perform this routine once a month to keep your hair full, shiny, and beautifully manageable.

23

Vinegar

Historians reckon that vinegar was discovered by accident at least 10,000 years ago, when a wine vat was opened early. Instead of maturing into a delicious beverage, the fruit "morphed" into a not-so-tasty, but much more versatile liquid. Ever since then, vinegar has played an impressive role in history. Hippocrates, the father of medicine, prescribed it for numerous ailments. Helen of Troy bathed in it to relax. World War I medics used it to treat soldiers' wounds. And active folks from samurai warriors to Sam Houston drank it as a fortifying tonic. Today, in natural-health and beauty circles, vinegar is more popular than ever!

Vim and Vinegar

✔ Kill the Poison

Poison ivy, oak, and sumac are no match for apple cider vinegar. So the next time you have a run-in with any of these noxious weeds, split a brown paper bag open, soak it in some apple cider vinegar, and lay it on the rash. It'll draw out the toxins in no time flat.

✔ Heal Sore, Chapped Hands

You say you spent too much time working bare-handed in frigid weather, and now your hands are red, raw, and burning? Not to worry! Just mix some ultra-rich hand cream with an equal amount of vinegar (any kind will do), and smooth it on your paws every time you wash them. Within days, your skin will be as good as new.

✔ Get Ready for Ol' Sol

When summertime rolls around, stash a bottle of apple cider vinegar in the refrigerator. Then whenever you spend too much time in the sun, pull out the bottle and pat your skin every 20 minutes with the cold liquid. It'll take the pain away fast and (as long as you don't rinse it off), it'll prevent your burned skin from blistering and peeling. **Note:** This trick also works well for very minor burns from the stove, the barbecue grill, or a hot iron.

✔ Relief When You're Already Scorched

You say the sun has already done a number on your skin, and you haven't any refrigerated vinegar? No problem! Just head for the bathroom, and pour 1 cup of room-temperature apple cider vinegar into a tub of warm water. Then ease on in, and heave a soothing sigh of relief.

✔ Heal Bites and Stings

When you combine the drawing power of plantain (yes, that pesky weed) and the anti-inflammatory action of apple cider vinegar, what do you get? A tincture that not only relieves the symptoms of a bite or sting, but also actually heals the wound! Here's how to make your own supply of this super summertime helper:

STEP 1. Gather up a bunch of plantain leaves that have not been treated with pesticides or herbicides. Wash them, tear them into pieces, and

---

POTENT POTION

TIMELY TICK REPELLENT

Ticks are not simply summertime nuisances; they can also spread life-threatening diseases. So make up a batch of this powerful, but gentle, repellent and keep it on hand throughout the bad-bug season.

2 cups of white vinegar
1 cup of water
20 drops of eucalyptus essential oil
20 drops of lavender essential oil
20 drops of peppermint essential oil

Mix all of the ingredients together, and pour the mixture into pocket-size spray bottles. Then, whenever you're in tick territory, spritz your clothes and exposed skin (but not your face!) thoroughly. The tiny terrors will keep their distance—guaranteed!

YIELD: 24 OUNCES

crush them to extract the volatile oils. (The bottom of a jar works well for this purpose.)

STEP 2. Pack the leaves into a large glass jar that has a tight-fitting lid, and cover them with apple cider vinegar. Store the jar in a cool, dark place for two weeks, shaking it daily.

STEP 3. When time's up, strain the liquid through cheesecloth into a clean glass jar with a tight-fitting lid, label it, and store it in the refrigerator. As needed, pour some of the tincture into smaller, dark-colored bottles to carry in your pocket, backpack, or golf bag.

To use the potion, immediately dab it generously onto the site of a bite or sting. You should feel almost-instant relief. **Note:** If the culprit was a poisonous spider or snake, apply the tincture and then get medical help pronto!

✔ Eradicate the Itch

An apple cider vinegar bath is excellent for relieving the discomfort of psoriasis, hives, or pruritus (the medical term for itching that's generally

ACV + H$_2$O = Relief!

Apple cider vinegar (ACV) and water can help solve a myriad of nagging health problems. Reach for this classic combo whenever one of these conditions strikes.

HEALTH PROBLEM	THE R$_X$
Bladder infection	2 tsp. of ACV in a glass of water three times a day*
Dizzy spell	½ tsp. of ACV in a glass of water
Hot flashes	1 tbsp. of ACV in 8 oz. of ice water as needed
Indigestion	2 tsp. of ACV in a glass of water once an hour until you feel better
Morning sickness	1 tsp. of ACV in a glass of water as soon as you get up
Sinusitis or facial neuralgia	½ tsp. of ACV in a glass of water once an hour for seven hours

* Get your doctor's okay first.

associated with an illness of some kind). In this case, use 2 cups of cider vinegar per tub full of warm water, and soak your itch away.

✔ A Head Start on Psoriasis Relief

To relieve the itch of psoriasis on your scalp, don't soak your head! Instead, gently massage it with a half-and-half mixture of apple cider vinegar and water. It'll not only stop the itching, but will also help reduce the inflammation and heal any associated infections.

✔ Whittle Your Waistline

Trying to lose a little weight? Here's a trick that may help: Before each meal, mix 1 teaspoon of apple cider vinegar in a glass of warm water (make sure it's warm!), and drink up. If you're like most folks, this elixir will decrease your appetite, so you'll just naturally want to eat less, and that—combined with getting more exercise—is the healthiest way there is to shed unwanted pounds!

✔ Nail Athlete's Foot

Vinegar is a surefire weapon for killing the fungi that cause athlete's foot, and it also keeps them from coming back. Here's the routine:

■ Rinse your afflicted feet several times a day with either white or apple cider vinegar.

■ To avoid reinfecting yourself, soak your socks and/or panty hose in white vinegar for 20 minutes or so before washing them. Also, moisten a cotton ball or pad with white vinegar, and use it to wipe out any shoes or boots you've worn since contracting the condition.

■ If you swim or work out at a gym or health club, keep a spray bottle of vinegar in your tote bag or locker. Then each time you get out of the shower, spray your toes thoroughly, rinse them with clear water, and dry them well.

CAUTION

Vinegar is strong stuff, so to avoid upsetting your stomach, never drink it straight. Always mix it with a milder carrier like water, fruit juice, or honey. Also, over time, the acid in vinegar can damage your tooth enamel, so whenever you use it as a gargle or dental aid, rinse your mouth thoroughly with clear water immediately afterward.

Like many healers (homemade and otherwise), vinegar interacts with some medications, including digoxin (Lanoxin®), insulin, and diuretic drugs. So if you're taking any of those meds, check with your doctor before you use vinegar in medicinal quantities. Finally, if you are pregnant or think you might be pregnant, ask your obstetrician how much vinegar is safe for you to consume.

✔ End Nail Fungus Naturally

There are powerful prescription medications that can cure finger- and toenail fungi from the inside—and quickly. There's just one problem: These meds can deliver side effects, including kidney damage, that are a lot worse than the pain and itch of your infected digit. So why take chances? Instead of popping pills, soak your affected hand or foot for 15 to 20 minutes every day in a solution made from 1 part white or apple cider vinegar to 2 parts warm water. Granted, it will take longer to work than a doctor's prescription, but it will kill the foul fungi with no damage to your innards.

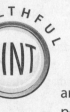

HEALTHFUL HINT

Bring on the Clouds

For medicinal and beauty purposes, always use raw, organic, unfiltered apple cider vinegar (available in health-food stores and in the health-food sections of most supermarkets). Avoid the clear, filtered kind generally found with the salad dressings in the main grocery aisles. When you look at a bottle of the good stuff, you'll see that it has a cloudy consistency, with some strand-like sediment floating at the bottom. Those clouds and strands (a.k.a. "the mother") contain all the enzymes and friendly bacteria that give apple cider vinegar its miraculous healing power.

✔ Stop a Bloody Nose

This old-time cure works like a charm: Soak a cotton ball in apple cider vinegar, and gently insert it into the dripping nostril. Then, holding both nostrils closed with your fingers, breathe through your mouth for about five minutes. Slowly remove the cotton. If the bleeding hasn't stopped, repeat the procedure. **Note:** If you have recurring nosebleeds, it could signify an underlying health condition, so see your doctor. And if blood is flowing from both nostrils, hightail it to the ER!

✔ Give Headaches the Heave-Ho

As kooky as it sounds, the old-timers in my family swore by this headache remedy, and I still do today. Here's all there is to it: Dip a large white cotton cloth in vinegar (either white or apple cider), and wring it out. Put it against your forehead, and tie it tightly in the back. Keep it there until the pain backs off, which should be within 30 minutes. If your head is still pounding after half an hour, repeat the process.

✔ Make Varicose Veins Vamoose

If you're plagued by varicose veins, you know that their unsightly appearance is the least of the problem. They're also painful as the dickens— and even dangerous because they can trigger blood clots. But before you resort to drugs or surgery, try this simple trick. Soak a couple of cloths in apple cider vinegar, and wrap them around your legs. Then lie down with your feet propped up about a foot, and hold that pose for half an hour or so. Do this twice a day until those ugly blue road maps hit the trail.

✔ Clobber Coughs and Colds . . .

And sore throats, too, with this classic triple-threat combo: Mix equal parts of apple cider vinegar, honey, and warm water, and stir in about ¼ teaspoon of mashed fresh ginger per cup of the mixture. Store it at room temperature in a covered glass jar, and take 1 teaspoon three times a day. Before you know it, your colds and coughs will be history!

✔ A Tangy Sore Throat Solution

If your painful throat is not associated with a cold, give this trick a try: Mix 2 teaspoons of apple cider vinegar in 8 ounces of warm water, and proceed as follows: Gargle a mouthful of the solution, and spit it out. Then swallow a mouthful. Keep it up, alternating gargling and swallowing, until the glass is empty. Wait 60 minutes, and perform the routine again. Continue as needed until

Fabulous Food Fix

SUPER JUICE

Don't be fooled by the delicious, sweet-tart taste of this beverage. It's actually a powerful cold killer, crackerjack hangover cure—and an efficient delivery mechanism for all the health-giving benefits of apple cider vinegar.

½ cup of unfiltered apple cider vinegar
¼ cup of 100 percent organic grape or apple juice
1 tbsp. of lemon juice
1 tsp. of raw honey (or more to taste)
½ tsp. of ground cinnamon
2 cups of water

Mix all of the ingredients thoroughly in a pitcher or large jar. Store it, tightly covered, in the refrigerator. Serve it in ice-filled glasses anytime you want a super-refreshing *and* super-healthy pick-me-up.

YIELD: ABOUT 5 SERVINGS, BUT YOU CAN DOUBLE OR EVEN TRIPLE THE RECIPE IF YOU LIKE BECAUSE IT'LL KEEP FOR SEVERAL WEEKS IN THE FRIDGE.

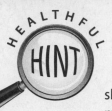

A Triumphant Triad

Worldwide studies show that a mixture made of apple cider vinegar, honey, and garlic can cure or help prevent almost every ailment under the sun, including arthritis, asthma, high blood pressure, obesity, and ulcers, as well as ease muscle aches and colds. The simple formula: Mix 1 cup of apple cider vinegar, 1 cup of raw honey, and 8 peeled garlic cloves in a blender on high speed for 60 seconds. Pour the blend into a glass jar with a tight-fitting lid, and let it sit in the refrigerator for five days. Then every day (ideally before breakfast) take 2 teaspoons of the tonic stirred into a glass of water or fruit juice. Researchers especially recommend using fresh orange or 100 percent grape juice. Now, I can't guarantee that this will cure what ails you, but it's worth a try.

you've put your pain to rest. **Note:** If your throat is still sore after a week or so, and you have no other symptoms, see your doctor to rule out a more serious condition.

✔ Beef Up Your Chicken Soup

We all know that chicken soup is a powerful weapon in the fight against cold and flu germs. Well, here's a way to add even more oomph to your favorite recipe (or even instant chicken broth): Heat up 1 cup of soup or broth, and stir in 1 tablespoon of apple cider vinegar, 1 crushed garlic clove, and a dash of hot-pepper sauce to taste. Pour it into a bowl or mug, and sip yourself to good health. Repeat as necessary until you're back in the pink again.

✔ Open Your Sinuses

Clogged sinuses driving you crazy? Apple cider vinegar can solve the problem lickety-split. How you put it to work is your call. Two or three times a day, use one of these remarkable remedies—or, if you like, try all three and see which one works best for you:

■ Drink a glass of warm water with 2 teaspoons of cider vinegar mixed in it.

■ Mix 2 tablespoons of cider vinegar and 1 tablespoon of raw honey in 8 ounces of lukewarm water, and drink it down.

■ Mix 1 cup of cider vinegar and 1 cup of water in a pan. Heat it on the stove, then bend over the pan and inhale the steamy vapors while keeping your mouth and eyes closed. Have tissues at hand because this should get things flowing fast. Just be careful not to burn yourself!

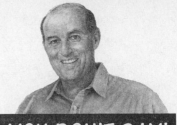

✔ Jump-Start Your Inner Plumbing

Constipation got you down? Mix 2 tablespoons of apple cider vinegar in a glass of water or 100 percent apple or grape juice. Drink this mixture three times a day, and things should start moving merrily along.

✔ Relieve Arthritis Pain

It seems that every arthritis sufferer either has a favorite remedy or is searching high and low for one that *really* works. Well, according to everyone I know who's tried it, this one's a jim-dandy: Combine equal parts of apple cider vinegar and raw honey, and store the mixture in a lidded glass jar at room temperature. Then once a day, stir 1 teaspoon of the combo and 1 teaspoon of unflavored Knox® Gelatine into 6 ounces of water, and drink it down. Before you know it, your joints should be jumpin'!

✔ Ease Your Workout Woes

You say you got a little carried away with your new workout routine, and now your muscles are so sore you can hardly move? Well, don't just lie on the couch moaning and groaning. Instead, saturate a soft cloth with apple cider vinegar, and wrap it around your aching area. Leave it on for 20 minutes. If you still feel achy, repeat the procedure every three to four hours until the pain is gone for good. It should be soon because the vinegar helps to draw out the lactic acid that causes your muscles to feel stiff and sore in the first place.

✔ Leapin' Liniment!

No matter what's caused the pain in your muscles or joints, a gentle rubdown with this vintage recipe will ease it fast. Mix 2 egg whites with ½ cup of apple cider vinegar and ¼ cup of olive oil. Massage the lotion into the painful areas, and wipe off the

YOU DON'T SAY!

In the 17th century, the bubonic plague swept across Europe, killing at least half the population, and thus becoming known as the Black Death. French folklore tells us that in Marseilles, four men repeatedly looted the homes of deceased victims but, miraculously, never got sick. According to one version of the story, after the thieves were arrested, they were forced to bury the dead, with the promise that if they survived, they would go free. Well, survive they did—apparently thanks to an herbal vinegar tincture concocted by one of the bad guys, who happened to be an herbalist. As the gang's resistance to the disease became obvious, other folks began using the potion. Today, natural-health gurus still swear by the amazing healing power of Four Thieves Vinegar (see the recipe on page 322 and "Good Things from Bad Guys" on page 323).

excess with a soft cotton cloth. (Be careful not to get any of the stuff on sheets, clothes, or upholstery fabric!)

✔ Battle Chronic Fatigue

We all get tired every now and then. But if you feel constantly fatigued, the reason may be that lactic acid has built up in your system. (That tends to happen during periods of stress or strenuous exercise.) If that's the case, this simple trick may help: At bedtime each night, take 3 teaspoons of apple cider vinegar mixed in ⅛ cup of honey. Continue the routine until your old vim and vigor return. **Note:** If that doesn't happen within a few weeks, call your doctor.

✔ Calm Down!

Whether your nerves are frayed from a busy day at the office followed by a bumper-to-bumper commute, or the state of world affairs has your anxiety level soaring off the charts, this de-stressing cocktail can help you relax: Put 1 tablespoon of apple cider vinegar and a chamomile tea bag

POTENT POTION

FOUR THIEVES VINEGAR

Numerous variations of this recipe have evolved over the centuries, but this is one of the most popular and easiest to make and use (see page 323).

2 tbsp. of dried food-grade lavender
2 tbsp. of dried mint
2 tbsp. of dried rosemary
2 tbsp. of dried sage
2 tbsp. of dried thyme
4–8 fresh garlic cloves, minced
32-oz. bottle of apple cider vinegar

Put the first six ingredients in a glass jar, and pour the vinegar over them. Cover the jar tightly, and leave it in a cool, dark place for six to eight weeks, shaking it daily. When time's up, strain the tonic into smaller containers for easier use. Store them away from heat and light.

* If your jar has a metal lid, cover the opening with plastic wrap before you screw on the cap; otherwise, the vinegar will react with the metal.

YIELD: 1 QUART

into 1 cup of boiling water. Reduce the heat, and let it simmer for three or four minutes. Then remove the pan from the stove, pull out the tea bag, and pour the tea into a mug. When the brew has cooled a bit, sit back, and sip your cares away.

✔ Good Things from Bad Guys

Ever since the 17th century, savvy folks have been tapping into the remarkable healing power of Four Thieves Vinegar, which, according to legend, was first formulated by a convicted robber. (You'll find the recipe at left and the colorful saga in the You Don't Say! box on page 321.) Here's a quartet of ways to use this wonder "drug":

CURE COLDS, FLU, AND OTHER ILLNESSES. Adults should take 1 tablespoon of Four Thieves Vinegar three times a day. The dosage for children is 1 teaspoon three times a day. How you take it is your call. For example, you can sip it from a spoon, add it to salad dressing, or mix it with water, fruit juice, or herbal tea.

HEAD OFF COLDS AND FLU. Use the same quantities (1 tablespoon for adults, 1 teaspoon for children), but for prevention purposes, taking the potion once a day should do the trick. For additional resistance, you can add a tablespoon or so to your bathwater, and breathe in the healing vapors while you're soaking your cares away.

KILL GERMS. Fend off airborne viruses as well as surface bacteria by filling a small spray bottle with equal parts of Four Thieves Vinegar and water and spraying it into the air and onto surfaces throughout your home and office. It also makes a dandy hand sanitizer.

REPEL DISEASE-SPREADING INSECTS. Or any other kind, for that matter! Pour ¼ cup of Four Thieves Vinegar into a spray bottle, and fill the balance with water. Spray the potion onto your skin and clothes whenever you venture outside into bug-infested territory.

De-Pollute Your Produce

HEALTHFUL HINT

The best way to stay healthy is to eat good food. To ensure that all of your fruits and veggies are free of pesticides, chemical fertilizers, and other toxic substances, call out the big guns (or a small spray bottle). Fill it with 2 tablespoons of vinegar (any kind), 1 tablespoon of lemon juice, and 1 cup of water. Keep the bottle by the sink, and spray your fruit and veggies thoroughly. Then rinse 'em with clear water, and you're good to go!

A Bottle of Beauty

✣ Strengthen—and Whiten—Your Nails

You can make your fingernails stronger and whiter with this terrific trick: Once a week, soak your nails in lemon juice for 10 minutes. Then, using a nailbrush, scrub them with a half-and-half solution of white vinegar and warm water, and rinse with clear H₂O. The result: nails that you'll be proud to show off anywhere!

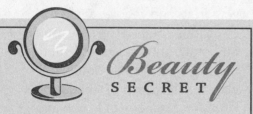

Beauty SECRET

MAKE YOUR POLISH LINGER LONGER

It's frustrating, all right—you carefully paint your fingernails or toenails and patiently wait for them to dry. Then before you know it, the polish starts chipping off. Well, don't get all hot and bothered about it. Instead, just adopt this simple prep routine: Soak your nails in vinegar (either white or apple cider) for about 60 seconds. Wait until they've dried thoroughly, and paint the surfaces as usual. The vinegar will remove the natural oils from the surface of your nails, so instead of sliding off, your polish will hang on tight!

✣ Ditch the Dirt

When working in the garden or puttering in your workshop leaves your hands as grubby as all get-out, it's time for drastic (but gentle) action. March into your kitchen, and pour a teaspoon or two of cornmeal into your palm, add a few drops of apple cider vinegar, and scrub-a-dub-dub. Rinse with cool water, and admire the results: Your hands will be as clean as a whistle and softer to boot.

✣ Ditch the Aroma, Too

This tip is just for the gardeners in our audience. You know that there is nothing better for your plants than frequent servings of compost tea or manure tea. And you also know that when you get the stuff on your hands, it smells to high heaven. To get rid of the odor, wash your hands with dishwashing liquid, then rinse them with vinegar (any kind will do). And from now on, wear plastic or rubber gloves at garden teatime!

✤ Get Rid of Warts

Annoying and unsightly warts will vanish when you use this simple old-time remedy. At bedtime, dab the bump with apple cider vinegar. (But *don't* rub it in—that could cause more warts to form.) Then soak a gauze pad in apple cider vinegar, put it over the wart, and cover it with a bandage to hold in the moisture. Leave it on overnight. In the morning, remove the bandage, but don't rinse off the vinegar. Repeat the treatment each night until the wart is gone.

✤ Brighten Your Choppers Cheaply

Teeth-whitening treatments don't come any easier—or cheaper—than this one: Simply saturate a cotton pad with apple cider vinegar, rub it across your teeth, and rinse thoroughly with clear water. Then go out and have fun with the money you *didn't* have to spend at the dentist's office!

✤ This Aftershave Gets an A+

Commercial aftershave lotions are designed to do four things: act as an antiseptic to clean any nicks or cuts, moisturize your skin, close your pores, and soothe razor burn. Well, guess what? The acetic acid in apple cider vinegar can perform those same feats at a fraction of the cost—on gents' faces or ladies' legs. All you need to do is fill a clean bottle or jar with equal parts apple cider vinegar and water, and shake it to blend them. Then splash the mixture onto your skin as you would any other aftershave. And don't fret about the aroma because it'll vanish when the vinegar dries.

Fabulous Food Fix

SENSATIONAL SALAD DRESSING

You don't have to drink vinegar straight up to enjoy its numerous beautifying effects. Simply adding more of it to your diet—for instance, with this delicious salad dressing—can help banish cellulite, soften your skin, eradicate blemishes, and generally reduce signs of aging.

¼ cup of unfiltered apple cider vinegar
2 tbsp. of raw honey
2 tbsp. of water
Salt and pepper to taste
¾ cup of extra virgin olive oil

Mix the first four ingredients in a blender or food processor. Then, with the machine still running, slowly drizzle in the olive oil. Use it to dress your favorite salad, or splash it onto steamed vegetables or baked potatoes.

YIELD: ABOUT 1 CUP

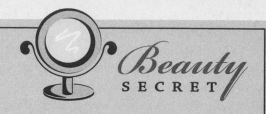

CUSTOMIZE YOUR HAIR CONDITIONER

*F*or centuries, women have been using vinegar to shine and condition their hair. But with a few herbal additives, you can tailor the treatment to do more than that. Simply add 1 cup of dried herbs to 1 quart of high-quality vinegar (either white or apple cider). Let it steep for a few weeks, strain out the solids, and pour the liquid into a clean, unbreakable bottle. As for the type of herbs to use, that depends on the effect you're looking for.

Here's the rundown:

■ *Calendula is a good all-round conditioner.*

■ *Chamomile puts highlights in blonde or light brown hair.*

■ *Lavender and lemon verbena add enticing fragrance.*

■ *Nettles control dandruff.*

■ *Parsley and rosemary make dark hair come alive.*

■ *Sage darkens graying hair.*

Use the potion as a final rinse after shampooing, at a ratio of roughly 1 tablespoon of herbal vinegar per gallon of water.

✤ Fight Cellulite Two Ways

Trying to get rid of unsightly "cottage cheese" patches on your skin? Apple cider vinegar can help in two ways:

FROM THE INSIDE. Once a day, drink an 8-ounce glass of water with 2 tablespoons of apple cider vinegar and 1 tablespoon of honey mixed into it. The dynamic duo will help your body burn fat more efficiently, thereby streamlining the lumpy areas.

FROM THE OUTSIDE. Mix 3 tablespoons of apple cider vinegar with 1 tablespoon of olive oil, and massage it into the problem spots for 10 minutes twice a day. This will increase circulation and help reduce the fatty deposits—before you know it.

✤ De-Gunk Your Hair

Over time, hair sprays, gels, and other styling products can build up in your hair, making it dull, drab, and tangle-prone. Fortunately, there's a fast, simple way to rout out that residue. Mix equal parts apple cider vinegar and water in a spray bottle. After shampooing, spritz the mixture onto your hair, and massage it into your scalp. Let it sit for three minutes or so, then rinse with clear water. You'll soon have soft, shiny, silky-smooth hair that's easy to manage. How often you need to use this treatment depends (of course) on when and in what quantities you use styling products. Your mirror will tell you when it's time for another round.

✤ De-Gunk Your Hairbrushes, Too

Getting built-up residue out of your hair is one thing. To make sure it stays out, you also have to keep your brushes clean and fresh. Here's an easy way to do it: After removing as much hair as possible from the brush, soak it for 15 minutes in a basin of warm water with ¼ cup of white vinegar and 2 teaspoons of shampoo mixed into it. Then pull off any remaining hair, and use an old toothbrush or nailbrush to scrub any stubborn residue from the bristles. Rinse the brush under warm running water, and lay it on a clean towel to dry. That's all there is to it!

To keep your brushes sanitary—and extend their lives—perform this routine two or three times a week. Or if you don't use commercial styling products at all, clean your brushes about once a month to get rid of airborne dirt that your hair picks up.

✤ Clean Your Makeup Brushes

To remove built-up powder, blusher, and other grime from your makeup brushes, mix equal parts of white

Do Away With Dandruff

HEALTHFUL HINT

The same half-and-half mixture of apple cider vinegar and water that removes hair-care-product residue from your tresses (see "De-Gunk Your Hair," above) can also help you bid good-bye to your white-flake woes. The vinegar will restore the proper pH balance of your scalp to make it flake- and itch-free. Just spray the potion onto your head, work it into your scalp, and leave it on for one to two hours before rinsing with clear water. After that, to keep your dandruff from coming back, use this treatment at least once a week, keeping it on for three minutes before rinsing.

POTENT POTION

SUMMERTIME CLARIFYING MASK

When Mother Nature turns up the heat, sweat, dirt, and melting makeup all add up to one thing: clogged pores. But this terrific trio will clear out the nasty crud, fend off blemish breakouts, and leave your skin soft and radiant.

4 tbsp. of canned pumpkin puree*
3 tbsp. of apple cider vinegar
1½ tbsp. of rose water**

Mix all of the ingredients in a bowl. Spread the mixture onto your face, and leave it on for 15 to 20 minutes. Rinse with warm water, and follow up with your usual cleansing and moisturizing routine. Repeat as needed to fend off summer's dirty tricks.

* Not pumpkin pie filling.
** For a simple DIY version, see "Grandma Knew Best" on page 182.

vinegar and warm water in a basin, and add a couple drops of baby shampoo to soften the bristles. Swirl the brushes around in this mixture until all the yucky residue comes off, and then rinse them under warm running water. Reshape the bristles with your fingers, and stand the brushes upright in a mug or jar to dry. They'll be as clean and fresh as the day you bought them!

✤ A Beautiful Balancing Act

You could pay an arm and a leg for a toner that will moisturize, refresh, and purify your skin. Or you could mix 1 part apple cider vinegar with 2 parts water, and dab it onto your face with a cotton ball. It'll lock in moisture, reduce any inflammation, and help restore your skin's natural pH balance, so it's better able to shed dead skin cells and fend off blemish-causing bacteria. **Note:** If your skin is very sensitive, use more water. Start with 3 parts water to 1 part vinegar, and experiment until you find the ratio that's right for you.

✤ Punch It Up

To add even more oomph (and a more enticing aroma) to your toner, use rose water instead of plain water in your vinegar solution. Or make a strong infusion using one or more of your favorite herbs, and use that to replace the H_2O (see Tea Times Two on page 99). As with hair conditioner (see "Customize Your Hair Conditioner" on page 326), your best choice depends on what you want to accomplish. The herbs listed below are all packed with complexion-improving power. You can find fresh versions at many farmers' markets, natural-food stores, and large supermarkets, and dried forms are available in herb shops and online.

CHAMOMILE (flowers). Reduces inflammation, soothes, cleanses, and supplies antifungal agents.

ELDER (flowers). Cleanses, tones, and acts as a gentle astringent.

LAVENDER (flowers). Soothes, cleanses, and reduces inflammation.

LINDEN (flowers). Supplies the same benefits as chamomile (above), but in a milder form that's especially good for aging skin.

MALLOW. Soothes irritated skin.

MINT. Cools and refreshes.

POT MARIGOLD, A.K.A. CALENDULA (flowers). Cleanses, soothes, and reduces inflammation; often used in a half-and-half mixture with chamomile or lavender.

ROSEMARY. Tones, revitalizes, and improves blood circulation to your skin's capillaries.

THYME. Fights bacteria; is especially effective on acne and eczema.

YARROW. Tones, cleanses, and heals; particularly good for sensitive, aging, or damaged skin.

Best of the Rest

★ Balsamic Blasts Belly Fat

Balsamic vinegar—the tastiest of all vinegars—can help eliminate one of the most dangerous kinds of fat: the "spare tire" around the belly that can lead to conditions like heart disease, sleep apnea, and type 2 diabetes. It works by activating genes that cause your body to distribute fat more evenly, rather than store it at your waist. The jury is still out on exact dosages, but a good amount to aim for is 5 teaspoons a day, which is the amount that researchers have found to increase insulin sensitivity in diabetics.

Fabulous Food Fix

ROASTED BALSAMIC ONIONS

If you think of balsamic vinegar as only a tasty ingredient in salad dressings, think again. There are scads of simple and delicious ways to add its health- and beauty-giving powers to your diet. This is one of my favorites.

3 large, sweet white onions, peeled and quartered*
¼ cup of balsamic vinegar
3 tbsp. of extra virgin olive oil
½ tsp. of sugar
Kosher salt and freshly ground black pepper to taste

Mix all of the ingredients together in a large bowl. Spread them out in an even layer in a large oven-proof skillet. Cover it with aluminum foil, and roast at 350°F for 20 to 25 minutes. Remove the foil, toss the onions to coat them with the sauce, and return the skillet to the oven, uncovered, for another 20 to 25 minutes. Serve the sweet and tangy onions warm as a side dish, or as a topping for pasta or baked potatoes.

* Or substitute red onions.

YIELD: 4 SERVINGS

★ Great Grapes Alive!

Thanks to the Trebbiano and Lambrusco grapes that it's made from, balsamic vinegar is loaded with compounds that fight cancer, strengthen your immune system, and destroy the free radicals that cause premature aging and hardening of the arteries. So here's a hot tip for all you pasta fans: The next time you order a big dinner at your favorite Italian restaurant, make sure you include balsamic vinegar on your salad. It'll keep your blood sugar from spiking, thereby preventing the sudden fatigue (a.k.a. "sugar crash") that can set in a few hours later. By the way, this trick works just as well for runners who load up on carbs before a big race.

★ Secret of the Samurais

Japan's famous samurai warriors claimed they owed their strength and power to a tonic called *Tamago-su*, or egg vinegar. Folks throughout Japan still take it to maintain good health and slow down the aging process. Of course, the samurais didn't know why it worked, but we do: It prevents both the formation of damaging free radicals and the buildup of LDL (bad) cholesterol in your body. Here's how to make your own supply:

1. Immerse a whole raw egg in 1 cup of rice vinegar, and let it sit, covered, for seven days.

2. When the week's up, you'll find that everything has dissolved into the vinegar except the transparent membrane that was just inside the shell. Discard the membrane, and stir the egg-infused vinegar thoroughly. Store the tonic in a glass jar that has a tight-fitting lid.

3. Three times a day, stir 1 or 2 teaspoons of the vinegar in a glass of hot water, and drink to a long, healthy life.

★ Make Your Hair Glow

Want to make your hair so shiny that it gleams (maybe for a special occasion)? Just mix 2 tablespoons of malt vinegar in a quart of water, and use it as a final rinse. Your luxuriant locks will sparkle like the stars!

★ Rice and Soft

When your heels are dry and cracked, reach for some rice vinegar. Mix 1 tablespoon of it with 1 table-spoon each of raw honey and coarse sea salt to make a watery paste, and scrub away. Then slather on a rich hand or foot cream, put on a pair of cotton socks to help the cream sink in, and leave them on overnight. The next morning, your heels will be noticeably softer. Repeat the procedure each night until all the thickened, dead skin is gone with the wind.

★ Soak Your Way to Softness

If you prefer a less hands-on approach to foot treatments, mix equal parts of rice vinegar and water in a basin, and soak your feet for 20 to 30 minutes. Again, repeat the routine until your skin is smooth and silky again. **Note:** This vinegar-water remedy will also help prevent or clear up any lingering nail fungus.

Beauty SECRET

GIVE BODY ODOR THE BOOT

Few things are more embarrassing than body odor, a.k.a. BO. Here's what to do about it: Shortly before bedtime, saturate a cloth with malt vinegar, and wipe your whole body down with it. Then let your skin air-dry before you hit the sack. The acid will change your skin's pH, thereby deactivating the odor-causing bacteria. Come morning, hop in the shower, and you should come out smelling like a rose—more or less. **Note:** *If your BO persists, see your doctor. The problem may be a sign of ill health or a poor diet.*

24

Witch Hazel

Unlike many homemade healers, witch hazel (*Hamamelis virginiana*) is a genuine Yankee Doodle Dandy. It's been growing in the woodlands of eastern North America since long before recorded time. Various Indian tribes distilled the leaves, roots, and bark and used the brew for everything from soothing sore muscles to treating burns, colds, coughs, and dysentery. Fast forward to 1846, when it became the first mass-marketed toiletry to be made in America. (It was first called Golden Treasure and later renamed Pond's Extract.) Today, witch hazel remains a health and beauty superstar from sea to shining sea.

Calling Dr. Hazel

✔ Relieve External Hemorrhoids

Don't let this annoying affliction get you down. Witch hazel can greatly reduce the pain and itch and help dry up any bleeding. Simply mix equal parts of witch hazel with either aloe gel, glycerin, or petroleum jelly (to improve the sticking power), and gently rub the mixture onto the trouble spots. Trust me, sitting will be a whole lot more comfortable!

✔ Ease Sunburn Pain Fast

Just dip gauze or cheesecloth in witch hazel, and gently wrap it around the affected area. As the cloth dries, repeat the procedure until you feel relief—which will be a lot sooner than you think. Follow up with a rich moisturizing lotion. If the sun has done its number on a part of your body that cannot be easily wrapped, pour some witch hazel into a spray bottle, and spritz your sore skin.

✔ Sack Psoriasis Scales

Witch hazel can work wonders to send the painful, itchy, and unsightly scales (a.k.a. plaques) packing. Put it to work by mixing equal parts of alcohol-free witch hazel and glycerin USP (available in pharmacies) in a wide-mouthed container. After your shower or bath, pat your skin dry, and rub the mixture thoroughly into the affected areas— avoiding any open lesions. (The potion should disappear entirely; if your skin is greasy, it means that you've used too much.) Repeat the procedure daily. Within about three weeks, redness and scaling should be reduced by 80 to 90 percent. After that, use the treatment once a week or as often as needed to help prevent flare-ups. **Note:** Use a lotion applicator to treat patches on your back or other hard-to-reach areas.

To relieve psoriasis flare-ups on your head, shampoo your hair as usual, and then massage the mixture into your scalp until it is completely absorbed.

Ways and Means

H E A L T H F U L
HINT

All witch hazel extract is produced from the leaves, roots, and bark of the same shrub, *Hamamelis virginiana*. But there are a couple of different manufacturing methods, so when shopping, read the product labels very carefully. Some processes use isopropyl alcohol (in fact, some brands actually contain more alcohol than witch hazel). But for health and beauty purposes, look for a label that says "food grade" and/or "100 percent organic witch hazel hydrosol." This indicates that it was distilled slowly under low pressure using pure water, which helps preserve all the beneficial properties of the plant. What's more, unlike the alcoholic versions, the hydrosol is gentle enough to use on even the most sensitive skin.

✔ Mind Your Mouth

The antiseptic, anti-inflammatory, and astringent powers of witch hazel make it a first-class healer for gingivitis and other gum problems. Mix ½ to 1 teaspoon of food-grade witch hazel and 2 or 3 drops of clove oil in 1 cup of lukewarm water. Use the mixture three or four times a day, as you would mouthwash, until your gums are back to normal. **Note:** If you're being treated for gingivitis, consult your dentist before using this remedy.

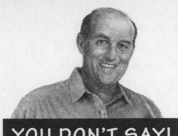

YOU DON'T SAY!

Have you ever wondered how our native North American witch hazel plant (*Hamamelis virginiana*) got its common name? Well, no one knows for sure, but it has nothing to do with witches or witchcraft. Most likely, the first part came about because our Pilgrim fathers (taught by the Indians) used the shrub's forked branches to dowse for underground water. In the language of the day, the word *wych* meant small and lively, which precisely described the dowsing rod as it bobbed up and down in the diviner's hands. Over the years, the spelling *wych* evolved to *witch*. As for who Hazel was, your guess is as good as mine!

✔ Go Deeper

To treat either laryngitis or a sore throat, make the same witch hazel–clove oil solution as described in "Mind Your Mouth" (see page 333). But instead of simply swishing the potion around in your mouth, gargle with it three or four times a day (but don't swallow it!). Before you know it, you'll be as right as rain again.

✔ Colonoscopy Prep Made Easy

Make that *easier*. Prepping for a colonoscopy is far more unpleasant than the procedure itself. It entails a 24-hour process of cleaning out your colon by drinking only clear fluids and a foul-tasting "beverage," and the routine can make your rear end as sore as the dickens. You can buy commercial hemorrhoid pads to relieve the discomfort, but here's a better (and cheaper) idea: The evening before you start prepping, mix together a few drops of lavender essential oil per ounce of witch hazel. Dip a dozen or so cotton pads in the solution, put them into a ziplock freezer bag, and then stash them in the freezer. The next day, use them right out of the bag as often as needed to bring powerful relief to your sitting area. **Note:** If you have any pads left over, save them in the freezer for soothing future cuts, scratches, or insect bites, and as handy wipes for hemorrhoid relief.

✔ Cool Aid for Hot Muscles

When you've been working or playing hard in the hot sun, give your aching muscles a nice cooling treat. Here's how: Mix 2 cups of witch hazel, 2 teaspoons of light corn syrup, ½ teaspoon of castor oil, and 3 or 4 drops of essential oil in a jar with a tight-fitting lid. Shake well, and massage the potion into your sore body parts for almost-instant relief. **Note:** Rosemary, peppermint, wintergreen, and eucalyptus oils are all excellent choices for cooling and relaxing sore, stiff muscles and joints.

✔ Very Good Varicose Vein Relief

Millions of folks suffer from this circulation problem—and if you're one of them, you know that it can be pure agony. Fortunately, witch hazel can help. The simple routine: Chill a bowl of witch hazel in the refrigerator for an hour or two, then soak washcloths in it. Sit back in a comfortable chair, put your legs up, and lay the cold compresses on the affected areas. Keep them in place for 15 minutes or so, and the pain should be gone, or at least greatly diminished. Repeat the procedure as often as necessary to maintain your comfort level. **Note:** The amount of witch hazel you need to use depends on the size of the area you need to cover.

✔ Solo Acts

Straight from the bottle, witch hazel can perform heaps of health-care feats. Here's a handful of everyday problem solvers:

BLACK EYE. Soak a washcloth in witch hazel, and hold it over your eye. The pain and swelling will vamoose. Just make sure you don't get any in your eye, though, because it will sting like crazy!

BRUISES. Dab witch hazel on the mark three times a day, and it'll be gone in no time.

CUTS AND SCRAPES. Pour a generous amount of witch hazel on the wound, let it air-dry, and then cover it with a bandage.

DIAPER RASH. Gently smooth witch hazel onto baby's bottom using a cotton ball or pad. You should see improvement almost immediately.

Foot and Leg Refresher

HEALTHFUL HINT

When you've been standing up all day or walking farther than you're used to, a gentle gel can give your muscles a refreshing treat. To make it, mix ½ cup of aloe vera gel, 1 tablespoon of witch hazel, and 1½ teaspoons of cornstarch in a microwave-safe container. Nuke it on high for 1 to 2 minutes, stirring every 30 seconds, until the mixture is about the consistency of honey. Let it cool, stir in 3 or 4 drops of peppermint extract, and store the gel at room temperature in an airtight container. Smooth it on your tired, aching feet and legs, wait 10 to 15 minutes, then rinse with warm water. Believe it or not, you'll feel like running a marathon! (Or at least walking to the mailbox.)

SORE, STRAINED EYES. Soak two small cotton pads in witch hazel, and put one over each closed eye. Lie back and relax for 10 minutes or so.

✔ Say "No!" to Nosebleeds

Almost everybody gets a nosebleed from time to time. So make like a Boy Scout and be prepared with this classic remedy: Mix 6 drops of cypress essential oil (available in health-food stores) per 2 tablespoons of witch hazel in a bottle, and stash it in the medicine chest. Then whenever the need arises, shake the bottle well, moisten a cotton ball with the potion, and gently insert it into the bleeding nostril. Sit up straight, with your head tilted just slightly forward. Within two or three minutes, the blood should stop flowing. **Note:** To speed up the process, squeeze the soft tissue of your nose firmly, but gently, between your thumb and forefinger.

✔ Keep Bugs at Bay

Here's an insect repellent that will fend off bad bugs like mosquitoes, as well as tiny no-see-'em nuisances. Plus, it contains none of the harsh chemicals found in most commercial products and smells a lot better to boot! To make it, follow this simple four-step procedure:

POTENT POTION

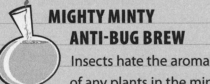

MIGHTY MINTY ANTI-BUG BREW

Insects hate the aroma of any plants in the mint family. So whip up a batch of this excellent elixir, and spritz it on your skin and clothing whenever you head outdoors.

1½ tbsp. of peppermint leaves*
1½ tbsp. of spearmint leaves*
1 tbsp. of dried or fresh lavender
1 cup of distilled water, boiling hot
1 cup of witch hazel

Put the herbs in a heat-proof container, and pour the boiling water over them. Mix well, and cover the top. Let the mixture steep until it has cooled to room temperature, then strain out the solids. Add the witch hazel, and pour the solution into two 8-ounce spray bottles or three or four pocket-size versions. Store them in the refrigerator, and put them to use all summer long.

* Either dried or fresh, chopped.

YIELD: ABOUT 16 OUNCES

STEP 1. Round up witch hazel, distilled or boiled water, your choice of essential oils (see the list in Step 4 for suggestions), vegetable glycerin (optional), and an 8-ounce spray bottle.

STEP 2. Fill the bottle halfway with the water, and pour in enough witch hazel to reach almost to the top.

STEP 3. Add ½ teaspoon of vegetable glycerin if desired. (It will help the spray cling longer to your skin.)

STEP 4. Mix in 30 to 50 drops of essential oils. (The more oil you use, the more potent the repelling action will be.) Citronella, clove, eucalyptus, lavender, and rosemary are all good bug-chasing choices, either alone or in any combination that strikes your fancy.

All-American Beauty

✤ Spray Foot Odor Away

Bothered by smelly feet? If so, here's a simple deodorizing solution: Mix 40 drops of geranium essential oil and 20 drops of peppermint essential oil with 1 cup of witch hazel. Pour the mixture into a spray bottle, and shake it well before each use. Then first thing each morning, spritz your feet, and let them dry thoroughly before you put on your socks and shoes. Repeat the procedure when you get home from work (or play) and again at bedtime. Your tootsies are guaranteed to stay odor-free!

✤ Chill Out

When the weather turns steamy, keep your cool by misting your skin with this elixir: Mix 2 teaspoons of witch hazel, 10 drops of peppermint essential oil, and 12 drops of lavender essential oil in an 8-ounce spray bottle, and fill the balance of the bottle with water. Keep it in the refrigerator, and reach for it anytime you feel too darn hot.

✤ Lovely Liquid Chlorophyll

When used on its own, liquid chlorophyll makes a highly effective deodorant. But it'll also give a major power boost to any DIY formula. To make it, loosely pack a large glass canning jar with chopped, washed grass clippings, and pour in enough witch hazel to cover them completely. Close the jar and set it in a cool, dark place for 7 to 10 days, shaking it every now and then. When the time's up, strain out the grass, and pour the liquid into a clean bottle with a tight-fitting cap. To use the chlorophyll, dab it onto your underarms with a cotton ball, or measure out whatever amount you need for a deodorant recipe. **Note:** Only use grass clippings that have not been treated with herbicides, pesticides, or chemical fertilizers.

✤ Ahhh! Aftershave

Commercial aftershave lotions are chock-full of alcohol and all kinds of chemicals. As a result, instead of relieving the burning and irritation on your freshly shaved skin, they can actually make it worse. So do your face a favor and switch to my favorite feel-good formula: Mix ½ cup of distilled water, ¼ cup of alcohol-free witch hazel, 1 tablespoon of olive oil,

POTENT POTION

SUPER SPRAY DEODORANT

The aluminum that's used in commercial antiperspirants can leave hard-to-remove stains on your clothing, but this formula will eliminate your laundry-day challenges. Plus, it contains none of the unpronounceable chemicals found in both brand-name and generic products.

½ cup of witch hazel
¼ cup of aloe vera gel or juice
¼ tsp. of baking soda
10 drops of clary sage essential oil*

Combine all of the ingredients in a spray bottle. Shake it before each use, and spritz the deodorant on your underarms, as you would any other antiperspirant.

* If you are pregnant or think you might be pregnant, substitute either lavender oil or liquid chlorophyll. (It's available in health-food stores and online from sites that specialize in herbal products or essential oils. Or you can make your own using the simple formula above.)

YIELD: 6 OUNCES

and ¼ cup each of dried cedar and dried sage in a glass jar. Cover it, and set it in a cool, dark place for two to three weeks, shaking it once or twice a day. Then strain out the herbs, and pour the liquid into a clean bottle with a tight-fitting cap. Use it as you would any other after-shave for a refreshing finish to your shaving routine.

✤ Amazing Face Firmer

Although this skin pleaser dates back to the 1600s, it's more popular today than ever before. And that's no wonder because it's cheap, easy to make, and works like a dream to smooth and firm any type of skin. The simple procedure: Mix 3 table-spoons of alcohol-free witch hazel and 1 teaspoon of raw apple cider vinegar in a bowl, then lightly beat in one egg white. Whip the mixture until it's foamy, and pop it into the refrigerator for five minutes or so. Apply the mixture to your warm, moist skin using a cotton pad. Leave it on for at least 30 minutes (the longer, the better). For best results, repeat the procedure at least once a week.

✤ Stop the Problem-Skin Merry-Go-Round

When you're battling acne and similar skin problems, it may seem logical to use commercial astringents. But these products dry out your skin, making it produce more oil. So then you use more astringent, and

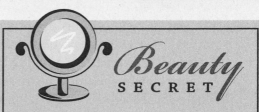

Beauty S E C R E T

TONE DOWN THE SHINE

Summer's heat and humidity can leave any type of skin looking shiny and oily. But instead of buying commercial de-shining products (most of which dry out your skin even more), mix ⅓ cup of witch hazel with 1 cup of rose water and 1 cup of spring water, and store the solution in the re-frigerator. (It'll keep for up to two weeks in a glass jar with a tight-fitting lid.) Then each morning and evening—or anytime in between—gently wipe the potion onto your face and neck using a cotton pad. It will reduce any shine while keeping your skin healthy and moisturized. **Note:** *You can buy rose water in health-food and herbal-product stores, as well as online. But it's a snap (and cheaper) to make your own. For the easy procedure, see "Grandma Knew Best" on page 182.*

you start a vicious circle of no-win action. Fortunately, there is a gentle, natural alternative that will fight the bacteria without upping your oil production. Just mix 1 cup of witch hazel, ½ teaspoon of tea tree extract, and ½ cup of strong chamomile infusion (see Tea Times Two on page 99) in a bottle with a tight-fitting cap, and store it at room temperature for up to nine months. Use it each morning and evening to keep your skin clear and soft. **Note:** This potion also makes an excellent everyday toner for oily skin that's problem-free.

✢ Two Terrific Toners

Store-bought toners are generally alcohol based, and some even contain acetone—the key ingredient in nail polish removers. Do you really want to use that stuff on your face? I don't think so! Instead, depending on your skin type, opt for one of these complexion-friendly formulas that get the job done, naturally:

NORMAL SKIN. Ingredients: ½ cup each of witch hazel, water, and peppermint infusion (see Tea Times Two on page 99).

POTENT POTION

ENERGIZING BATH OIL

There are plenty of bath oil blends that will relax your muscles or lull you into a good night's sleep. This one, however, is especially formulated to rev up your energy!

Mix all of the ingredients in a bottle that has a tight-fitting cap. At bath time, fill the tub with warm water, and pour in 1 tablespoon of the mixture. Stir the water vigorously with your hand to disperse the oils. Then settle in, and feel your get-up-and-go power soar!

½ cup of witch hazel
20 drops of lavender essential oil
8 drops of peppermint essential oil*
8 drops of rosemary essential oil*
4 drops of basil essential oil

If you are pregnant or think that you might be pregnant, substitute juniper berry, lime, patchouli, or rosewood oil.

YIELD: ENOUGH FOR 8 BATHS

DRY AND MATURE SKIN. Ingredients: ½ cup each of witch hazel and water and 4 tablespoons each of aloe vera gel, rose water, and glycerin.

To make either type, mix the ingredients in a bottle that has a tight-fitting cap. Store the container at room temperature, shaking it occasionally and before each use. Apply the toner to your face and neck with a cotton ball or pad. It will keep well for 8 to 10 months—and your face will thank you!

Best of the Rest

★ Keep Help on Ice

You never know when you might need to use ice to ease pain, swelling, or irritation. So be prepared by keeping a reusable, all-purpose ice pack on hand. To make it, mix 1 part rubbing alcohol with 2 parts water, and pour the solution into a heavy-duty ziplock freezer bag (but don't fill it; leave room for expansion). Squeeze out all of the air, seal the bag, and put it in the freezer. Alcohol doesn't freeze, so the contents will be slushy rather than rock hard—and all the more comfortable on any part of your achin' body.

★ Mouthing Off

Antiseptic mouthwash is good for more than just freshening your breath and keeping your gums healthy. Reach for it whenever any of these common problems arises:

BLISTERS. Moisten a cotton ball with antiseptic mouthwash, and dab it onto your blisters three times a day until the blasted things dry out.

CUTS AND SCRAPES. After you clean a wound, pour some antiseptic mouthwash over it. It kills germs on your skin just as well as it does in your mouth.

MOSQUITO BITES. Moisten a cotton pad or paper towel with antiseptic mouthwash, hold it on the bite for about 15 seconds, and you'll kiss the itch good-bye.

SCALP IRRITATION. If your head is itchy and irritated from eczema or contact dermatitis, use antiseptic mouthwash as an after-shampoo rinse. Massage it into your scalp, then rinse thoroughly with clear water.

★ Let's Ear It for Alcohol

Attention, frequent (or even occasional) swimmers! The next time you're plagued by that annoying—and often painful—condition called swimmer's ear, mix equal parts rubbing alcohol and vinegar (either the white or apple cider kind). Dribble 2 or 3 drops of the solution into your afflicted ear. The alcohol will help dry up the trapped water, and the vinegar will kill any bacteria that may be present.

To prevent the problem, take along an eyedropper and a small bottle of the mixture anytime you head off for a dip in a lake or any other body of non-chlorinated water. As soon as you're through swimming for the day, dry your ears well, and put 2 drops of the solution into each ear. It'll stop bad bacteria dead in their tracks.

> ## CAUTION ⚠️
>
> Once upon a time, hydrogen peroxide was considered the be-all and end-all for cleaning wounds. But no more. In fact, medical science now tells us that applying hydrogen peroxide to cuts, scrapes, and sores actually does more harm than good because it damages healthy tissue surrounding the wound and delays the healing process. The same goes for rubbing alcohol. Although it is excellent for sterilizing instruments (like scissors or tweezers), you should keep it away from open wounds.
>
> The best way to clean an "owie" is to wash the site thoroughly with soap and water. Then follow up with an antibiotic ointment or one of the homemade healers found throughout this book.

★ Waxing and Waning

Swimmer's ear isn't the only annoying ailment that can afflict our hearing apparatus. For those of a certain age, wax tends to build up in our ears. Not only does it interfere with our ability to hear, but it can also be quite painful. One easy remedy: Squirt 3 or 4 drops of 3% hydrogen peroxide into each ear. Leave it there for four minutes or so, then flush it and the wax out with warm water. If some wax remains, repeat the process. **Note:** If the wax has hardened so much that it's blocking your ear canal, have your doctor clear it out.

★ Dodge Blisters

It doesn't take much time for a pair of tight shoes to cause painful blisters. So what do you do if the new shoes you bought for a can't-miss event are too tight? Try this old-time solution: Saturate a cotton ball with rubbing alcohol, and rub it on the inside of each shoe at the tight spots. Then head off to the big do. The next day, get permanent relief by taking that footgear to a cobbler for professional stretching.

★ Prevent Athlete's Foot . . .

And toenail fungus, too. How? After every shower, soak a cotton ball with antiseptic mouthwash, and swab the bottoms of your feet, the spaces between your toes, and the skin around your toenails. (This is especially important when you're using the locker-room facilities at a gym, swimming pool, or health club.) **Note:** This trick only works with traditional mouthwashes that have a high alcohol content.

★ Hair's to Mouthwash

This oral-care staple can also work wonders for your hair in a couple of ways, namely these:

PREVENT DANDRUFF. Simply wash your hair with antiseptic mouthwash every two weeks or so, and you'll bid your white-flake woes good-bye.

MAKE YOUR HAIR SHINE. Mix ¼ cup of your favorite mouthwash (any kind will do) with 1 cup of water. After shampooing as usual, pour the mixture through your hair. Massage it in for a minute or two, and then rinse with clear water. The result: lusciously luminous locks.

★ BO Stopper

If you're looking for an aluminum-free deodorant, try this refreshing formula: Simply swab your armpits with a cotton ball soaked in mouthwash (choose your favorite scent). Give it a minute or so to dry before you get dressed. One word of caution: Wait at least a day before using this remedy if you've recently shaved.

Forget the Flu

HEALTHFUL HINT

This cold- and flu-evasion technique may sound kooky, but folks who've tried it swear it's kept them fit as fiddles even during the fiercest flu seasons. The simple routine: The minute you feel the first sign of symptoms, use a small eyedropper to insert 4 or 5 drops of 3% hydrogen peroxide into one ear. (It may sting a little, but don't worry—that's normal.) Wait until the bubbling and stinging subside, which may be anywhere from 3 to 10 minutes. Then drain the solution onto a tissue, and repeat the procedure with the other ear. It works because, as medical scientists first discovered in the late 1920s, the viruses that cause colds and flu can enter your body through your ear canal. As long as you've acted quickly enough, you should be able to kill the germs before they get a toe-, er, ear-hold. But remember, it's still important to wash your hands frequently during flu season, and steer clear of anyone who's coughing and sneezing.

★ Highlight Your Hair

For generations, women have been using hydrogen peroxide to put lustrous highlights in their hair, and for several good reasons. First and foremost, it works like a charm. Unlike commercial products, it has no harsh chemicals that can irritate your scalp, which, over time, make your hair dull, drab, and feeling like steel wool. Plus, it costs a tiny fraction of the price you pay at beauty salons. And it couldn't be simpler to use: Just mix equal parts of 3% hydrogen peroxide and water in a spray bottle, and spritz the solution onto your damp hair. Comb it through, and leave it on for 10 to 15 minutes. Then shampoo and condition your hair as usual. **Note:** Hydrogen peroxide stronger than 3% can bleach your hair, so read the label carefully.

★ Lip Service

If you're troubled (and embarrassed) by dark hair on your upper lip, fret no more. Just try this simple vanishing act: Mix ¼ cup of 6% hydrogen

---

POTENT POTION

FABULOUS FACIAL MIST

A quick spritz of facial mist can give your whole body a cooling pickup when you're on the go. Plus, it hydrates your skin and enhances its color. Try this DIY version and see for yourself!

1 black-tea bag
2 cups of water
¼ cup of hydrogen peroxide*
1 tsp. of lime extract

Steep the tea bag in 1 cup of just-boiled water for 60 minutes. Let the tea cool to room temperature, then mix ¼ cup of the brew with the hydrogen peroxide, lime extract, and 1 cup of water. Pour the solution into pocket-size spray bottles. Take one wherever you go, and give your face a quick spritz—even on top of your makeup—whenever you need an energy boost. (Just be careful not to get it in your eyes.) Store the other bottles in the refrigerator for up to a week.

* Use 2.5% or less.

YIELD: 12 OUNCES

peroxide with 1 teaspoon of ammonia (no more!). Dip a cotton ball into the solution, and dab it onto the hair. Let it sit for 30 minutes, then rinse it off with cool water. End of problem!

★ Whiten Your Nails

Wearing nail polish for long periods of time can make your nails dull, drab, and dark. To brighten them up, make a paste by mixing 1 tablespoon of hydrogen peroxide and 2 tablespoons of baking soda. Rub it generously onto your fingernails and/or toenails, and leave it on for five minutes or so. Rinse with clear water, and bingo—bright, shiny nails!

★ Whiten Your Teeth, Too!

Forget whitening strips, uncomfortable trays, and expensive trips to the dentist. Simply use 3% hydrogen peroxide instead of your current mouthwash. It will not only kill the germs that cause bad breath, but also make your teeth whiter and brighter. **Note:** Whatever you do, don't swallow any of the peroxide. When you're done swishing it around, spit it out and rinse your mouth thoroughly with clear water.

★ No More Zits

Everybody's been there at least once: On the morning of a big event, you wake up with an ugly pimple. No worries! Just use a cotton swab to dab a little hydrogen peroxide on the blemish. It should be gone by the time you get where you need to go. If not, at least it will be far less noticeable.

Beauty S E C R E T

NO SWEAT!

*Here's a take-along spritzer that'll leave you feeling cool, clean, and dry whenever you're working or playing outdoors in the summertime. Mix 1 teaspoon of hydrogen peroxide (2.5% or less), 1 teaspoon of cucumber juice, and 1 teaspoon of lemon extract in 1 cup of water. Pour the mixture into one 8-ounce or two 4-ounce spray bottles, and shake each one for 10 seconds or so. Spray the potion onto your face and body periodically to keep yourself calm. (Just don't get it in your eyes.) In between uses, store the potion in the refrigerator for up to four days. **Note:** To make cucumber juice, puree a cucumber in a blender, and strain the pulp through cheesecloth for 15 minutes.*

25

Yogurt

Remember those old TV commercials featuring cavorting Russian peasants who claimed that they owed their century-plus life spans to heaping helpings of yogurt? Well, it turns out they weren't so far off the mark. While eating yogurt may not guarantee that you'll live well into your hundreds, study after study has shown that a serving or two of yogurt a day can boost your immune system, help fend off colds and allergies, lift your spirits, lower bad cholesterol levels—and the list goes on. Of course, whether you eat yogurt or smooth it onto your skin, it can also help you keep your youthful looks a whole lot longer.

The Tangy Taste of Health

✔ Keep Colds at Bay . . .

And hay fever, too. Studies have shown that folks who eat as little as 6 ounces of yogurt a day sail right through the cold and allergy seasons. For best results, though, you need to begin your prevention plan before the viruses start circulating and the pollen flies, and keep at it all the way through the peak season.

✔ Save the Good Guys

Anyone who's ever taken antibiotics knows that these meds can deliver side effects in the form of diarrhea, an upset stomach, or a yeast infection. The simple solution: Eat ½ to 1 cup of yogurt about two hours before or after taking each dose of your medication. Then, after you finish your prescription, eat 1 cup of yogurt each day for two to four weeks. This way, you'll restock your body with a full load of the bacteria that are essential for good health.

✔ Yo, Fight the Fungus!

The active cultures in yogurt make a terrific topical treatment for these two common fungal infections:

ATHLETE'S FOOT. Rub plain yogurt directly onto the affected skin. For good measure, eat a cup or two of yogurt each day until the pain and itch are gone.

NAIL FUNGUS. Coat the infected nail with a generous layer of plain yogurt, cover it with a piece of gauze or bandage, and let it soak in overnight. Come morning, rinse off any residue. Repeat the procedure each night until your fungus has flown the coop. **Note:** If you're treating several nails, put on cotton socks or gloves before you hit the sack.

✔ Defeat Canker Sores

Got a painful canker sore? Reach for (you guessed it) yogurt. Eat at least 8 ounces of plain yogurt each day until the painful ulcer is gone. For extra healing power, swirl the dairy dynamo around in your mouth before swallowing it. This way, it'll coat your gums, tongue, throat, and the roof of your mouth with beneficial bacteria, which will kill the bad bacteria that may be causing your dilemma—or at least contributing to it.

After that, to prevent future outbreaks, eat at least 4 tablespoons of plain yogurt each day. **Note:** If you don't care for the taste of plain yogurt,

---

Live and Active

HEALTHFUL HINT

The magic bullets that give yogurt its remarkable healing (and beautifying) power are living organisms with the tongue-twisting names of *Lactobacillus bulgaricus* and *Streptococcus thermophilus*. This duo converts pasteurized milk to yogurt during the fermentation process. Unfortunately, after fermentation, some brands of yogurt undergo a heat treatment, which kills off most of the beneficial cultures. So how do you know you're getting the real thing? It's simple. Whether you're shopping for plain or flavored yogurt, frozen or refrigerated, make sure the carton sports the *Live & Active Cultures* seal bestowed by the National Yogurt Association (NYA). It guarantees that the product contains a full load of these beneficial bugs.

mix it with a teaspoon or so of raw honey, or use it in a recipe like the Triple-Delight Smoothie (below).

✔ Slather Away Your Sunburn

When too much time in the sun leaves your skin red and sore, grab the coldest container of plain yogurt that you can lay your hands on—preferably the whole-milk kind. Stir in 1 to 2 teaspoons of aloe vera gel, and slather the mixture generously onto the burned area(s). Leave it on for 15 to 20 minutes, or until it dries. Then *gently* wipe it off with a soft, damp cloth. If your pain persists, repeat the procedure as many times as necessary. When your skin is sore no more, step into the shower and rinse any residue off with tepid water. And next time, remember to use sunscreen!

✔ Relieve Sunburn Another Way

If slathering isn't your style, and the burn covers a fairly small area, try this neater remedy: Make the yogurt-aloe vera mixture as described above, spread it on a piece of cheesecloth, and lay it on your affected skin. When the compress warms up, replace it with a fresh, cool one. Continue this routine until you feel relief, and then gently rinse off any remaining salve with cool water.

✔ Arthritis-Relief Remedy

If you suffer from arthritis, treat your stiff, aching joints to this potent, penetrating, and pain-soothing cream. Here's how to make it:

STEP 1. Round up ½ cup of wheat germ oil, 1 ounce of beeswax, ¼ cup of plain yogurt, four 400 IU vitamin E capsules, and 10 drops of bay leaf es-

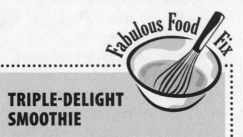

Fabulous Food Fix

TRIPLE-DELIGHT SMOOTHIE

Whether your aim is to heal a canker sore, ramp up your immune system, dodge the side effects of antibiotics—or simply enjoy a delicious, healthy drink—this bracing beverage can't be beat.

2 cups of frozen mixed berries*
2 cups of plain yogurt
3 tbsp. of raw honey

Put all of the ingredients in a blender and hit the high-speed button. When you've got a rich, smooth consistency, pour the cocktail into a glass and drink to your good health!

* Or substitute another fruit, such as frozen bananas or fresh mango or apple slices.

YIELD: 2 SERVINGS

sential oil. You'll also need a double boiler, a blender, and a glass jar with a tight-fitting lid.

STEP 2. Heat the wheat germ oil and beeswax in the top of a double boiler until the wax melts, but the mixture is cool enough to touch. (Don't let it get too hot, or you'll damage the healing compounds in the oil.)

STEP 3. Put the yogurt and vitamin E oil (squeezed from the capsules) in the blender, and turn it on its lowest setting. With the motor running, slowly pour in the warm wax and oil mixture, and add the bay leaf oil. Continue blending until you've got a smooth cream.

STEP 4. Pour the cream into the jar, and let it cool to room temperature before putting the lid on. Store it in the refrigerator, where it will keep for about 30 days.

Once a day, or more often as needed, rub the cream into your afflicted joints and feel the pain float away!

✔ Take It Easy!

You say you've got a speech to make, and you're so nervous that you'll surely blow it? Or maybe an upcoming job interview has butterflies performing acrobatics in your stomach. No matter what's given you a case of the jitters, here's good news: With a slight tweak, the same topical treatment that eases joint pain

---

POTENT POTION

WINTER WONDER CREAM

In the winter, your skin can turn as itchy as the dickens in no time flat—thanks to the moisture-draining duo of cold, dry air outside and warm, dry air inside. But this remarkable remedy will keep your body's "outer wrapper" hydrated and itch-free all season long.

8 oz. of plain yogurt
¼ cup of raw honey
2 tsp. of bee pollen powder*
2 tsp. of lemon juice
1 tsp. of hot-pepper sauce (any kind)

Mix all of the ingredients in a blender or food processor. Pour the mixture into a container with a tight-fitting lid, and store it in the refrigerator, where it will keep until the expiration date on the yogurt container. To use the cream, gently rub it onto any dry, itchy patches as needed, and let your skin absorb its soothing goodness.

* Available in health-food stores and online.

YIELD: ABOUT 10 OUNCES

can soothe your frazzled nerves. Just make and store the cream according to the directions in "Arthritis-Relief Remedy" (see page 348), but substitute juniper essential oil for the bay leaf oil. Several times a day, rub the cream onto your hands (yes, you read that right). The juniper's calming properties will penetrate your skin, making you feel relaxed and ready for action!

Tart and Lovely

❖ Put the Brakes on Bad Breath

If you have chronic halitosis (rather than the temporary kind that comes from a thick slice of onion on your burger), yogurt may help sweeten the air. That's because it can polish off the nasty bacteria in your digestive system that frequently cause bad breath. So start eating a serving or two of yogurt each day. **Note:** If your breath isn't beginning to freshen up after a couple of weeks, see your doctor to rule out any underlying medical condition.

❖ Ditch Dandruff

Flake-removal methods don't come any simpler than this one: After washing your hair, massage 1 cup of plain yogurt onto your scalp. Give it 15 minutes or so to penetrate your skin, and then rinse thoroughly. Repeat the procedure daily, and within a week your dandruff should disappear. After that, use this treatment every couple of weeks, or as often as needed to keep the white stuff at bay.

❖ Restore the Luster

Styling products and air pollution can sap moisture from your hair and leave a residue that dulls its shine. To make it gleam again, simply massage ½ cup of plain yogurt into your damp hair, and leave it on for 20 minutes. Rinse it off with warm water, then with cool

CAUTION !

When an all-natural food gains the kind of superstar status that yogurt has, it only stands to reason that manufacturers would co-opt its healthy image to market their own products. But don't be fooled by things like yogurt-based salad dressings or yogurt-coated pretzels, candies, and cookies—or cosmetic creams and lotions that pitch yogurt as a key ingredient. They contain no live and active cultures whatsoever. So go ahead and eat 'em or rub them onto your body if you want to, but don't expect to snag any of yogurt's health or beauty benefits!

water. Follow up with your normal shampoo and conditioner. Perform this routine every other week to keep the lights in your locks.

✤ Rev Up the Color

Yogurt can help make your tresses' tones richer and more radiant. How you need to use it depends on your natural hair color.

FOR BRUNETTES. Mix ½ cup of plain yogurt, ½ cup of cocoa powder, 1 teaspoon of honey, and 1 teaspoon of apple cider vinegar to form a smooth paste. Apply the mixture to your freshly shampooed hair, and leave it on for two to three minutes. Then rinse and style as usual.

FOR REDHEADS. In a blender or food processor, mix 3 tablespoons of plain yogurt, 2 tablespoons of honey, and three medium-size chopped carrots (or ½ cup of cranberries if you want copper undertones) to get a coarse paste. After shampooing, work the mixture through your hair. Leave it on for one to two minutes, and then rinse it out. Follow up with your usual styling routine.

✤ Intensive Conditioning Treatment

Dry, damaged hair all but cries out for this rich and robust healer: Beat ½ cup of plain whole-milk yogurt, ½ cup of full-fat mayonnaise, and 1 egg white in a bowl. Slather it onto your head, and thoroughly coat all of your hair strands, concentrating on the ends. Put on a shower cap, and

---

POTENT POTION

HAIR-GROWTH TONIC

It happens to most women at least once: You impulsively opt for a new short, perky hairstyle, only to find that it doesn't suit you at all. Well, don't fret. Your hair will grow back to a more flattering length, and this formula can help speed up the process.

1½ tbsp. of plain yogurt
1½ tbsp. of raw organic honey
1 tbsp. of coconut oil
1 tsp. of extra virgin olive oil

Mix all of the ingredients together. Gently brush your hair, then apply the mixture to your scalp, and work it through to your hair tips. Put on a shower cap, or cover your head with a plastic bag, and keep it on for at least 60 minutes—the longer, the better! Then wash and condition your hair as usual. Repeat the procedure once a week or so until you're happy with the length of your locks.

tuck tissues or cotton balls around the edges to catch the drips. Leave it on for 30 minutes or so. Rinse thoroughly with cool to lukewarm water. (Don't use hot water, or you'll wind up with a head full of scrambled eggs!) You can follow up with a shampoo, or just dry and style your hair as usual.

✤ Nourishing Facial Scrub

To deep-cleanse, soften, and rejuvenate dry skin, use this gentle formula once a week. Here's all you need to do: Mix 6 ounces of plain whole-milk yogurt, ¼ cup of ground uncooked oatmeal (use a coffee grinder or food processor), 2 teaspoons of raw honey, and 1 teaspoon of lemon or orange juice in a bowl. Massage the mixture onto your freshly washed face and neck using small circular motions. Let it dry, then rinse it off with warm water. Pat your skin dry, and follow up with your normal moisturizer.

✤ Anti-Acne Cleanser

Are you (or your resident teenagers) waging an ongoing war against acne? If so, then make this treatment a part of your daily cleansing routine: Mix 4 tablespoons of plain whole-milk yogurt with 4 tablespoons of freshly squeezed lemon juice. Spread a thin layer of the mixture on the affected areas, leave it on for about five minutes, and then rinse with lukewarm

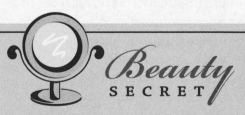

DEEP-CLEANING ALL-OVER SCRUB

*T*his mighty mixture is a powerful, but oh-so-gentle, facial cleanser, especially good for blemished or irritated skin. But even the parts of your body that are not facing a daily assault of airborne dirt and pollutants benefit from a periodic "house" cleaning. So once every week or two, mix 2 tablespoons of plain yogurt, 1 tablespoon of un-cooked oatmeal, and 1 tablespoon of cornmeal in an unbreakable container. Let the mixture warm up to room temperature, then step into the shower and massage the scrub onto your skin using circular motions. Rinse it off, towel yourself dry, and apply your favorite moisturizing lotion.

Beauty SECRET

water. The lemon juice helps remove excess oil from your skin, and the lactic acid in yogurt prevents breakouts. Between uses, store the cleanser in a covered container in the refrigerator.

✤ Less Stress = Better Looks...

And, of course, better health, too! Believe it or not, an ultra-simple facial mask can actually help lower your stress level. Here's how to make it happen: Mix 2 parts plain whole-milk yogurt with 1 part honey, and spread the mixture over your face. Then lean back and relax for 15 minutes or so. Rinse the combo off with warm water, and enjoy the results: calmer spirits and softer skin!

✤ Be a Masked Woman

Yogurt-based facial masks can work wonders for any type of skin. Here's a trio of fine examples:

MOISTURIZE DRY SKIN. Mix 2 tablespoons of plain whole-milk yogurt, 1 tablespoon of raw honey, and 1 to 2 tablespoons of cooked and cooled oatmeal to form a smooth paste.

EXFOLIATE OILY SKIN. Using a fork, mash four clean, ripe strawberries in a bowl, and stir in 1 teaspoon of plain low-fat yogurt.

SOOTHE IRRITATED SKIN. Puree ½ cup of plain whole-milk yogurt, 2 tablespoons of aloe vera gel, 1 tablespoon of raw honey, half a chopped cucumber, and 3 drops of chamomile essential oil in a blender.

In each case, spread the mixture over your freshly washed face, and leave it on for 10 to 15 minutes. Rinse the mask off with lukewarm water, pat dry, and apply your favorite moisturizer.

Fabulous Food Fix

CURRIED YOGURT DIP

You don't have to slather yogurt onto your face to make your skin softer, smoother, and younger looking. The powerful probiotics work their magic just as well from the inside. Here's one delicious and ultra-simple way to start the process.

1 cup of plain yogurt
1 medium-size tomato, diced
1 scallion, thinly sliced
1 tsp. of curry powder
1 tsp. of lemon juice
¼ tsp. of prepared horseradish

Mix all of the ingredients in a blender or food processor, and pour the dip into a bowl. Serve it with raw veggies, crackers, or Melba toast rounds, or as a terrific topping for steamed vegetables or baked potatoes.

YIELD: ABOUT 1 CUP

❖ Hold Back the Years: A Solo Performance

All by itself (thanks to its potent load of lactic acid), yogurt can delay or reduce signs of aging such as fine lines, wrinkles, and age spots. It will also dissolve dead skin cells that clog your pores and make your complexion look dull. Plus, it closes large pores and gives your skin a younger appearance. To turn on this fountain of youth, apply a thick layer of plain whole-milk yogurt to your face, leave it on for 20 minutes or so, and rinse it off with lukewarm water. Repeat the process at least once a week—more often if you have the time. With this treatment, you can never have too much of a good thing!

Best of the Rest

★ Egg-zactly the Ticket for Sunburn Relief!

When the weather turns hot, make up a supply of these comforting sticks, and keep them on hand to supply instant relief whenever sunburn strikes. Here's the simple three-step procedure:

STEP 1. In a small bowl, beat an egg until it's frothy. Then slowly whisk in ½ cup of warm (but not hot) coconut oil and 1 tablespoon of raw honey until the mixture is the consistency of mayonnaise.

STEP 2. Set an empty toilet paper roll on end in another bowl, spoon the blend into the tube, and set it (still in the bowl) in the freezer until it's frozen solid.

STEP 3. When it's skin-soothing time, peel away the top ¼ inch of the cardboard, and gently rub the top of the frozen stick over the burned area. Wait 5 to 10 minutes, and rinse with cool water. Repeat as needed until you've banished the burn.

Between uses, cover the cream stick with plastic wrap, and keep it frozen. It will last indefinitely. By the way, this handy tool works just as well on minor kitchen burns, and it makes an egg-cellent skin-softening treatment.

★ A Milky Way to Ease Eczema Agony

When a flare-up strikes, help is as close as your refrigerator. Just mix cold whole milk in a bowl with an equal amount of water, and saturate a gauze pad or soft cotton cloth with the solution. Hold it on the affected area for about three minutes. Perform this procedure two to four more times in quick succession. Then repeat as needed throughout the day. Just be sure to rinse your skin with cool water after each treatment—otherwise, before you know it, you'll smell like sour milk!

★ Dismiss Psoriasis

You can find major psoriasis relief in your fridge—from buttermilk. Here's your trio of options:

■ Pour 2 to 4 cups of buttermilk into a tub of warm water, and soak for 20 minutes. Gently pat your skin dry, and smooth on a rich, natural moisturizing lotion.

■ If you prefer showers to baths, fill a clean plastic squirt bottle with buttermilk, and use it as a body wash. Again, follow up with an intensive-care moisturizer.

■ To treat psoriasis on your scalp or a small area of your body, saturate a soft all-cotton cloth with buttermilk, apply it directly to the site, and hold it there until the pain and itch subside.

In each case, repeat the process as needed. Also, start drinking more buttermilk. There is no specific dose (at least not yet), but studies do show that it seems to relieve psoriasis pain. **Note:** If what you think is a psoriasis patch suddenly appears, and you have not been diagnosed with the disease, see your doctor immediately. It could be a more serious, look-alike condition.

★ Give a Boil Some Skin

Got a boil that's driving you nuts? Try this old-time remedy: Remove the shell from a hard-boiled egg, and then gently peel off the delicate skin that's

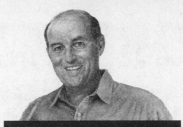

YOU DON'T SAY!

Historians reckon that people started drinking milk about 10,000 years ago, when animals were first domesticated. Records show that the British were milking cows at least 6,000 years ago, and they brought cattle to our shores in the 1600s. To say that milk drinking has become a Yankee institution is putting it mildly. Surveys show that if you open the refrigerator in 96 percent of American households, you'll find a carton of milk. Twenty states have designated milk as their official beverage (or, as some of them call it, their official state drink). And here's an amazing fun fact for you: The United States is the only country in the world where cow's milk is the most popular kind. Elsewhere, dairy fans favor the offerings of other critters, including goats, donkeys, reindeer, sheep, yaks, and water buffalo.

POTENT POTION

DE-STRESSING BATH BLEND

Scientific studies have proven that stress can put you at high risk for just about every ailment under the sun, and make you accident-prone to boot. So make up a big batch of this calming blend, and use it every time you feel your stress level rising.

4 cups of dry whole-milk powder
2 cups of cornstarch
4–5 drops of your favorite essential oil*

Mix all of the ingredients in a blender or food processor. When it's time to unwind, add ½ cup of the mixture to hot bathwater, sink into the tub, and relax. Store the remaining blend in an airtight container at room temperature.

* Geranium, jasmine, lavender, orange, and vanilla are all good stress-busting choices.

YIELD: 12 BATHS

left on the egg. Wet it, and lay it over the boil. It should draw out the pus and reduce the inflammation pronto. **Note:** If the pain gets steadily worse, or you see a red streak in the boil, get medical help immediately!

★ Halt a Hangover

Before you take off for a cocktail party or an after-work happy hour, mix a pinch of nutmeg in a glass of milk, and sip it slowly. It should coat the lining of your stomach, slowing the absorption of alcohol into your system, thereby helping to lessen the damage if you have one drink too many. **Note:** This trick will only help ease morning-after miseries. It will do nothing to alleviate the effects of alcohol on your reflexes or your mental processes.

★ Butter Up!

Dry-skin treatments don't come any simpler, or more effective, than this one: Just mix 1 teaspoon of soft, unsalted butter with 1 teaspoon of warm water. Rub the mixture thoroughly into all the dry areas of your face. Leave it on for 15 to 20 minutes, and then rinse it off with cold water.

★ Be a Sour Puss

Sour cream may not be so great for your diet, but it can perform miracles for your face. Here it plays a leading role in a mask that exfoliates, brightens, and moisturizes your skin, and also refines your pores, heals any irritation, prevents breakouts, and fades acne scars. (WOW!) The simple formula: Mix 2 tablespoons of sour cream, 2 tablespoons of raw honey, and 1 tablespoon of either unfiltered apple cider vinegar or fresh-squeezed lemon juice. Spread the mixture onto your freshly washed face, and leave it on for 20 minutes. Rinse with tepid water, then cool (not cold) water. Perform this procedure twice a week to keep your skin looking like a million bucks!

★ Hand It to Buttermilk

Your face isn't the only part of your body that can benefit from a leave-on "mask." The next time your hands could use a little TLC, treat them to this nourishing routine: Mix ¼ cup of buttermilk and ½ cup of dry milk to form a smooth paste. Using a small, soft paintbrush or pastry brush, spread an even layer of the mixture onto each hand. Leave it on for 15 minutes or so, or until it's dried completely. Rinse it off with cool water, and pat dry. Your skin should be soft and smooth, with a nice healthy glow.

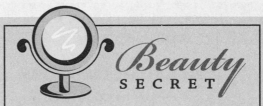

Beauty
S E C R E T

GET EGG ON YOUR FACE

Looking for a quick, easy, and economical way to tighten your skin and reduce the appearance of wrinkles? If so, you've come to the right place. Here's all you need to do: Let an egg warm up to room temperature, then crack it open and separate it. Set aside the yolk and whip the white just enough to make it easily spreadable. Smooth it over your face, and lie down (with no pillow under your head) for 15 to 20 minutes. As the egg white dries, it'll pull your skin back, just as a plastic surgeon would do in a facelift. When the mask has hardened completely, rinse your face with cool water. (Whatever you do, don't perform this maneuver sitting up, or gravity will drag the egg whites down and take your skin with it.) Of course, this cosmetic "surgery" is only temporary, but it's a darn sight cheaper and safer than the real deal!

POTENT POTION

LEMON-FRESH FACE CREAM

Use this luxurious cream every night to keep your skin satiny soft.

1 lemon

¼ cup or so of heavy whipping cream

Contents of 1 (400 IU) vitamin E capsule

Piece of muslin or other light cloth

From the center of the lemon, cut a slice that's about ¼ inch thick. Lay it flat in a clean glass jar that has a tight-fitting lid. Pour in enough cream to cover the lemon slice, cover the container with the cloth, and let it sit at room temperature for 24 hours, or until the mixture is about the thickness of face cream. Stir in the vitamin E, replace the cloth with the regular jar lid, and put the jar in the refrigerator. Rub the cream into your skin every night at bedtime. The mixture will eventually spoil, so you'll need to make a new batch every week or so.

YIELD: ABOUT ¼ CUP

★ Soak It to 'Em

Here's an easy, foolproof way to strengthen your fingernails. Beat 1 egg yolk, ¼ cup of buttermilk, and 1 tablespoon of raw honey in a bowl. Soak your nails in the mixture for 10 minutes, and then rinse well with cool water. The buttermilk will soften dry cuticles, and the protein in the egg will make your nails as hard as, well, nails.

★ Here's Egg in Your Hair!

Fresh out of styling mousse or gel? No problem! There's a super substitute in your fridge. Simply separate two eggs, and beat the whites until they hold stiff peaks. Rub them into your damp hair, and style it as usual. Just be sure to rinse the egg out with cool water before you shampoo!

★ Great-Grandma's Hair Conditioner

Our grandmothers and *their* grandmothers used this all-natural conditioner to shine and soften their hair, and it works every bit as well today as it did back then. Here's all you need to do: Beat two egg yolks until they're frothy, and then beat in 1 cup of water and 1 teaspoon of baby oil or olive oil. Work the mixture through your hair as you would any other conditioner, wait for a minute or two, and rinse thoroughly with cool water. The result: sleek, silky hair with no chemical residue!

Index